Diverticulitis

Marylise Boutros • Richard Garfinkle
Sameh Emile • Patricia Sylla
Editors

Diverticulitis

A Comprehensive, Evidence-Based Guide to Diagnosis and Management

Springer

Editors
Marylise Boutros
Colorectal Surgery
Cleveland Clinic Florida
Weston, FL, USA

Sameh Emile
Colorectal Surgery
Cleveland Clinic Florida
Weston, FL, USA

Richard Garfinkle
Colon and Rectal Surgery
Jewish General Hospital
McGill University
Montreal, QC, Canada

Patricia Sylla
Colon and Rectal Surgery
Icahn School of Medicine at Mount Sinai
New York, NY, USA

ISBN 978-3-032-21719-6 ISBN 978-3-032-21720-2 (eBook)
https://doi.org/10.1007/978-3-032-21720-2

This Springer imprint is published by the registered company Springer Nature Switzerland AG
The registered company address is: Gewerbestrasse 11, 6330 Cham, Switzerland

To the patients living with diverticular disease, whose experiences, questions, and trust have continually challenged traditional thinking and inspired a more thoughtful, evidence-based approach to care. This work is also shaped by the mentors who instilled rigor, curiosity, and humility in surgical practice, and by the trainees and collaborators whose commitment to asking better questions continues to advance the field. Finally, to our families, whose unwavering support has been our constant anchor throughout this academic and clinical journey.

Preface

We wrote *Diverticulitis: A Comprehensive, Evidence-Based Guide to Diagnosis and Management* because, despite how common diverticulitis is, there remains a great deal of uncertainty in how it is diagnosed, discussed, and treated in everyday practice. Over the years, we have seen wide variation in management decisions—often driven by habit or historical teaching rather than evidence—and we felt there was a need for a resource that reflects how our understanding of this disease has truly evolved.

Our interest in diverticulitis developed through direct patient care. We have looked after patients at every stage of the disease, from uncomplicated first episodes to recurrent and complicated presentations requiring urgent or elective surgery. Many of the questions patients ask—about recurrence, the role of antibiotics, when surgery is necessary, and what outcomes they can realistically expect—do not have simple or uniform answers. These same questions have also come up repeatedly in our research, involvement in guideline and consensus work, and in discussions with trainees and colleagues.

Much of our academic work in this area has focused on outcomes, recurrence, and decision-making, with the goal of helping clinicians move away from rigid rules and toward individualized, evidence-informed care. Teaching and mentoring have further reinforced the importance of clarity and balance when translating data into practice, particularly in a condition where patient quality of life plays such a central role.

This book brings together passion and clinical and academic experience in diverticular disease. It is intended to provide a clear, practical, and evidence-based approach to the diagnosis and management of diverticulitis, while acknowledging areas where uncertainty remains. Above all, it is written with the hope of supporting thoughtful decision-making and improving care for patients living with this disease.

Diverticulitis: A Comprehensive, Evidence-Based Guide to Diagnosis and Management is a clinically focused reference intended for healthcare professionals involved in the evaluation and treatment of diverticular disease. This book synthesizes the latest research and guidelines to provide a practical, multidisciplinary approach to diverticulitis—from pathophysiology and diagnostic strategies to outpatient care, hospital management, complications, and surgical interventions.

Designed for use in both training and practice, the text offers:

- Concise, evidence-based recommendations
- Clinically relevant algorithms and decision pathways
- Summaries of key controversies and evolving practices
- Guidance on long-term management and recurrence prevention

This resource aims to support consistent, high-quality, and patient-centered care across the spectrum of diverticulitis presentations.

Weston, FL, USA Marylise Boutros
Montreal, QC, Canada Richard Garfinkle
Weston, FL, USA Sameh Emile
New York, NY, USA Patricia Sylla

Acknowledgments

We extend our heartfelt thanks to Elektra McDermott, our Developmental Editor and Editorial Services partner, whose dedication and support were essential to bringing this book to life. From the earliest drafts to the final revisions, Elektra provided thoughtful guidance, keen editorial insight, and steady support. Her commitment to excellence kept this project moving forward, even through its most demanding stages. We are deeply grateful for her partnership, trust, and belief in this work.

Contents

Contributors

Ahmed Alkhamis Kuwait University, Health Science Center, Jabriya, State of Kuwait

Alberto Arezzo Department of Surgical Sciences, Molinette Hospital and University of Torino School of Medicine, Turin, Italy

Simone Arolfo Department of Surgical Sciences, Molinette Hospital and University of Torino School of Medicine, Turin, Italy

Tan Arulampalam School of Medicine, Anglia Ruskin University, Chelmsford, UK

Willem A. Bemelman Department of Surgery, Amsterdam University Medical Center, Amsterdam, The Netherlands

Karalyn R. Bentley Baton Rouge General Hospital, Advanced Robotics Institute of Louisiana, Baton Rouge, LA, USA

Sebastiano Biondo Colorectal Unit, Bellvitge University Hospital, University of Barcelona, Barcelona, Spain

Liliana G. Bordeianou Department of Surgery, Massachusetts General Hospital and Harvard Medical School, Boston, MA, USA

Neyla Boukhili Department of Surgery, McGill University, Montreal, QC, Canada

Marylise Boutros Colorectal Surgery, Cleveland Clinic Florida, Weston, FL, USA

Nicole D. Bouvy Faculty of Health, Medicine and Life Sciences, Maastricht University, Maastricht, The Netherlands

Department of General Surgery, Maastricht University Medical Center, Maastricht, The Netherlands

W. Donald Buie Foothills Medical Center, University of Calgary, Department of Surgery and Oncology, Calgary, AB, Canada

V. R. W. Di Leonardo Faculty of Health, Medicine and Life Sciences, Maastricht University, Maastricht, The Netherlands

Department of General Surgery, Maastricht University Medical Center, Maastricht, The Netherlands

Scott C. Dolejs Franciscan Health Indianapolis, Indiana Colon and Rectal Specialists, Indianapolis, IN, USA

Sameh Emile Colorectal Surgery, Cleveland Clinic Florida, Weston, FL, USA

Ryan Flanagan Division of Gastroenterology, Hepatology and Endoscopy, Brigham and Women's Hospital, Boston, MA, USA

Richard Garfinkle Colon and Rectal Surgery, Jewish General Hospital, McGill University, Montreal, QC, Canada

Muhammad Ghanem Orlando Health Weight Loss and Bariatric Surgery Institute, Orlando, FL, USA

Thomas Golda Colorectal Unit, Bellvitge University Hospital, University of Barcelona, Barcelona, Spain

Jason Hall Tufts Medical Center, Boston, MA, USA

Jon M. Harrison Department of Surgery, Massachusetts General Hospital, Boston, MA, USA

Alexander T. Hawkins Division of General Surgery, Section of Colon & Rectal Surgery, Vanderbilt University Medical Center, Nashville, TN, USA

Traci L. Hedrick Department of Surgery, University of Virginia Health System, Charlottesville, VA, USA

Sook C. Hoang Department of Surgery, University of Virginia Health System, Charlottesville, VA, USA

Nir Horesh Cleveland Clinic Florida, Ellen Leifer Shulman and Steven Shulman Digestive Disease Center, Weston, FL, USA

Department of Surgery and Transplantations, Sheba Medical Center, Ramat Gan, Israel

Tel Aviv University, Tel Aviv, Israel

Cameron W. Hunt Department of Surgery, Massachusetts General Hospital, Boston, MA, USA

Andreas M. Kaiser Department of Surgery, Division of Colorectal Surgery, City of Hope National Medical Center, Duarte, CA, USA

Paul A. Kolarsick Monmouth Medical Center, Department of Surgery, Long Branch, NJ, USA

Sarah E. Koller Department of Surgery, Division of Colorectal Surgery, Keck School of Medicine of the University of Southern California, Los Angeles, CA, USA

Sebastien Lachance Hopital Cite-de-la-Sante de Laval, 1755, Boul. Rene-Laennec, Laval, QC, Canada

Daniël P. V. Lambrichts Department of Surgery, Erasmus University Medical Center, Rotterdam, The Netherlands

Department of Surgery, Amsterdam University Medical Center, Amsterdam, The Netherlands

Johan F. Lange Department of Surgery, Erasmus University Medical Center, Rotterdam, The Netherlands

Lawrence Lee Steinberg-Bernstein Centre for Minimally Invasive Surgery and Innovation, Department of Surgery, McGill University Health Centre, Montreal, QC, Canada

Colon and Rectal Surgery, Department of Surgery, McGill University Health Centre, Montreal, QC, Canada

Mark E. Lipson Peter Lougheed Centre, Alberta Health Services, University of Calgary, Calgary, AB, Canada

Rohin Mittal Department of Surgery Unit 2 (Colorectal Surgery), Christian Medical College and Hospital, Vellore, Tamil Nadu, India

Allison J. Pang Division of Colon and Rectal Surgery, Jewish General Hospital, Montreal, QC, Canada

Mythili P. Pathipati Department of Gastroenterology, Palo Alto Medical Foundation/Sutter Health, Palo Alto, CA, USA

Terrah J. Paul Olson Division of Colorectal Surgery, Emory University, Atlanta, GA, USA

Vincent Pelsser Department of Radiology, Jewish General Hospital, Montreal, QC, Canada

Andrea Petrucci Department of Surgery, Cite de la Sante Hospital, Laval, QC, Canada

Virginia Shaffer Department of Surgery, University of Chicago, Chicago, IL, USA

Harris B. Shumacker Department of Surgery, Indiana University School of Medicine, Indiana University Health North Hospital, Carmel, IN, USA

Kyle Staller Division of Gastroenterology, Massachusetts General Hospital, Boston, MA, USA

Dimitrios Stefanidis Department of Surgery, Indiana University School of Medicine, Indiana University Health North Hospital, Carmel, IN, USA

Paul Strombom Northwell Health Physician Partners Surgical Specialties at Phelps, Sleepy Hollow, NY, USA

Patricia Sylla Colon and Rectal Surgery, Icahn School of Medicine at Mount Sinai, New York, NY, USA

Jean-François Toupin Department of Diagnostic Radiology, McGill University Health Center, Montreal, QC, Canada

Maude Trepanier Steinberg-Bernstein Centre for Minimally Invasive Surgery and Innovation, Department of Surgery, McGill University Health Centre, Montreal, QC, Canada

Michael S. Truitt Department of Surgery, TCU School of Medicine, Medical City Plano, Plano, TX, USA

Carol-Ann Vasilevsky Division of Colon and Rectal Surgery, Jewish General Hospital, Montreal, QC, Canada

Steven D. Wexner Ellen Leifer Shulman and Steven Shulman Digestive Disease Center, Cleveland Clinic Florida, Weston, FL, USA

Samuel A. Younan Division of General Surgery, Section of Colon & Rectal Surgery, Vanderbilt University Medical Center, Nashville, TN, USA

1 Relevant Anatomy and Pathophysiology

Virginia Shaffer and Terrah J. Paul Olson

Introduction

Diverticulosis is a common condition that impacts a large proportion of the population. While most patients with diverticulosis do not develop symptoms, diverticular disease—which includes inflammation (diverticulitis) and bleeding (diverticular bleeding)—can be morbid and burdensome for both patients and the healthcare system. This chapter will describe the anatomy relevant to diverticular disease and will review some of the proposed theories in pathophysiology of diverticulosis and symptomatic diverticular disease.

Anatomy and Physiology of the Colon

The colon is a partially peritonealized structure in the abdomen and pelvis. The cecum, ascending colon, and descending colon are partially affixed to the retroperitoneum posteriorly, while the anterior surface is within the abdomen and covered with peritoneum. The transverse and sigmoid colon are attached by their respective mesenteries to the retroperitoneum and are fully peritonealized. The sigmoid colon transitions to the rectum, which is covered with peritoneum for a variable length anteriorly before the rectum becomes an extraperitoneal structure as it enters the pelvis. Posteriorly, the mesorectum extends toward the pelvic brim extraperitoneally.

The colon wall has an inner circular and an outer longitudinal muscular layer. This outer layer, which is circumferentially complete around the colon and rectum, is noticeably thickened in three bands named the taenia coli, running along the colon from the appendix to the rectosigmoid junction, where the taenia splay out and coalesce, marking the transition from colon to rectum. The taenia are slightly shorter than the length of the colon, which contributes to areas of outpouching along the colon termed haustra. The haustra are divided along the length of the bowel by the plicae semilunares.

Histologically, the wall of the large intestine consists of mucosal epithelium, which lines the luminal surface of the colon and rectum. The submucosa is deep to the epithelium, which is where blood supply, enteric ganglia, and lymphatics are located. The inner circular and outer longitudinal muscular layers are deep to the submucosa. Subserosal tissue separates the muscular layer from the colonic serosa, which is the outer layer of the colon wall. Finally, the peritoneal surfaces of the colon are then covered by visceral peritoneum overlying the serosa.

V. Shaffer (✉)
Department of Surgery, University of Chicago, Chicago, IL, USA
e-mail: virginia.shaffer@bsd.uchicago.edu

T. J. Paul Olson
Division of Colorectal Surgery, Emory University, Atlanta, GA, USA
e-mail: terrah.paul.olson@emoryhealthcare.org; tpaulol@emory.edu

M. Boutros et al. (eds.), *Diverticulitis*, https://doi.org/10.1007/978-3-032-21720-2_1

The blood supply to the right colon arises from the ileocolic, right colic, and middle colic arteries, which are branches of the superior mesenteric artery. These arteries supply the cecum, ascending colon, and transverse colon, respectively. The left colic artery and sigmoid branches arise from the inferior mesenteric artery, which becomes the superior hemorrhoidal or superior rectal artery as it crosses the left iliac vessels. The venous drainage of the colon parallels that of the arterial supply, with the left colon and sigmoid colon draining via the inferior mesenteric vein before joining the splenic vein to drain into the portal venous system. The inferior mesenteric vein does not run next to the inferior mesenteric artery, but rather can be found at the base of the left colon mesentery lateral to the ligament of Treitz. The superior mesenteric vein drains the cecum, ascending colon, and transverse colon, and similarly joins the portal venous system. The terminal branches of the blood supply, or vasa recta, penetrate the colon wall to reach the colonic submucosa and epithelium [1].

The enteric nervous system is comprised of specialized nerve cells located within the wall of the colon which serve to regulate colonic motility, blood flow within the colon wall, and mucosal absorption and secretion. Meissner's plexus is located in the submucosa of the colon and regulates ion transport through the mucosa. Auerbach's plexus, or the myenteric plexus, is located between the inner circular and outer longitudinal layers of the colon. This plexus regulates smooth muscle function in the colon, including vascular smooth muscle. The interstitial cells of Cajal serve as pacemaker cells to regulate colonic motility. These cells generate electrical activity which is then propagated through the smooth muscle cells of the colon wall in a coordinated fashion. Repetitive, cyclical depolarizations arising from the interstitial cells of Cajal lead to colonic slow waves [1, 2].

Colonic motility occurs in short phasic and longer tonic contractions. These contractions produce propulsive and nonpropulsive waves which serve to mix luminal contents to increase exposure to absorptive surfaces and slowly move colonic contents distally through the colon. Nonpropagating pressure waves or contractions occur simultaneously throughout the colon. These bursts of activity can be seen with a frequency of three times per minute. Propagating pressure waves are those that move distally through the colon over at least 10 cm and have a velocity of 0.5 cm/s. Additionally, about six times per day, high amplitude propagated contractions—which can generate pressures higher than the pressure waves—migrate through the colon and propel stool toward the rectum [1, 3].

Pathophysiology of Diverticulosis

Outpouchings in the colon wall are termed diverticula. These can be true diverticula, where all three layers of the colon wall are included in the saccule, or false diverticula, where only the mucosa and muscularis mucosa layers are included in the diverticulum. Most left-sided colonic diverticula are false diverticula, or pulsion diverticula. They tend to occur where the vasa recta penetrate the circular muscular layer of colon wall, which are areas of relative weakness (Fig. 1.1). The formation of diverticula is termed diverticulosis. While diverticulosis is frequently asymptomatic and incidentally found on imaging or during colonoscopy, colonic diverticula can manifest with inflammation, termed diverticulitis, or bleeding. Multiple

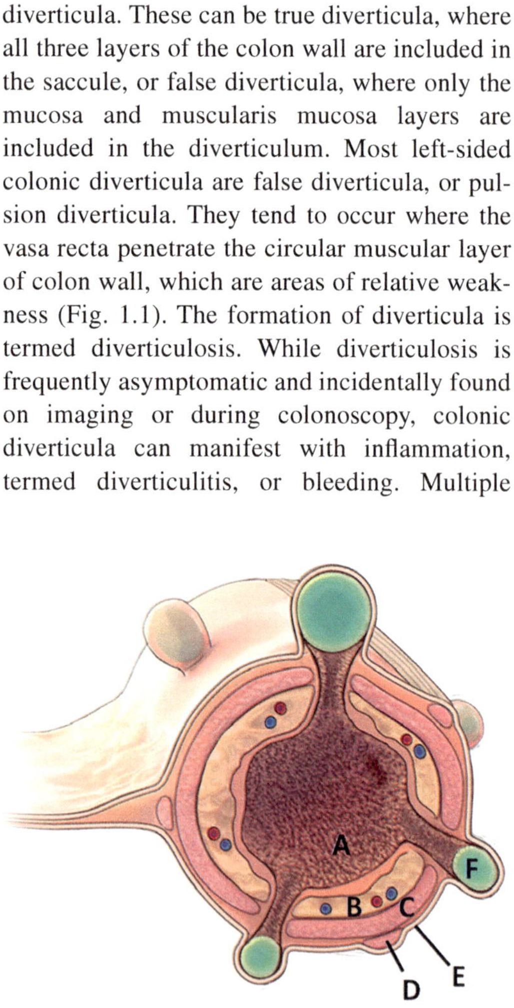

Fig. 1.1 Pathophysiology of diverticulosis
Cross-sectional diagram of colon. A: mucosa of colon, B: submucosa, C: circular muscular layer; D: longitudinal muscle layer/taenia coli, E: serosa, F: colonic diverticulu

researchers have proposed numerous underlying factors that allow these herniations through the colon wall to develop. Ultimately, the development of diverticulosis is a multifactorial process, with contributions from a number of environmental, degenerative, and genetic factors (Tables 1.1 and 1.2) [4–9].

Table 1.1 Proposed factors associated with diverticulosis

Dietary fiber
Altered colonic motility
Increased intraluminal pressure
Aging/connective tissue degeneration
Connective tissue disorders
Altered colon wall architecture
Increased elastin in taenia
Increased elastin in muscularis propria
Altered smooth muscle cells
Enteric nervous system dysregulation
Increased enterochromaffin cells
Altered serotonin receptors
Abnormal myenteric plexuses
Decreased interstitial cells of Cajal
Genetic factors

Table 1.2 Proposed factors associated with diverticular disease (diverticulitis, diverticular bleeding, symptomatic uncomplicated diverticular disease)

Protective factors associated with lower rates of diverticular disease
High fiber diet
Decreased red meat intake
Vegetarian diet
Nut and popcorn intake
Vigorous physical activity
Statin use
Factors associated with increased diverticular disease
Smoking/tobacco use
Elevated BMI/obesity
Medications
Nonsteroidal anti-inflammatory drugs
Aspirin
Corticosteroids
Opioids
Calcium channel blockers
Increased intestinal inflammatory markers
Alterations in microbiome

BMI body mass index

Dietary Factors

Dietary fiber has been implicated in the etiology of diverticulitis since Painter and Burkitt postulated that the shift in western European diets away from unprocessed foods toward refined flour and sugar was underlying the increased incidence in diverticular disease. They noted that populations who had less processed diets had softer stools that were easier to eliminate, and speculated that having softer, larger caliber stools would generate lower intraluminal pressures in the sigmoid colon, leading to less diverticula formation. They hypothesized that increased segmentation and high pressures within the colon could cause elevated wall pressures, making herniation of mucosa through the colon wall at the sites of vasa recta more likely [10]. Subsequent studies have shown mixed correlations between dietary fiber intake and incidence of diverticular disease. Several large prospective observational studies have shown an inverse relationship between the amount of dietary fiber intake and rates of diverticular disease [11–13]. Other studies, however, have found no association between dietary fiber and the incidence of diverticulosis noted on screening colonoscopy [14]. Increased dietary fiber and more frequent bowel movements have also been associated with increased rates of diverticular disease [15]. Therefore, while there is likely some association between dietary fiber intake and diverticular disease, the relationship is not as straightforward as previously thought.

Colonic Motility and Intracolonic Pressure

Following Painter and Burkitt's hypothesis about the etiology of diverticular disease [10], researchers investigated whether there was evidence for alterations in colonic motility and intraluminal pressures that correlated with diverticular disease. It was observed that in patients with diverticular disease, the affected segment of colon—typically the sigmoid or descending colon—had increased haustral markings that could be demonstrated on barium enema, perhaps demonstrating altered pressure or motility. However, this radiologic observation did not reliably correlate with increased pressure readings in the diseased segment of colon [16]. Other groups demonstrated increased pressures in the sigmoid colon in patients with diverticular disease compared to those without; however, they did not see a difference in overall motility at baseline and with the physiologic stimulus of eating between the two groups [17]. When colon motility was observed over 24 h, there was increased baseline motility in segments of colon affected by diverticulosis relative to unaffected segments with no difference in the response to eating. Additionally, when high-amplitude progressive contractions occurred in diseased segments, they were more likely to move retrograde rather than toward the rectum [18]. However, a systematic review of manometric data revealed only weak evidence for abnormal pressures in the sigmoid colon in patients with diverticulosis. Many studies have been hampered by inconsistencies in methodology or poor resolution in manometric data [3]. As such, the data supporting abnormal motility in the development of diverticulosis is suggestive but inconsistent, and often weak in quality.

Degenerative Processes and Connective Tissue Disorders

The incidence of diverticular disease increases with age, which suggests a degenerative aspect to diverticulosis. This can be explained by both increased weakness in the connective tissue of the colon wall, making it easier for diverticula to form, as well as dysregulation and degeneration in the enteric nervous system [8, 19]. In addition to degenerative changes, there may be an underlying predisposition to weakness in connective tissue in those who develop diverticulosis. In one study, patients who underwent surgery for diverticulitis were more likely to develop incisional hernias than those how underwent partial colectomies for other etiologies such as cancer [20]. A large population-based study found that subjects with diverticulosis were more likely to have other disorders associated with connective tissue alterations. Diverticular disease was shown to be significantly associated with rectal prolapse (adjusted odds ratio [OR] 3.9), polycystic kidney disease (OR 3.8), heritable syndromes such as Marfan's or Ehlers-Danlos (OR 2.4), female genital prolapse (OR 2.3), nonaortic aneurysm (OR 2.3), aortic aneurysm (OR 2.2), inguinal hernia (OR 1.9), and dislocation of shoulder and other joints (OR 1.7) [21].

Colon Wall Architecture

A number of alterations in the structure of the colon wall have been described and may be related to the development of diverticulosis. Pathologic studies of colons with diverticular disease have revealed abnormalities in the muscularis propria. Studies have demonstrated thickening of the taenia with increased elastin, along with foreshortening of the bowel. Microscopic examination of colons with diverticular disease has shown increased thickness of both the circular and longitudinal layers of the muscularis propria. However, there was significant overlap in these measurements between normal and diverticular colon walls, so this cannot be used as a reliable marker of diverticular disease. The increased thickness of the muscularis propria appears to be from increased amounts of connective tissue such as elastin rather than hypertrophy of the myocytes [22]. Increased elastin can be seen in the longitudinal muscle layer of the colon wall [23]. Examination of the smooth muscle cells showed altered and disordered architecture within the colon wall, although it is unclear if this is the underlying etiology of the changes seen in diverticular disease or a response to abnormal gene expression and protein function. There were also changes in gene expression which may be related to deficiencies in the smooth muscle contractile proteins, such as reductions in smooth muscle myosin heavy chain gene expression [22].

In addition to these findings, abnormal responses to neurotransmitters have been described in the diverticular colon. Colons affected by diverticular disease are hypercontractile, and have been shown to be over-responsive to acetylcholine with upregulation of specific subtypes of smooth muscle muscarinic receptors [24]. Nitric oxide contributes to smooth muscle relaxation in the bowel wall by direct action as well as by inhibiting acetylcholine. In diverticular colon tissue, there is less response to nitric oxide in the longitudinal muscle layer of the colon, leading to decreased relaxation of affected segments of colon [23].

The serotonergic system is also abnormal in diverticular disease. Increased enterochromaffin cells, which produce serotonin, can be seen in colons with diverticula [25]. Serotonin receptor mRNA is downregulated in the muscle and upregulated in the mucosa of diverticular colons [26]. However, serotonin changes may be more closely linked to diverticulitis rather than diverticulosis, as there were decreases in serotonin transporter transcription levels in colons affected by diverticulitis, but not in those affected by asymptomatic diverticulosis, compared to normal controls [27]. These findings may explain some of the motility changes associated with diverticulosis. It is unclear whether these changes are part of the underlying etiology of diverticulosis or represent responses to alterations in colonic motility or inflammation.

The enteric nervous system in general appears to be abnormal in diverticulosis. In addition to the changes in serotonin described above, enteric nerves appear abnormal in diverticular disease. There is reduced neuronal density in enteric nerve plexuses, with decreased ganglionic cells in the myenteric and submucosal plexuses and decreased glial cell content and density in the myenteric plexus [28]. There is also downregulation of glial cell line-derived neurotrophic factor in the muscularis propria of diverticular colons [29], and decreased enteric glial cells [2]. The interstitial cells of Cajal (ICC), which mediate input from the enteric nervous system on the colon wall smooth muscle and generate slow wave activity in the colon, are reduced in colonic diverticulosis as well. These findings may explain altered colonic motility, but again, it is unknown if these changes are the cause of motility changes or are responses to other pathology.

Genetic Factors

Genetic factors contribute to the development of diverticular disease. Two large twin studies have examined the degree of heritability in the development of diverticular disease. Granlund et al. [30] queried the Swedish Twin Registry and linked this to the national inpatient registry. They demonstrated that there is an increased hazard ratio for developing diverticular disease in monozygotic twins relative to dizygotic twins with no evidence for shared environmental effects. They estimated the heritability of diverticular disease to be 43% [30]. Strate et al. performed a similar study with the Danish Twin Registry and estimated heritability of diverticular disease to be 53%. They also found that siblings of patients with diverticular disease were three times more likely than the general population to develop diverticular disease [31].

Specific genetic variants that correlate with diverticular disease have also been described. A genome-wide association study performed by Sigurdsson et al. [32] showed significant associations of variants in specific genes with the development of diverticular disease and with diverticulitis in Icelandic and Dutch populations. Intronic variants rs4662344 in gene *ARHGAP15* (Rho GTPase-activating protein-15) and rs7609897 in gene *COLQ* (collagen-like tail subunit of asymmetric acetylcholinesterase) have been linked with diverticular disease. Intron variant rs67153654 in *FAM155A* (family with sequence similarity 155A) was also associated with diverticulitis. However, there were no differences in the expression of these genes found in samples of blood, adipose tissue, or other tissues in an available tissue bank; therefore, it is unclear *how* these variants may affect the development of diverticular disease [32]. Connelly et al. [33] demonstrated that the single-nucleotide polymorphism (SNP) rs7848647 in gene *TNFSF15* (tumor necrosis factor superfamily 15) was associated with the development of diverticulitis requiring surgery. Other SNPs have been associated with diverticulosis in white males (rs3134646 in *COL3A1*—collagen type III alpha 1 chain) [34] as well as in a family with a strong predilection to develop diverticulitis (D435N substitution in *LAMB4*—laminin beta 4) [35].

Pathophysiology of Diverticulitis

The development of diverticulosis appears to be the result of a complex interaction between genetics, dietary factors, alterations in colonic wall architecture and the enteric nervous system, and degeneration of connective tissue. Diverticulitis is inflammation associated with diverticular segments of the colon and tends to be in the sigmoid colon. The most common explanation for the development of acute diverticulitis is occlusion or irritation of the mucosa of a diverticulum, possibly by stool, which leads to inflammation, congestion, and possible perforation. However, recent research has challenged this concept. Several additional etiologic factors have been associated with the development of diverticulitis and are discussed further below.

Dietary Factors

Several dietary factors may be associated with the development of diverticulitis. While there is conflicting data about the role of dietary fiber in the development of asymptomatic diverticulosis [11–15], there is better evidence that high fiber diets are protective against the development of symptomatic diverticulitis. A large cohort study of male health professional demonstrated an inverse relationship between higher intake of insoluble fiber and rates of self-reported diverticular disease [11]. Another large study of men and women also showed a reduced risk of symptomatic diverticular disease associated with higher intake of dietary fiber, particularly with fiber from cereal/grain and fruit sources [13]. Decreased red meat intake and eating a vegetarian diet have also been associated with lower rates of diverticulitis in population studies [12, 36]. Finally, contrary to historical belief, there is no association between consumption of nuts, corn, or popcorn and increased risk of diverticulitis. In fact, a large cohort study of 47,228 men with 18 years of follow-up data showed an inverse relationship between the two, demonstrating decreased rates of diverticulitis associated with a higher intake of nuts and popcorn [37].

Vitamin D

Other environmental factors have also been associated with diverticulitis occurrence. Vitamin D plays an important but incompletely characterized role in colonic homeostasis [38, 39]. In a large retrospective review of a clinical database, Maguire et al. demonstrated a correlation between serum vitamin D levels and complicated diverticulitis. They compared serum vitamin D levels between those hospitalized for diverticulitis complications and those with a diagnosis of diverticulitis but no complications. Those who required hospitalization had significantly lower vitamin D levels prior to diagnosis than those with uncomplicated diverticulitis [40]. This same group also studied seasonal variations in non-elective admissions for diverticulitis and the correlation between complicated diverticulitis and UV light exposure. In areas with lower UV light exposure, there were higher rates of admission for complicated diverticulitis. They also noted seasonal variation in admissions, with higher rates of admissions in the summer months relative to winter months. This variation was more pronounced in low UV light exposure regions. They speculate that lower vitamin D from lower UV light exposure in the winter months leads to a delayed effect on colon health [38].

Smoking

Smoking has been associated with higher rates of symptomatic diverticular disease. Additionally, smokers have more complicated disease and are at higher risk for postoperative complications. While one large prospective cohort of males showed a weak and inconsistent association between smoking and symptomatic diverticulitis [36], a number of other studies have demonstrated a stronger association between tobacco use and diverticulitis. In a large prospective cohort of patients, Crowe et al. [12] demonstrated a dose-dependent increase in symptomatic diverticulosis in smokers. Relative to nonsmokers, former smokers had a 31% higher risk of diverticular disease, those who smoked half a pack per day or less had a 34% higher risk, and those using more than a half a pack per day had a 86% higher risk. In a large population study of Scandinavian women, smokers had a significantly increased risk of symptomatic diverticular disease even when controlling for age, fiber intake, medical comorbidities, medications, body mass index (BMI), and physical activity [41]. Smokers were also more likely to develop more significant diverticular complications such as colon strictures or diverticular perforation or abscess [41, 42].

Medications

A variety of medications have been evaluated for an association with the development of diverticulitis, diverticular bleeding, or complicated diverticulitis. Using a multivariate model that accounted for age, BMI, activity level, and dietary factors, Strate et al. found increased risk of diverticulitis in patients who used aspirin more than twice per week compared to those who did not use aspirin regularly, with a multivariate odds ratio (OR) of 1.25 (95% CI 1.05–1.47). They also demonstrated increased risk of diverticulitis with regular nonsteroidal anti-inflammatory drug (NSAID) use, with a multivariate OR of 1.72 (95% CI 1.40–2.11). A higher risk of diverticular bleeding was also associated with regular aspirin use (OR 1.70, 95% CI 1.21–2.39) and regular NSAID use (OR 1.74, 95% CI 1.15–2.64) [43].

Multiple other studies have looked at associations between medications and perforated diverticulitis or diverticular bleeding. Kvasnovsky et al. [44] performed a meta-analysis looking specifically at aspirin, NSAIDs, corticosteroids, opioids, warfarin, and calcium channel blockers. They found increased risk of diverticular perforation associated with NSAIDs (pooled OR 2.49, 95% CI 1.98–3.14), corticosteroids (pooled OR 9.08, 95% CI 3.49–23.62), and opioids (pooled OR 2.52, 95% CI 1.77–3.57). There was no significant association with aspirin use or calcium channel blockers. This meta-analysis also examined associations with diverticular bleeding. NSAIDs (pooled OR 2.69, 95% CI 1.65–4.40), aspirin (pooled OR 3.24, 95% CI 1.59–6.59), and calcium channel blockers (pooled OR 2.50, 95% CI 1.44–4.35) were associated with diverticular bleeding, while warfarin (pooled OR 0.94, 95% CI 0.38–2.37) and corticosteroids (pooled OR 1.95, 95% CI 0.63–5.93) were not. Statins have also been shown to be associated with a lower risk of perforated diverticulitis as well (OR 0.42, 95% CI 0.20–0.94) [45].

For many of these medications, the biological association with the development of diverticulitis has been theorized. The association between aspirin and NSAIDs and diverticular bleeding is perhaps the most evident, given the known bleeding diathesis that these medications induce. NSAIDs may be associated with increased rates of diverticulitis and diverticular perforation due to either to injury to the mucosa or via impaired prostaglandin synthesis, which can negatively affect mucosal integrity in the colon [7]. Corticosteroids may predispose patients to diverticular perforation due to alterations in the body's inflammatory response [46]. The association between opioid use and diverticulitis, however, is not as well understood. Opioids may be a marker of more severe disease rather than a causative agent for diverticular perforation.

Activity and Obesity

Another set of factors that have been investigated in relation to diverticulitis and diverticular bleeding is physical activity and obesity. One large prospective cohort study of men demonstrated an inverse relationship between levels of physical activity and incidence of diverticulitis and diverticular bleeding. After 18 years of follow-up, Strate et al. [47] showed that vigorous physical activity, such as running, was inversely correlated with self-reported rates of diverticulitis and diverticular bleeding in a large cohort of male health professionals. Their multivariate model adjusted for dietary and lifestyle factors and showed that the highest quintile of physical activity compared to the lowest quintile had a relative risk of 0.75 (95% CI 0.58–0.95) for diverticulitis and 0.54 (95% CI 0.38–0.77) for diverticular bleeding.

Two large prospective cohort studies demonstrated a relationship between BMI and rates of diverticulitis. In a population study with 28 years of follow-up, Rosemar et al. [48] showed that as BMI increased, the risk of developing diverticular disease that required hospitalization also increased. Increased BMI, waist circumference, and waist-to-hip ratio all correlated with increased rates of diverticulitis and diverticular bleeding in men. Over 18 years of follow-up, men in the highest quintile of waist circumference had a higher rate of diverticulitis (relative risk 1.56, 95% CI 1.18–2.07) and diverticular bleeding (relative risk 1.96, 95% CI 1.30–2.97) compared to those in the lowest quintile. A similar relationship was seen between waist-to-hip ratio for diverticulitis (relative risk 1.62, 95% CI 1.23–2.14) and bleeding (relative risk 1.91 (1.26–2.90) [49]. A systematic review of studies looking at the relationship between BMI and complications of diverticular disease reinforced the association between rising BMI and rates of symptomatic diverticular disease. This review included 1,636,777 subjects and 28,915 cases of diverticular disease and showed a relative risk of diverticular disease of 1.78 (95% CI 1.48–2.14) in the highest BMI group relative to the lowest BMI group. The study also demonstrated increasing relative risk with increasing BMI, with a dose-response analysis that reported a 1.28 (95% CI 1.18–1.40) times increase in the risk of diverticular disease for every 5 BMI units increased. With a BMI of 22.5, the relative risk was 1.15 (95% CI 1.07–1.23), whereas the relative risk increased to 3.01 (95% CI 2.06–4.39) with higher BMI values [50].

The reasons for this linkage between BMI and diverticular disease are still being clarified. This relationship exists even when controlling for differences in dietary factors such as fiber or red meat intake, rates of smoking, and rates of physical activity. Several mechanisms have been proposed. Obesity is known to be a chronic inflammatory state, which may impact inflammation within the colon as well. Additionally, differences in the colonic microbiome have been described between lean and obese subjects, as well as in the microbiome of those with diverticulitis and those without. Both of these possible etiologies are areas of active ongoing research [9, 39, 48–50].

Inflammation and Immune System

There does not appear to be a clear association between inflammation and the development of diverticulosis. Peery et al. [51] examined mucosal biopsies in patients incidentally found to have diverticula on routine screening colonoscopy. There was no difference in CD4, CD8, or CD57 immunostaining or mast cell tryptase—markers of altered immune response in the colonic mucosa—between subjects with diverticulosis and normal controls. There were reduced mucosal concentrations of the pro-inflammatory cytokine IL-6 and the anti-inflammatory cytokine IL-10 in colonic mucosa with diverticulosis. There were also no differences in TNF-α, an important mediator of inflammation, between diverticulosis and control subjects.

However, inflammation is the hallmark of diverticulitis. Acute uncomplicated diverticulitis is associated with infiltrates of both neutrophils and lymphocytes, although lymphocytic infiltrates can be seen in other forms of diverticular disease [52, 53]. Neutrophilic infiltrates are only seen with acute diverticulitis [52]. The degree of inflammation in the colon can be reflected by elevated serologic markers of inflammation such as CRP, ESR, and elevated WBC; more abnormal lab values correlate with higher degrees of lymphocytic infiltrates [53]. Elevated levels of TNFα are seen in the mucosa of colons with acute uncomplicated diverticulitis relative to normal controls [54].

These findings are not particularly surprising or controversial. However, there is quite a bit more controversy about the role of inflammation and its effect on the enteric nervous system and visceral sensation in more chronic forms of diverticular disease. Tursi et al. have correlated increasing severity of lymphocytic infiltrates in colonic mucosa with severity of abdominal symptoms reported by patients, with increasing levels in asymptomatic diverticulosis, SUDD (symptomatic uncomplicated diverticular disease), and acute uncomplicated diverticulitis [52]. This group also demonstrated increased expression of TNFα in colonic mucosa with increased abdominal symptoms, with elevated levels in SUDD and acute uncomplicated diverticulitis patients compared to healthy controls [54]. Humes et al. also found elevated levels of TNFα as well as the neuropeptide NK1 in patients with SUDD relative to patients with known diverticulosis but no abdominal pain. They also demonstrated heightened visceral sensation in patients with SUDD, which may impact presentation and suggests a role for chronic inflammation in the etiology of symptoms [55]. Barbara et al. showed that patients with diverticula, regardless of the presence or absence of symptoms, had >70% increase in levels of colonic macrophages relative to normal controls. They also found elevated levels of metabolic products linked with pathways involved in inflammation and in gut neuromotor dysfunction, pointing to a role for underlying inflammation in the etiology of diverticulitis and symptomatic diverticulosis [56].

In contrast, Simpson et al. showed no evidence of chronic low-grade inflammation in the colonic mucosa of patients with chronic abdominal symptoms after diverticulitis, but did demonstrate elevated levels of neuropeptides such as galanin and tachykinins, which are known to affect visceral sensation. They also described active remodeling of myenteric nerves and muscular hypertrophy in the colon wall. They proposed that mucosal inflammation from acute diverticulitis can destroy or damage enteric nerves, and as these regenerate, there is a proliferation of tachykinin-containing axons [57]. Peery et al. also demonstrated no difference in levels of TNFα or other markers of inflammation in the colonic mucosa of subjects with diverticulosis and either chronic abdominal pain or IBS-like symptoms [51]. Both of these findings argue against low-grade chronic inflammation as the underlying etiology of SUDD or postdiverticulitis functional bowel disorders.

Alterations in Gut Microbiome

The microbial species that colonize the gut play a crucial role in health and response to illness. The microbiome is established early in life, and alterations in microbiome are linked to chronic inflammatory conditions, such as asthma and atopy [39]. Many of the factors that have been linked to increased risk of diverticulitis have also been associated with dysbiosis of the gut microbiome. Obesity, another condition associated with chronic inflammation, appears to affect microbiome alterations. Vitamin D levels may interact with the gut microbiome to alter the immune response and affect inflammatory conditions [39]. Fiber intake is associated with changes in the composition of the microbiome. In populations with higher dietary fiber intake, there can be higher populations of species that ferment fiber to short-chain fatty acids. These compounds have been found to have anti-inflammatory properties [58].

Currently, there is no compelling evidence that alterations in the gut microbiome are associated with asymptomatic diverticulosis. In a large cohort study of patients undergoing screening colonoscopies, 226 subjects with incidentally found colonic diverticulosis were compared with 309 normal controls. Biopsies were taken during colonoscopy, and the microbiota were compared. There were no significant differences between the microbial species in subjects with asymptomatic diverticulosis and those without diverticula [59]. Diverticulitis, however, has been associated with alterations in the composition of the gut microbiome. In a study looking at the microbiota of patients with acute uncomplicated CT-proven diverticulitis compared to those without diverticulitis, there was higher diversity of *Proteobacteria* phylum in subjects with diverticulitis. The ratio of the phyla *Bacteroidetes* and *Firmucutes*, which can be an indicator of gut dysbiosis, was similar between groups [60]. Another study looked at normal controls and subjects with SUDD. They found a lower abundance of bacteria in genus *Akkermansia* in the areas of the colon affected by diverticula in subjects with SUDD relative to normal controls or those with asymptomatic diverticulosis. In subjects with SUDD or asymptomatic diverticulosis, biopsies of the colon in areas affected by diverticula as well as from distant, nonaffected sites in the colon had a lower abundance of Enterobacteriaceae than normal controls, in particular the *Clostridium* cluster IV bacterial group. *Akkermansia* is a genus of bacteria that degrades colonic mucus and has been linked with anti-inflammatory and anti-obesity effects. When levels of *Akkermansia* are depleted, this has been associated with gut inflammation. Likewise, *Clostridium* cluster IV bacteria include a number of species with anti-inflammatory properties [56]. Finally, differences in the microbiome and fungal species have been demonstrated in areas of the colon affected by chronic diverticulitis and distant unaffected segments of colon. The diseased segments of colon had increased *Microbacteriaceae* and fungal *Ascomycota*, while the unaffected colon segments were enriched for *Pseuodomonas* and fungal *Basidiomycota*. It is unclear if these findings are correlated with non-specific colonic inflammation or if they are related to the development of diverticulitis. *Pseudomonas* species in particular can release collagenases in response to tissue injury, and may be implicated in the development of diverticulitis [61].

Conclusion

Diverticulosis of the colon arises from a complex interplay between genetic susceptibility and alterations in colon wall structure and function. The development of diverticulitis is multifactorial and also has genetic, environmental, inflammatory, and microbial underpinnings. The pathophysiology of diverticulosis and of diverticulitis is an area of active and ongoing research, and a better characterization of pathophysiology may lead to improved preventative and therapeutic strategies in diverticulitis.

References

1. The ASCRS textbook of colon and rectal surgery. 3. New York: Springer; 2016.
2. Bassotti G, Battaglia E, Bellone G, Dughera L, Fisogni S, Zambelli C, et al. Interstitial cells of Cajal, enteric nerves, and glial cells in colonic diverticular disease. J Clin Pathol. 2005;58(9):973–7.
3. Jaung R, Robertson J, O'Grady G, Milne T, Rowbotham D, Bissett IP. Limited evidence of abnormal intra-colonic pressure profiles in diverticular disease – a systematic review. Color Dis. 2017;19(6):O168–O76.
4. Feuerstein JD, Falchuk KR. Diverticulosis and diverticulitis. Mayo Clin Proc. 2016;91(8):1094–104.
5. Rezapour M, Ali S, Stollman N. Diverticular disease: an update on pathogenesis and management. Gut Liver. 2018;12(2):125–32.
6. Tursi A, Papa A, Danese S. Review article: the pathophysiology and medical management of diverticulosis and diverticular disease of the colon. Aliment Pharmacol Ther. 2015;42(6):664–84.
7. Collins D, Winter DC. Modern concepts in diverticular disease. J Clin Gastroenterol. 2015;49(5):358–69.
8. Spiller RC. Changing views on diverticular disease: impact of aging, obesity, diet, and microbiota. Neurogastroenterol Motil. 2015;27(3):305–12.
9. Schieffer KM, Kline BP, Yochum GS, Koltun WA. Pathophysiology of diverticular disease. Expert Rev Gastroenterol Hepatol. 2018;12(7):683–92.
10. Painter NS, Burkitt DP. Diverticular disease of the colon: a deficiency disease of Western civilization. Br Med J. 1971;2(5759):450–4.
11. Aldoori WH, Giovannucci EL, Rockett HR, Sampson L, Rimm EB, Willett WC. A prospective study of dietary fiber types and symptomatic diverticular disease in men. J Nutr. 1998;128(4):714–9.
12. Crowe FL, Appleby PN, Allen NE, Key TJ. Diet and risk of diverticular disease in Oxford cohort of European Prospective Investigation into Cancer and Nutrition (EPIC): prospective study of British vegetarians and non-vegetarians. BMJ. 2011;343:d4131.
13. Crowe FL, Balkwill A, Cairns BJ, Appleby PN, Green J, Reeves GK, et al. Source of dietary fibre and diverticular disease incidence: a prospective study of UK women. Gut. 2014;63(9):1450–6.
14. Peery AF, Sandler RS, Ahnen DJ, Galanko JA, Holm AN, Shaukat A, et al. Constipation and a low-fiber diet are not associated with diverticulosis. Clin Gastroenterol Hepatol. 2013;11(12):1622–7.

15. Peery AF, Barrett PR, Park D, Rogers AJ, Galanko JA, Martin CF, et al. A high-fiber diet does not protect against asymptomatic diverticulosis. Gastroenterology. 2012;142(2):266–72 e1.
16. Weinreich J, Moller SH, Andersen D. Colonic haustral pattern in relation to pressure activity and presence of diverticula. Scand J Gastroenterol. 1977;12(7):857–64.
17. Parks TG, Connell AM. Motility studies in diverticular disease of the colon. Gut. 1969;10(7):534–42.
18. Bassotti G, Battaglia E, Spinozzi F, Pelli MA, Tonini M. Twenty-four hour recordings of colonic motility in patients with diverticular disease: evidence for abnormal motility and propulsive activity. Dis Colon Rectum. 2001;44(12):1814–20.
19. Phillips RJ, Walter GC, Powley TL. Age-related changes in vagal afferents innervating the gastrointestinal tract. Auton Neurosci. 2010;153(1–2):90–8.
20. Pogacnik JS, Messaris E, Deiling SM, Connelly TM, Berg AS, Stewart DB, et al. Increased risk of incisional hernia after sigmoid colectomy for diverticulitis compared with colon cancer. J Am Coll Surg. 2014;218(5):920–8.
21. Broad JB, Wu Z, Clark TG, Musson D, Jaung R, Arroll B, et al. Diverticulosis and nine connective tissue disorders: epidemiological support for an association. Connect Tissue Res. 2019;60(4):389–98.
22. Hellwig I, Bottner M, Barrenschee M, Harde J, Egberts JH, Becker T, et al. Alterations of the enteric smooth musculature in diverticular disease. J Gastroenterol. 2014;49(8):1241–52.
23. Golder M, Burleigh DE, Ghali L, Feakins RM, Lunniss PJ, Williams NS, et al. Longitudinal muscle shows abnormal relaxation responses to nitric oxide and contains altered levels of NOS1 and elastin in uncomplicated diverticular disease. Color Dis. 2007;9(3):218–28.
24. Golder M, Burleigh DE, Belai A, Ghali L, Ashby D, Lunniss PJ, et al. Smooth muscle cholinergic denervation hypersensitivity in diverticular disease. Lancet. 2003;361(9373):1945–51.
25. Banerjee S, Akbar N, Moorhead J, Rennie JA, Leather AJ, Cooper D, et al. Increased presence of serotonin-producing cells in colons with diverticular disease may indicate involvement in the pathophysiology of the condition. Int J Color Dis. 2007;22(6):643–9.
26. Bottner M, Barrenschee M, Hellwig I, Harde J, Egberts JH, Becker T, et al. The enteric serotonergic system is altered in patients with diverticular disease. Gut. 2013;62(12):1753–62.
27. Costedio MM, Coates MD, Danielson AB, Buttolph TR 3rd, Blaszyk HJ, Mawe GM, et al. Serotonin signaling in diverticular disease. J Gastrointest Surg. 2008;12(8):1439–45.
28. Wedel T, Busing V, Heinrichs G, Nohroudi K, Bruch HP, Roblick UJ, et al. Diverticular disease is associated with an enteric neuropathy as revealed by morphometric analysis. Neurogastroenterol Motil. 2010;22(4):407–14. e93–4
29. Bottner M, Barrenschee M, Hellwig I, Harde J, Egberts JH, Becker T, et al. The GDNF system is altered in diverticular disease – implications for pathogenesis. PLoS One. 2013;8(6):e66290.
30. Granlund J, Svensson T, Olen O, Hjern F, Pedersen NL, Magnusson PK, et al. The genetic influence on diverticular disease – a twin study. Aliment Pharmacol Ther. 2012;35(9):1103–7.
31. Strate LL, Erichsen R, Baron JA, Mortensen J, Pedersen JK, Riis AH, et al. Heritability and familial aggregation of diverticular disease: a population-based study of twins and siblings. Gastroenterology. 2013;144(4):736–42 e1. quiz e14
32. Sigurdsson S, Alexandersson KF, Sulem P, Feenstra B, Gudmundsdottir S, Halldorsson GH, et al. Sequence variants in ARHGAP15, COLQ and FAM155A associate with diverticular disease and diverticulitis. Nat Commun. 2017;8:15789.
33. Connelly TM, Berg AS, Hegarty JP, Deiling S, Brinton D, Poritz LS, et al. The TNFSF15 gene single nucleotide polymorphism rs7848647 is associated with surgical diverticulitis. Ann Surg. 2014;259(6):1132–7.
34. Reichert MC, Kupcinskas J, Krawczyk M, Jungst C, Casper M, Grunhage F, et al. A variant of COL3A1 (rs3134646) is associated with risk of developing diverticulosis in white men. Dis Colon Rectum. 2018;61(5):604–11.
35. Coble JL, Sheldon KE, Yue F, Salameh TJ, Harris LR III, Deiling S, et al. Identification of a rare LAMB4 variant associated with familial diverticulitis through exome sequencing. Hum Mol Genet. 2017;26(16):3212–20.
36. Aldoori WH, Giovannucci EL, Rimm EB, Wing AL, Trichopoulos DV, Willett WC. A prospective study of alcohol, smoking, caffeine, and the risk of symptomatic diverticular disease in men. Ann Epidemiol. 1995;5(3):221–8.
37. Strate LL, Liu YL, Syngal S, Aldoori WH, Giovannucci EL. Nut, corn, and popcorn consumption and the incidence of diverticular disease. JAMA. 2008;300(8):907–14.
38. Maguire LH, Song M, Strate LL, Giovannucci EL, Chan AT. Association of geographic and seasonal variation with diverticulitis admissions. JAMA Surg. 2015;150(1):74–7.
39. Ly NP, Litonjua A, Gold DR, Celedon JC. Gut microbiota, probiotics, and vitamin D: interrelated exposures influencing allergy, asthma, and obesity? J Allergy Clin Immunol. 2011;127(5):1087–94. quiz 95–6
40. Maguire LH, Song M, Strate LE, Giovannucci EL, Chan AT. Higher serum levels of vitamin D are associated with a reduced risk of diverticulitis. Clin Gastroenterol Hepatol. 2013;11(12):1631–5.
41. Hjern F, Wolk A, Hakansson N. Smoking and the risk of diverticular disease in women. Br J Surg. 2011;98(7):997–1002.
42. Turunen P, Wikstrom H, Carpelan-Holmstrom M, Kairaluoma P, Kruuna O, Scheinin T. Smoking

increases the incidence of complicated diverticular disease of the sigmoid colon. Scand J Surg. 2010;99(1):14–7.
43. Strate LL, Liu YL, Huang ES, Giovannucci EL, Chan AT. Use of aspirin or nonsteroidal anti-inflammatory drugs increases risk for diverticulitis and diverticular bleeding. Gastroenterology. 2011;140(5):1427–33.
44. Kvasnovsky CL, Papagrigoriadis S, Bjarnason I. Increased diverticular complications with nonsteriodal anti-inflammatory drugs and other medications: a systematic review and meta-analysis. Color Dis. 2014;16(6):O189–96.
45. Humes DJ, Fleming KM, Spiller RC, West J. Concurrent drug use and the risk of perforated colonic diverticular disease: a population-based case-control study. Gut. 2011;60(2):219–24.
46. von Rahden BH, Kircher S, Thiery S, Landmann D, Jurowich CF, Germer CT, et al. Association of steroid use with complicated sigmoid diverticulitis: potential role of activated CD68+/CD163+ macrophages. Langenbeck's Arch Surg. 2011;396(6):759–68.
47. Strate LL, Liu YL, Aldoori WH, Giovannucci EL. Physical activity decreases diverticular complications. Am J Gastroenterol. 2009;104(5):1221–30.
48. Rosemar A, Angeras U, Rosengren A. Body mass index and diverticular disease: a 28-year follow-up study in men. Dis Colon Rectum. 2008;51(4):450–5.
49. Strate LL, Liu YL, Aldoori WH, Syngal S, Giovannucci EL. Obesity increases the risks of diverticulitis and diverticular bleeding. Gastroenterology. 2009;136(1):115–22 e1.
50. Aune D, Sen A, Leitzmann MF, Norat T, Tonstad S, Vatten LJ. Body mass index and physical activity and the risk of diverticular disease: a systematic review and meta-analysis of prospective studies. Eur J Nutr. 2017;56(8):2423–38.
51. Peery AF, Keku TO, Addamo C, McCoy AN, Martin CF, Galanko JA, et al. Colonic diverticula are not associated with mucosal inflammation or chronic gastrointestinal symptoms. Clin Gastroenterol Hepatol. 2018;16(6):884–91 e1.
52. Tursi A, Brandimarte G, Elisei W, Giorgetti GM, Inchingolo CD, Danese S, et al. Assessment and grading of mucosal inflammation in colonic diverticular disease. J Clin Gastroenterol. 2008;42(6):699–703.
53. Tursi A, Elisei W, Brandimarte G, Giorgetti GM, Aiello F. Predictive value of serologic markers of degree of histologic damage in acute uncomplicated colonic diverticulitis. J Clin Gastroenterol. 2010;44(10):702–6.
54. Tursi A, Elisei W, Brandimarte G, Giorgetti GM, Inchingolo CD, Nenna R, et al. Musosal tumour necrosis factor alpha in diverticular disease of the colon is overexpressed with disease severity. Color Dis. 2012;14(5):e258–63.
55. Humes DJ, Simpson J, Smith J, Sutton P, Zaitoun A, Bush D, et al. Visceral hypersensitivity in symptomatic diverticular disease and the role of neuropeptides and low grade inflammation. Neurogastroenterol Motil. 2012;24(4):318–e163.
56. Barbara G, Scaioli E, Barbaro MR, Biagi E, Laghi L, Cremon C, et al. Gut microbiota, metabolome and immune signatures in patients with uncomplicated diverticular disease. Gut. 2017;66(7):1252–61.
57. Simpson J, Sundler F, Humes DJ, Jenkins D, Scholefield JH, Spiller RC. Post inflammatory damage to the enteric nervous system in diverticular disease and its relationship to symptoms. Neurogastroenterol Motil. 2009;21(8):847–e58.
58. De Filippo C, Cavalieri D, Di Paola M, Ramazzotti M, Poullet JB, Massart S, et al. Impact of diet in shaping gut microbiota revealed by a comparative study in children from Europe and rural Africa. Proc Natl Acad Sci USA. 2010;107(33):14691–6.
59. Jones RB, Fodor AA, Peery AF, Tsilimigras MCB, Winglee K, McCoy A, et al. An aberrant microbiota is not strongly associated with incidental colonic diverticulosis. Sci Rep. 2018;8(1):4951.
60. Daniels L, Budding AE, de Korte N, Eck A, Bogaards JA, Stockmann HB, et al. Fecal microbiome analysis as a diagnostic test for diverticulitis. Eur J Clin Microbiol Infect Dis. 2014;33(11):1927–36.
61. Schieffer KM, Sabey K, Wright JR, Toole DR, Drucker R, Tokarev V, et al. The microbial ecosystem distinguishes chronically diseased tissue from adjacent tissue in the sigmoid colon of chronic, recurrent diverticulitis patients. Sci Rep. 2017;7(1):8467.

Epidemiology of Diverticulitis

2

Nir Horesh

Introduction

Diverticular disease is one of the most common gastrointestinal conditions affecting adult population around the world. The prevalence of diverticular disease, which will be discussed in this chapter, underscores its importance as a public health concern and justifies the need for a comprehensive understanding of its epidemiology.

In this chapter, we will review the epidemiology of diverticular disease, tracing it from a historical perspective to contemporary global patterns. Our analysis will encompass age and gender distribution, the burden and economic cost of the disease, and the effectiveness of global strategies for prevention and management. We will also delve into current trends and future predictions, culminating in a discussion on future directions in research and policy. This comprehensive exploration will not only provide a global overview but also highlight the personal impact of diverticular disease, leading to a deeper understanding crucial for shaping future healthcare strategies [1–4].

N. Horesh (✉)
Cleveland Clinic Florida, Ellen Leifer Shulman and Steven Shulman Digestive Disease Center, Weston, FL, USA

Department of Surgery and Transplantations, Sheba Medical Center, Ramat Gan, Israel

Tel Aviv University, Tel Aviv, Israel
e-mail: horeshn@ccf.org

Historical Perspective

Diverticular disease, while predominantly recognized as a disease of the twentieth and twenty-first centuries, was first described in the medical literature in the seventeenth century. Alexis Littre, a prominent French surgeon, is credited with one of the earliest descriptions of colonic saccular outpouchings around 1700 [5]. The term "divertikel," originating from a Latin word meaning "bypath," was first coined as an anatomical finding by Fleischman in 1815 [6]. Colonic diverticulum, described as herniations through gaps in the colon's muscular layer, was described by the French anatomist Jean Cruveilhier in 1849 [7]. The first hypothesis for the pathogenesis of diverticuli was mentioned by Klebs, a German microbiologist, who suggested that diverticula were acquired and possibly linked to constipation. Later, in 1899, Graser described the inflammation of these diverticula, coining the term "peridiverticulitis." Complications such as fistulas, adhesions, peritonitis, and stenosis were described by Beer in 1904 and the first report of surgical treatment for diverticular disease was made by Mayo and his colleagues in 1907. The first documented radiologic studies of diverticula were performed by Case in 1914 [8].

Radiological advancements revealed the commonality of diverticula, a realization further supported by postmortem and barium studies. Mayo, in 1930, estimated that about 5% of individuals over 40 years old had diverticula in their

M. Boutros et al. (eds.), *Diverticulitis*, https://doi.org/10.1007/978-3-032-21720-2_2

colons, aligning with findings from both Europe and America [9]. The 1940s marked a significant advancement in the treatment of diverticular disease, particularly with the widespread introduction of antibiotics. Smithwick in 1942 advocated for resection of the affected colon, which then became a standard surgical procedure [10]. Hartmann's perfection of the end-colostomy in 1923 played a pivotal role in this surgical evolution and is still considered by many as the standard of care for emergency cases [11]. The work of Painter and Burkitt in the mid-twentieth century, which matured into a pivotal publication in 1971, significantly advanced the understanding of colonic pressure in relation to the pathogenesis of diverticular disease, suggesting that fiber intake should be a principal measure for the prevention of diverticular complications [12]. Since then, many authors described the epidemiological, clinical, and therapeutic aspects related to diverticular disease, with challenges of the treatment dogmas arising mostly in the last two decades.

Global Epidemiology

Over the past century, there has been a significant increase in the incidence of diverticular disease. Early twentieth-century autopsy studies reported colonic diverticula rates of 2% to 10%. However, more recent data indicate that up to 50% of individuals over 60 years have colonic diverticula [13]. It has been estimated that 10% to 25% of people who have diverticulosis will develop symptoms and complications related to diverticulitis [14]. Hospitalization rates for diverticular disease have mirrored this trend, with a notable 26% increase in admissions observed in a pivotal study reviewing the National Inpatient Sample database (NIS) in the United States between 1998 and 2005 [15]. This pattern was later confirmed by large population studies conducted in Canada [16] and Europe [17].

The global landscape of diverticular disease has also undergone significant changes in recent decades, reflecting broader shifts in dietary patterns, population movements, and healthcare practices. Historically predominant in Western nations, where high-fat, low-fiber diets have long been the norm, diverticular disease has seen its prevalence escalate in regions previously less affected, such as Asian countries [18]. Recent reports suggest a notable increase in incidence rates in Asia, which are estimated to increase by 0.5% annually. This shift is closely linked to the global convergence towards Western dietary habits, compounded by widespread immigration, which has reduced the geographical disparities in disease prevalence [19]. A recent systematic review and meta-analysis conducted by Ray-Offor et al. [20] included 30 studies conducted from 1985 to 2022 examining the incidence and prevalence of colonic diverticulosis in Africa, showing a significant increase over the past decade. The pooled prevalence rate has surged to 9.7% between 2012 and 2022, up from 3.5% in the previous years. The increase was most prevalent among males over the age of 50. As with Asian populations, this increase is likely related to a few factors, mainly the increased exposure to western diet in the last few decades, but perhaps also demonstrating some bias as in the last decades patients probably had better access to healthcare and therefore higher rates of diagnosis.

These changes also influenced the anatomical variations in the manifestation of diverticular disease. In Western populations, diverticulosis predominantly affects the left colon, whereas in Asian countries, right-sided diverticula are more common. This geographical variation has sparked debates about the congenital versus acquired nature of diverticuli, with recent studies challenging the notion that right-sided diverticular disease in Asians is inherently congenital [21]. Furthermore, genetic research, including studies on the TNFSF15 single-nucleotide polymorphism (SNP), suggests that there are possible interactions between genetic factors in the susceptibility to diverticulitis to acquired factors including dietary habits [22].

As the incidence of diverticular disease continues to rise globally, the absence of comprehensive worldwide data from organizations such as the World Health Organization (WHO) or similar entities becomes a notable gap in the current understanding of the disease's prevalence and characteristics. This limitation highlights the need for extensive, coordinated studies that can provide a clearer picture of diverticular disease prevalence, its varying manifestations across different populations, and potential shifts in its demographic profile.

Age, Gender, and Race Distribution

The distribution of diverticular disease by age and gender shows that prevalence significantly increases with age, being uncommon in people under 40 years of age but rising sharply to affect 50–70% of individuals over 80 years. Early studies indicated a higher incidence in men, but recent findings suggest that the gender gap narrows with age, with older women exhibiting equal or greater prevalence [13].

Age is the most significant risk factor for developing diverticulosis, with rates increasing from below 20% at age 40 to 60% by age 60 in the United States. The prevalence in older populations suggests a progressive deterioration of the colonic wall as the main mechanism behind the creation of diverticuli over time [23]. The incidence of diverticulitis also escalates with age, peaking at a mean admission age of 63, though about 16% of cases occur in individuals under 45, indicating that while age is a pivotal factor, younger populations are not exempt from this condition [18].

The severity of diverticular disease and the risk for surgical intervention also increase with age, as older patients are more likely to develop complications that necessitate surgery. Gender differences also play a role, with men under 50 years more commonly affected by diverticulitis, but women show a higher incidence in older age groups. Although younger age was considered a risk factor for severe presentation, a recent meta-analysis encompassing 27 studies found no significant difference in the severity of acute diverticulitis or need for emergency surgery between young patients (aged 40–50) and elderly patients [24]. Younger patients showed a higher relative risk for recurrent diverticulitis in crude data analysis, but this association disappeared when a survival analysis was performed [25]. Consequently, the evidence, which supported surgical intervention for younger patients, has changed and current guidelines do not support a more aggressive treatment or a lower threshold for elective surgery in this population [26].

Race and ethnicity also play a significant role in the prevalence and outcomes of colonic diverticular disease. A recent cross-sectional analysis of patients presenting to the emergency department in the United States with diverticular disease demonstrated that the prevalence of the disease is notably higher among Black individuals, with Black men showing a prevalence of 53.9% and Black women 71.5%, compared to other racial and ethnic groups. While there is no significant difference in the severity of diverticular bleeding between men and women, women generally have lower odds of being admitted to the hospital for the condition (0.88; 0.80–0.97). Furthermore, racial disparities are evident in the management of the disease; Blacks, Hispanics, and Asian/Pacific Islanders have higher odds of requiring red blood cell (RBC) transfusions compared to White patients. Additionally, Asian/Pacific Islanders of both sexes and Black men specifically are more likely to be admitted to the hospital for diverticular disease. These disparities underscore the importance of considering race and ethnicity in the diagnosis, treatment, and management of colonic diverticular disease to ensure equitable healthcare outcomes [27].

Disease Burden and Costs

Diverticular disease presents a significant healthcare challenge, especially in industrialized nations like the United States. Approximately 3 million Americans are diagnosed with diverticulitis annually, and 1 in 4 are reported to suffer from recurrent episodes [28]. In 2014, complaints related to diverticulitis led to over 370,000 emergency department visits, nearly a million days of inpatient care, and incurred $5.5 billion in healthcare costs [23]. Notably, there has been an 82% increase in age-adjusted admissions for younger patients aged 18 to 44 from 1998 to 2005, highlighting a shift towards the admission of younger patients [15]. However, a study examining admission trends between 2006 and 2011 showed that the admission rates for low risk (defined as age <50 with no comorbidities) declined from 35.2% in 2006 to 26.8% in 2011 [29]. This shift is probably due to the evolving evidence on the treatment of diverticulitis, which created a shift towards less aggressive, more cost-effective management strategies. These included promoting community management for patients with acute diverticulitis, which were beneficial in reducing hospital admissions and treatment costs. Evidence from multiple studies supports the safety and efficacy of outpatient treatment for mild diverticulitis cases, particularly for patients without significant comorbidities, who can manage an oral diet and antibiotics [30]. The disease's burden varies widely across different regions, reflecting the need for targeted public health strategies and efficient management approaches to mitigate its impact.

These changes created significant variability in healthcare costs related to diverticular disease. A recent study by Isacson et al. [31] highlighted the economic benefits of ambulatory management of diverticulitis, showing a reduction in total healthcare costs related to diverticulitis from Euro 558,679 in 2011 to Euro 370,370 in 2014 after adopting selective outpatient management policies. However, the increased access to healthcare and the improvement in disease diagnosis had the contrary effect on healthcare costs related to diverticulitis. A study examining patients with a primary diagnosis of diverticulitis in the National Emergency Department Sample (NEDS) between 2006 and 2013, showed a significant increase in the rate of emergency department (ED) visits by 26.8%, rising from 89.8 to 113.9 visits per 100,000 population. Concurrently, the national cost for these visits doubled, escalating from approximately $822 million to over $1.6 billion. These costs were significantly elevated despite the fact that there was a notable decrease in the percentage of patients directly admitted to the hospital from the ED, dropping from 58.0% to 47.1%. Additionally, the rate of surgeries per 100,000 ED visits for diverticulitis saw a significant reduction of 33.7% during the same period [32]. To conclude, diverticular disease imposes a growing financial and healthcare burden, with increasing emergency visits and rising costs challenging healthcare systems. Efforts to optimize management strategies have proven effective and should be implemented to reduce the rates of hospital admissions and surgeries for this condition.

Current Trends and Future Predictions

The epidemiology and incidence of diverticulitis are currently characterized by several noteworthy trends. As mentioned before, there has been an increase in the incidence of diverticulitis among younger populations, challenging the traditional view of diverticulitis as a condition predominantly affecting the elderly [33]. This shift is partly attributed to changes in dietary habits, lifestyle factors, and increasing obesity rates globally and partly due to increased access to healthcare and diagnostic measures. Although this shift caused an increase in admission for diverticulitis in younger populations, it is likely that ambulatory management of diverticular disease will continue to rise especially within this population, which typically is at a lower risk for severe sequela. Furthermore, although slow to adapt, many studies published in recent years challenged the dogma of diverticulitis management increasing the shift towards more conservative management of uncomplicated and complicated diverticulitis. Increasing evidence supports the safety and efficacy of treating mild cases of diverticulitis without antibiotics, which is now recommended in some societies' guidelines across the globe [34]. This trend is driven by a growing awareness of antibiotic resistance and the potential for antibiotics to disrupt the gut microbiome. Future management strategies are likely to increasingly favor observation and symptomatic treatment for select patients, reserving antibiotics and surgical management for more severe cases or those with complicating factors. Furthermore, the trend towards personalized medicine is also making its way into diverticulitis care. Understanding the variability in how individuals respond to different treatments is leading to more customized treatment plans, which is also reflected in management guidelines [26]. Factors such as a patient's age, comorbidities, lifestyle, and quality of life are increasingly considered when deciding on management strategies. This patient-centered approach aims to optimize outcomes while minimizing unnecessary interventions.

The knowledge gained in the last few decades also improved our understanding about certain risk factors which can be play a role in disease prevention. The growing emphasis on the role of diet, physical activity, and weight management is likely to reduce the risk of complicated disease [35, 36]. Public health initiatives are likely to increase in number and intensity, aiming to educate the public about the importance of dietary fiber and healthy lifestyle choices in preventing diverticular disease. Future research may provide more data about the role of the microbiome and potential interventions related to the microbiota which might help with disease prevention and treatment [37].

Looking ahead, the increasing prevalence of diverticulitis as life expectancy is on the rise along with the increased prevalence in younger population suffering from the disease, should cause healthcare systems to address the needs of these demographics, including developing guidelines for younger patients and focusing on prevention and early intervention. As mentioned before, despite lower rates of surgical interventions and admissions, costs and disease burden are on the rise, which should lead decision makers in healthcare to adapt to these ongoing changes [34, 36].

Conclusions

The epidemiology of diverticulitis reveals a complex condition influenced by a myriad of factors, including age, gender, dietary habits, and lifestyle choices. Recent trends indicate a shift in the age distribution of affected individuals, with an increasing incidence among younger populations. This shift, alongside the established prevalence in older adults, underscores the need for a nuanced understanding of the disease's pathophysiology and risk factors. The role of diet, particularly fiber intake, and the impact of obesity highlight the importance of preventive measures and lifestyle modifications in managing the condition's burden. The evolving landscape of diverticulitis management, favoring conservative treatments and personalized care, reflects a broader trend towards optimizing patient outcomes while minimizing unnecessary interventions.

Future directions in the research and management of diverticulitis should focus on refining diagnostic criteria, enhancing noninvasive treatment options, and further exploring the genetic and microbiomic factors contributing to the disease. Additionally, public health initiatives aimed at promoting dietary changes and healthy lifestyle choices could play a crucial role in reducing the incidence and severity of diverticulitis. As the global population ages and dietary patterns continue to shift, the burden of diverticulitis is likely to increase, making it imperative for healthcare systems to adapt and for research to continue advancing our understanding of this condition. The collective efforts of clinicians, researchers, and public health professionals will be essential in addressing the challenges posed by diverticulitis and improving the quality of life for those affected.

References

1. Nallapeta NS, Farooq U, Patel K. Diverticulosis. In: StatPearls. Treasure Island: StatPearls Publishing; 2024.
2. Bailey J, Dattani S, Jennings A. Diverticular disease:epidemiology of: rapid evidence review. Am Fam Physician. 2022;106(2):150–6.
3. Hobson KG, Roberts PL. Etiology and pathophysiology of diverticular disease. Clin Colon Rectal Surg. 2004;17(3):147–53.
4. Diverticulitis: Practice Essentials, Background, Pathophysiology [Internet]. [cited 2024 Feb 8]. Available from: https://emedicine.medscape.com/article/173388-overview
5. Matrana MR, Margolin DA. Epidemiology and pathophysiology of diverticular disease. Clin Colon Rectal Surg. 2009;22(3):141–6.

6. Myers A, Jones OM. Diverticulitis, pelvic and other intra-abdominal abscesses (including laparoscopic management). Surgery (Oxford). 2011;29(8):391–4.
7. Jackman RJ, Buie LA. Diverticula of the colon. JAMA. 1943;121(14):1144.
8. Patterson SW. The history of diverticulitis of the intestine. Proc R Soc Med. 1950;43(11):785–9.
9. Mayo WJ. Diverticula of the sigmoid. Ann Surg. 1930;92(4):739–43.
10. Smithwick RH. Experiences with the surgical management of diverticulitis of the sigmoid. Ann Surg. 1942;115(6):969–85.
11. Sanderson ER. Henri Hartmann and the Hartmann operation. Arch Surg. 1980;115(6):792–3.
12. Painter NS, Burkitt DP. Diverticular disease of the colon: a deficiency disease of Western civilization. Br Med J. 1971;2(5759):450–4.
13. Weizman AV, Nguyen GC. Diverticular disease:epidemiology of: epidemiology and management. Can J Gastroenterol. 2011;25(7):385–9.
14. Horesh N, Wasserberg N, Zbar AP, Gravetz A, Berger Y, Gutman M, et al. Changing paradigms in the management of diverticulitis. Int J Surg. 2016;33(Pt A):146–50.
15. Etzioni DA, Mack TM, Beart RW, Kaiser AM. Diverticulitis in the United States: 1998–2005: changing patterns of disease and treatment. Ann Surg. 2009;249(2):210–7.
16. Warner E, Crighton EJ, Moineddin R, Mamdani M, Upshur R. Fourteen-year study of hospital admissions for diverticular disease in Ontario. Can J Gastroenterol. 2007;21(2):97–9.
17. Cammarota S, Cargiolli M, Andreozzi P, Toraldo B, Citarella A, Flacco ME, et al. Increasing trend in admission rates and costs for acute diverticulitis during 2005-2015: real-life data from the Abruzzo Region. Ther Adv Gastroenterol 2018;11:1756284818791502.
18. Imaeda H, Hibi T. The burden of diverticular disease and its complications: west versus east. Inflamm Intest Dis. 2018;3(2):61–8.
19. Bhatia M, Mattoo A. Diverticulosis and diverticulitis: epidemiology, pathophysiology, and current treatment trends. Cureus. 2023;15(8):e43158.
20. Ray-Offor E, Egboh SM, Ijah RFOA, Hany Emile S, Wexner SD. Colonic diverticulosis at colonoscopy in Africa: a systematic review and meta-analysis of pooled estimates. Dig Surg. 2024;41(2):63–78. https://doi.org/10.1159/000536587. Epub 2024 Feb 20
21. Turner GA, O'Grady MJ, Purcell RV, Frizelle FA. The epidemiology and etiology of right-sided colonic diverticulosis: a review. Ann Coloproctol. 2021;37(4):196–203.
22. Connelly TM, Berg AS, Hegarty JP, Deiling S, Brinton D, Poritz LS, et al. The TNFSF15 gene single nucleotide polymorphism rs7848647 is associated with surgical diverticulitis. Ann Surg. 2014;259(6):1132–7.
23. Hawkins AT, Wise PE, Chan T, Lee JT, Glyn T, Wood V, et al. Diverticulitis: an update from the age old paradigm. Curr Probl Surg. 2020;57(10):100862.
24. Peery AF, Keku TO, Galanko JA, Sandler RS. Sex and race disparities in diverticulosis prevalence. Clin Gastroenterol Hepatol. 2020;18(9):1980–6.
25. Edna T-H, Jamal Talabani A, Lydersen S, Endreseth BH. Survival after acute colon diverticulitis treated in hospital. Int J Color Dis. 2014;29(11):1361–7.
26. Hall J, Hardiman K, Lee S, Lightner A, Stocchi L, Paquette IM, et al. The American Society of Colon and Rectal Surgeons clinical practice guidelines for the treatment of left-sided colonic diverticulitis. Dis Colon Rectum. 2020;63(6):728–47.
27. Zheng NS, Ma W, Shung DL, Strate LL, Chan AT. Sex, race, and ethnicity differences in patients presenting with diverticular disease at Emergency Departments in the United States: a National Cross-Sectional Study. Gastro Hep Adv. 2023;3(2):178–80. https://doi.org/10.1016/j.gastha.2023.11.012. PMID: 39129950; PMCID: PMC11307830
28. Hantouli MN, Khor S, Strate LL, Lavallee DC, Mower WR, Porter AJ, et al. What's in a number? Assessing the burden of diverticular disease. Ann Surg Open. 2022;3(4):e202.
29. Greenwood-Ericksen MB, Havens JM, Ma J, Weissman JS, Schuur JD. Trends in hospital admission and surgical procedures following ED visits for diverticulitis. West J Emerg Med. 2016;17(4):409–17.
30. van Dijk ST, Bos K, de Boer MGJ, Draaisma WA, van Enst WA, Felt RJF, et al. A systematic review and meta-analysis of outpatient treatment for acute diverticulitis. Int J Color Dis. 2018;33(5):505–12.
31. Isacson D, Andreasson K, Nikberg M, Smedh K, Chabok A. Outpatient management of acute uncomplicated diverticulitis results in health-care cost savings. Scand J Gastroenterol. 2018;53(4):449–52.
32. Bollom A, Austrie J, Hirsch W, Nee J, Friedlander D, Ellingson K, et al. Emergency department burden of diverticulitis in the USA, 2006–2013. Dig Dis Sci. 2017;62(10):2694–703.
33. Strate LL, Morris AM. Epidemiology, pathophysiology, and treatment of diverticulitis. Gastroenterology. 2019;156(5):1282–1298.e1.
34. Sartelli M, Weber DG, Kluger Y, Ansaloni L, Coccolini F, Abu-Zidan F, et al. 2020 update of the WSES guidelines for the management of acute colonic diverticulitis in the emergency setting. World J Emerg Surg. 2020;15(1):32.
35. Carabotti M, Falangone F, Cuomo R, Annibale B. Role of dietary habits in the prevention of diverticular disease complications: a systematic review. Nutrients. 2021;13(4)
36. Patient education: Diverticular disease (Beyond the Basics)—UpToDate [Internet]. [cited 2024 Feb 8]. Available from: https://www.uptodate.com/contents/diverticular-disease-beyond-the-basics/print
37. Piccioni A, Franza L, Brigida M, Zanza C, Torelli E, Petrucci M, et al. Gut microbiota and acute diverticulitis: role of probiotics in management of this delicate pathophysiological balance. J Pers Med. 2021;11(4)

Symptoms and Diagnosis

3

Andrea Petrucci and Sebastien Lachance

Introduction

Diverticulosis is a common pathology in Western countries, affecting 60% of the general population by the age of 60 [1]. Owing to its important incidence, diverticular disease inflicts important costs to healthcare systems of Western Countries [2]. The lifetime risk of diverticulitis in a person with diverticulosis was reported to range from 10% to 25% [1, 2].

Various Symptomatic Presentations of Diverticulitis

Patients with diverticulitis can have different presentation patterns depending on whether they have acute or chronic disease. In patients with an acute presentation, they can have complicated or uncomplicated disease, with the latter being the most common of the two. Symptoms of diverticulitis will usually depend on the colonic location of the inflamed diverticulum, the degree of inflammation present in the colonic wall, and any complications associated with the disease.

Acute Uncomplicated Diverticulitis

Acute uncomplicated diverticulitis occurs when there is inflammation of the diverticula extending to the colonic wall without the formation of an abscess, fistula, stricture, or perforation [3]. In patients with acute uncomplicated diverticulitis, the most common symptom is left lower quadrant abdominal pain since the most common colonic segment affected is the sigmoid colon. This pain may or may not be accompanied by fever and leukocytosis [4]. With this classic presentation, a diagnosis of uncomplicated diverticulitis is the most likely, and treatment can be started accordingly. In cases where the sigmoid colon is very redundant, patients can present with right-sided abdominal pain, suprapubic pain or guarding and tenderness that can mimic other gastrointestinal presentations such as inflammatory bowel disease (IBD), acute appendicitis, or left-sided appendicitis; therefore, a focused history and physical exam are paramount in order to help guide workup and treatment. Less often, patients can present with nausea and vomiting, guarding and tenderness; however, this is usually associated with more advanced complicated disease causing an ileus or obstruction, to be discussed later [5, 6].

The original version of the chapter has been revised. A correction to this chapter can be found at https://doi.org/10.1007/978-3-032-21720-2_24

A. Petrucci (✉)
Department of Surgery, Cite de la Sante Hospital, Laval, QC, Canada

S. Lachance
Hopital Cite-de-la-Sante de Laval, 1755 Boul. Rene-Laennec, Laval, QC, Canada

M. Boutros et al. (eds.), *Diverticulitis*, https://doi.org/10.1007/978-3-032-21720-2_3

Acute Complicated Diverticulitis

Acute complicated diverticulitis occurs when the inflammation of the colon is associated with the formation of any of the following: abscess or phlegmon, fistula, obstruction, or perforation [4]. In patients with acute complicated diverticulitis, presentation can vary from one patient to the next depending on the severity of the disease, patient's immune system, and functional status. For example, a patient with a pericolic abscess may present with fever and localized left-sided abdominal pain while another patient may present with diffuse abdominal pain and signs of systemic toxicity. In the latter case, these symptoms are suggestive of the presence of perforation and these patients need to be evaluated and treated urgently.

For patients who develop a fistula, they will also have varying presentations depending on the location of the fistula and whether other adjacent organs are involved. The most common types of fistulas are colovesical (65%) and colovaginal (25%) fistulas. Other more rare fistulas include coloenteric (7%) colouetrine (3%), and colocutaneous fistulas (1%) [7, 8]. Up to 10% of patients may also present with multiple fistulas to different organs which can lead to multiple organ systems being simultaneously affected [7, 9]. Fistulizing disease is the reason for operative intervention in 20% of patients with complicated diverticulitis [10, 11]. Colovesical fistulas occur in up to 5% of patients with complicated disease [9]. In these cases, patients can present with pneumaturia, fecaluria, and recurrent urinary tract infections [9]. Colovaginal fistulas most commonly result from either having had a hysterectomy or report a history of diverticulitis. A common presentation includes a patient who reports passing stool and/or flatus per vagina, with or without persistent foul-smelling vaginal discharge [12]. Roughly half of these patients report abdominal pain [13]. They may also report vaginitis that is resistant to local or medical treatment [12]. Patients who have coloenteric fistulas, although rare, most commonly present with diarrhea as a result of the succus entericus bypassing the rest of the small bowel and emptying directly into the distal colon. Patients will commonly report large amounts of watery diarrhea and weight loss due to the inability to properly absorb water and nutrients in the small bowel [7, 14]. They may also have abdominal pain and the finding of an abdominal mass on physical exam [7, 15]. Colouterine fistulas are extremely rare due to the thickness of the uterine wall [16]. They are usually caused by complications from obstetrical trauma or intervention, malignancy, or radiation; however, significant inflammation of the colon can lead to necrosis that extends and erodes into the uterus causing a fistula [11, 17]. Symptoms can resemble those seen with a colovaginal fistula such as fecal or purulent vaginal discharge [11, 16] with or without fever or abdominal pain. Due to the vascularity of the uterine wall, colonic bacteria can easily translocate into the bloodstream causing septicemia without the formation of an abscess [17].

Lastly, enterocutaneous fistulas rarely develop spontaneously secondary to diverticulitis. They most commonly occur following complications from bowel resection for diverticulitis or any percutaneous intervention [8, 18]. Patients will present with foul smelling, feculent discharge from an opening in the skin, along with abdominal pain and may also have a palpable mass at the site [8].

Colonic obstruction in the acute setting is usually a result of partial narrowing of the colonic lumen either from thickening of the colon wall from acute inflammation or from extracolonic compression from a phlegmon or abscess. It is rare to have a high-grade large bowel obstruction during an acute attack and if this does occur, it is usually secondary to a stricture from chronic disease or a mass [7]. The inflammation at the site of an acute attack may also be significant enough to cause ileus [7]. There are also reports, albeit rare, of patients with small bowel obstruction (SBO) secondary to diverticulitis. In these cases, the small bowel becomes adherent to the inflammation on the sigmoid colon causing narrowing and kinking of the small bowel lumen [19]. These patients present with obstructive symptoms and can be treated using the same algorithm for a more typical adhesive SBO. Their symptoms may improve as the inflammation from the acute attack of diverticulitis is treated; however, if the adhesions persist and the small bowel remains obstructed, surgery may be necessary.

In the case of a perforation secondary to an acute attack, patients are typically very ill. Perforated diverticulitis results from either free perforation of a colonic diverticulum or perforation of an abscess causing purulent of fecal peritonitis. Patients will have significant diffuse abdominal pain possibly radiating to the shoulder with or without shortness of breath [6]. They can also be hemodynamically unstable due to the uncontrolled sepsis; therefore, it is important to quickly assess these patients as they will need emergent surgery.

Chronic Diverticulitis

Chronic diverticular disease occurs in patients whose symptoms do not resolve over a long period of time despite undergoing previous treatment. The length of time is not well defined in the literature; however, patients who continue to have longstanding left lower quadrant pain despite treatment are considered to have chronic manifestations of the disease. The term "smoldering" diverticulitis is used to describe a group of patients who are not responsive to medical management but do not progress to complicated disease [20]. These patients have documented diverticula either seen endoscopically or radiologically and commonly complain of unremitting left-sided abdominal pain with or without any signs of fever or leukocytosis [21, 22]. They are often defined as having a chronic disease due to the fact that their acute event does not fully resolve and continues to cause symptoms.

Recent studies have attempted to better characterize patients who had attacks of diverticulitis and continue to have abdominal pain and altered bowel habits after the acute attack has resolved. In a review by Boostrom et al. [22], these patients were classified as having "atypical" diverticulitis, where their symptoms had to last for a minimum of 3 months. One randomized clinical trial looking at antibiotics versus no antibiotics for the treatment of uncomplicated disease followed patients for a year after their diverticulitis attack and found that up to 40% of patients still had either mild or moderate abdominal pain and/or a change in bowel habits [23]. Another large retrospective study by Cohen et al. [24] looked at patients with acute attacks of diverticulitis and compared them to controls who did not have any diverticular disease. They found that patients who had previous bouts of diverticulitis were more likely to develop symptoms of irritable bowel syndrome (IBS) long after the attack had resolved. Symptoms included longstanding abdominal pain and an alteration in bowel habits, and the authors suggested naming this disorder "post-diverticulitis IBS." In the same study, they also found a greater than twofold increase in the development of depression and related mood disorders in patients who had previous attacks of diverticulitis [24].

Patients who have repeated attacks of diverticulitis in the same colonic segment can eventually develop colonic wall thickening secondary to inflammatory changes causing dense fibrosis and scarring [25]. This leads to narrowing of the lumen causing a stricture which can lead to patients experiencing partial obstructive symptoms such as chronic bloating and abdominal cramping after meals, constipation, and overall abdominal discomfort. Given that the segment of colon is narrowed due to fibrosis rather than acute inflammation, it is unlikely that symptoms will improve. Therefore, after ruling out any possible malignancy of the colon at this site, an elective sigmoid resection should be offered.

Special Cases

Immunocompromised Patients

An episode of acute diverticulitis may have a different clinical presentation in patients who are immunosuppressed compared to those who are immunocompetent. The definition of immunosuppressed patients according to the American College of Surgeons National Surgical Quality Improvement Program (ACS-NSQIP) database includes those who regularly take corticosteroids either orally or parentally, patients on immunosuppressive medications, including those used for chemotherapy or transplantation, and patients with chronic inflammatory conditions [26]. According to the literature, immunosuppressed patients present with more severe symptoms during their first diverticulitis attack compared to immunocompetent patients. Interestingly, this vulnerable group of patients usually presents with fever and hypotension and is less likely to present with abdominal pain and tenderness on physical exam due to their inability to mount an inflammatory response [27, 28]. Moreover, there is an increasing incidence of free peritoneal perforation or complicated disease in patients who are immunosuppressed compared to immunocompetent patients; therefore, regardless of the severity of the disease, the diagnosis of acute diverticulitis based on a patient's clinical presentation can be challenging [29]. It is critically important for physicians to have a high suspicion of a possible intra-abdominal process when evaluating this group of patients, even when their physical exam is not indicative because a missed diagnosis can lead to increased morbidity and mortality in this cohort of patients [29].

Unusual Presentation of Diverticulitis

Right-sided diverticulitis has a completely different presentation than the classic sigmoid diverticulitis. Diverticula of the cecum are extremely rare with an incidence of less than 2% [30]. They occur more frequently in younger patients, and more in the Oriental population, with equal sex distribution. Furthermore, the number of diverticula does not appear to progress with age [31]. The classic presentation of right-sided diverticulitis is right lower quadrant pain that can mimic acute appendicitis. Patients can also present with epigastric or right flank pain with associated fever, nausea, and vomiting, and leukocytosis [31]. Physical exam findings include guarding or rebound tenderness in the right lower quadrant [31]. There has also been a report of a middle-aged woman presenting with left-upper quadrant pain and constipation who was later diagnosed during laparotomy with a long redundant right colon, laying in her left-upper quadrant with an inflamed, gangrenous cecal diverticulum [32]. Because of the similar clinical presentations between acute right-sided diverticulitis and appendicitis, accurate diagnosis can be difficult. It can also be confused with cecal adenocarcinoma during surgery [30].

Other rare cases of diverticulitis include small bowel disease, such as jejunal diverticulitis. As an acquired diverticulum, this occurs later in life, usually around the fifth decade [33]. The incidence of jejunal diverticulitis is rare, ranging from 2 to 6%, and patients present with nonspecific symptomatology such as abdominal pain, fever, and occasional gastrointestinal bleeding usually related to ulceration. The presentation can be confusing as it may mimic acute appendicitis or cholecystitis [33]. Cases of jejunal diverticulitis are rarely studied and consist mostly of case reports; therefore, as with cecal diverticulitis, diagnosis can be challenging.

Diagnosis

History and Physical Exam

The initial evaluation of any patient with suspected acute diverticulitis should include a history and physical examination. The initial evaluation should not be limited to establishing the diagnosis of acute diverticulitis, but to rule out other etiologies of abdominal pain, which in women includes pelvic pathologies. The astute clinician should therefore consider other diagnoses such as constipation, irritable bowel syndrome (IBS), appendicitis, IBD, cancer, kidney stones, urinary tract infection, bowel obstruction, and gynecologic disorders in the differential diagnosis.

History and physical examinations raise suspicion of diverticulitis, as stated in the most recent American Society of Colon and Rectal Surgeons (ASCRS) and Society of American Gastrointestinal and Endoscopic Surgeons guidelines (SAGES) [34, 35]. Accordingly, laboratory tests should be used as an adjunct modality in the assessment of acute diverticulitis [36]. Computed tomography (CT) scan imaging has become the cornerstone for diagnosing and assessing the severity of acute diverticulitis.

Hinchey Classification

See Chap. 6.

Laboratory Findings

Typically, patients with acute diverticulitis may have an elevated white blood cell count. The leukocytosis is usually mild to moderate [23, 37]. In some series, the white blood cell count was normal in up to 45% of patients with diverticulitis [38]. Nevertheless, left sigmoid diverticulitis is commonly heralded by leukocytosis in the presence of left lower quadrant pain and fever [34, 35].

An elevated C-reactive protein (CRP) is another feature found in patients with acute diverticulitis and has been shown to have both a diagnostic and prognostic value [35, 39]. CRP values >50 mg/L have been shown to strongly support the diagnosis of acute diverticulitis. Furthermore, as opposed to other biomarkers, CRP correlates better with the severity in acute diverticulitis, the risk of perforation, and the response to therapy [39]. Accordingly, a value of >150 mg/L has been suggested to discriminate acute uncomplicated from complicated diverticulitis in patients with a first episode [40], while the value of >170 mg/L may predict a higher risk of treatment failure in Hinchey 1a diverticulitis [3]. Nonetheless, cut-off values vary in the literature as well as the quality of the studies upon which cut-off values are determined [40–43]. More recently, CRP was incorporated into a prediction model differentiating uncomplicated from complicated diverticulitis. With abdominal guarding and leukocytosis as cofactors, the model reached a negative predictive value of 96% for detecting complicated diverticulitis, thereby highlighting the value of CRP as an adjunct to any patient's diverticulitis assessment [35, 44].

Other potential laboratory predictors of acute diverticulitis severity that have been assessed in the literature include procalcitonin and fecal calprotectin. Jeger et al. [45] assessed 115 patients with acute diverticulitis using procalcitonin. They found that the highest values of procalcitonin on days 1 and 2 were able to distinguish between complicated versus uncomplicated disease, with a sensitivity and specificity of 81 and 91%, respectively. A cut-off value of 0.1 ng/L was reported. With regards to fecal calprotectin, a small study reporting on 48 patients established a potential role in predicting recurrent diverticulitis following an episode of acute diverticulitis [46].

Other laboratory investigations to consider when assessing patient with acute diverticulitis include urinalysis and urine culture. Urinalysis may reveal sterile pyuria as a result of nearby inflammation. Conversely, urine culture may be useful in identifying colonic flora, which may raise suspicion for a colovesical fistula as part of a more complicated process.

Despite the numerous tools at hand, there is not enough evidence to support a specific management algorithm for laboratory testing [46]. Therefore, it is well advised to consider each laboratory test as adjuncts when trying to rule in acute diverticulitis, stratify its severity and attempt to predict its course.

Imaging

Several features may be found on imaging in patients with diverticulitis. Similar to laboratory testing, imaging may help confirm the diagnosis of acute diverticulitis, while differentiating between an uncomplicated versus a complicated event. However, as opposed to laboratory testing, there is strong evidence to support the use of computed tomography (CT) scan over other modalities such as abdominal ultrasound (US), magnetic resonance imaging (MRI), and radiographs of the chest and abdomen [35, 36]. A more in-depth evaluation of each imaging modality in the assessment of acute colonic diverticulitis is explored in Chap. 5 [47–62].

Conclusion

Although most patients will present with classical symptoms of acute diverticulitis, it is important to have a high clinical suspicion of diverticulitis in certain patients who may not present with the classical picture. In these cases, knowledge of the different presentations along with the use of the wide range of diagnostic testing modalities available will help the treating physician appropriately diagnose and treat these patients and allow for prompt surgical treatment when necessary.

References

1. Peery AF, Barrett PR, Park D, Rogers AJ, Galanko JA, Martin CF, et al. A high-fiber diet does not protect against asymptomatic diverticulosis. Gastroenterology. 2012;142(2):266–72.e1.
2. Sandler RS, Everhart JE, Donowitz M, Adams E, Cronin K, Goodman C, et al. The burden of selected digestive diseases in the United States. Gastroenterology. 2002;122(5):1500–11.
3. Bolkenstein HE, Draaisma WA, van de Wall B, Consten E, Broeders I. Treatment of acute uncomplicated diverticulitis without antibiotics: risk factors for treatment failure. Int J Color Dis. 2018;33(7):863–9.
4. Steele SRHT, Read TE, Saclarides TJ, Senagore AJ, Whitlow CB. The ASCRS textbook of colon and rectal surgery, vol. 2. 3rd ed. New York: Springer; 2016. p. 649.
5. Pemberton J. Clinical manifestations and diagnosis of acute diverticulitis in adults UpToDate: UpToDate; 2019 [updated December 16, 2019. Available from: https://www.google.com/search?client=safari&rls=en&q=uptodate&ie=UTF-8&oe=UTF-8
6. Steele SRHT, Read TE, Saclarides TJ, Senagore AJ, Whitlow CB. The ASCRS textbook of colon and Rectal surgery. 3rd ed. New York: Springer; 2016. p. 1292.
7. Pemberton J. Diverticular fistulas UptoDate [updated March 26 2019.
8. Charalabopoulos A, Misiakos E, Macheras A. Colocutaneous fistula complicating sigmoid diverticulitis. Int J Surg Case Rep. 2011;2(5):68–70.
9. Bertelson NL, Abcarian H, Kalkbrenner KA, Blumetti J, Harrison JL, Chaudhry V, et al. Diverticular colovesical fistula: what should we really be doing? Tech Coloproctol. 2018;22(1):31–6.
10. Stollman NH, Raskin JB. Diagnosis and management of diverticular disease of the colon in adults. Ad hoc practice parameters Committee of the American College of Gastroenterology. Am J Gastroenterol. 1999;94(11):3110–21.
11. Choi PW. Colouterine fistula caused by diverticulitis of the sigmoid colon. J Korean Soc Coloproctol. 2012;28(6):321–4.
12. Berger MB, Khandwala N, Fenner DE, Burney RE. Colovaginal fistulas: presentation, evaluation, and management. Female Pelvic Med Reconstr Surg. 2016;22(5):355–8.
13. Hjern F, Goldberg SM, Johansson C, Parker SC, Mellgren A. Management of diverticular fistulae to the female genital tract. Color Dis. 2007;9(5):438–42.
14. Hool GJ, Bokey EL, Pheils MT. Diverticular colo-enteric fistulae. Aust N Z J Surg. 1981;51(4):358–9.
15. Woods RJ, Lavery IC, Fazio VW, Jagelman DG, Weakley FL. Internal fistulas in diverticular disease. Dis Colon Rectum. 1988;31(8):591–6.
16. Vilallonga R, Baena JA, Fort JM, Gonzalez O, Gemar E, Armengol CM. Colouterine fistula complicating diverticulitis in elderly women. Int J Color Dis. 2009;24(5):599–600.
17. Chaikof EL, Cambria RP, Warshaw AL. Colouterine fistula secondary to diverticulitis. Dis Colon Rectum. 1985;28(5):358–60.
18. Melchior S, Cudovic D, Jones J, Thomas C, Gillitzer R, Thuroff J. Diagnosis and surgical management of colovesical fistulas due to sigmoid diverticulitis. J Urol. 2009;182(3):978–82.
19. Kim AY, Bennett GL, Bashist B, Perlman B, Megibow AJ. Small-bowel obstruction associated with sigmoid diverticulitis: CT evaluation in 16 patients. AJR Am J Roentgenol. 1998;170(5):1311–3.
20. Bolshinsky VS, SR. Colonic Diverticular Disease http://www.clevelandclinicmeded.com/2018
21. Horgan AF, McConnell EJ, Wolff BG, The S, Paterson C. Atypical diverticular disease: surgical results. Dis Colon Rectum. 2001;44(9):1315–8.
22. Boostrom SY, Wolff BG, Cima RR, Merchea A, Dozois EJ, Larson DW. Uncomplicated diverticulitis, more complicated than we thought. J Gastrointest Surg. 2012;16(9):1744–9.
23. Chabok A, Pahlman L, Hjern F, Haapaniemi S, Smedh K, Group AS. Randomized clinical trial of antibiotics in acute uncomplicated diverticulitis. Br J Surg. 2012;99(4):532–9.
24. Cohen E, Fuller G, Bolus R, Modi R, Vu M, Shahedi K, et al. Increased risk for irritable bowel syndrome after acute diverticulitis. Clin Gastroenterol Hepatol. 2013;11(12):1614–9.
25. Onur MR, Akpinar E, Karaosmanoglu AD, Isayev C, Karcaaltincaba M. Diverticulitis: a comprehensive review with usual and unusual complications. Insights Imaging. 2017;8(1):19–27.
26. Al-Khamis A, Abou Khalil J, Demian M, Morin N, Vasilevsky CA, Gordon PH, et al. Sigmoid colectomy for acute diverticulitis in immunosuppressed vs immunocompetent patients: outcomes from the ACS-NSQIP database. Dis Colon Rectum. 2016;59(2):101–9.

27. Perkins JD, Shield CF 3rd, Chang FC, Farha GJ. Acute diverticulitis. Comparison of treatment in immunocompromised and nonimmunocompromised patients. Am J Surg. 1984;148(6):745–8.
28. Al-khamis A AKJ, Nazi T, et al. Operative management of acute diverticulitis in immunosuppressed compared to immunocompetent patients: a systematic review. WJSP 2015(5):155–166.
29. Brandl A, Kratzer T, Kafka-Ritsch R, Braunwarth E, Denecke C, Weiss S, et al. Diverticulitis in immunosuppressed patients: a fatal outcome requiring a new approach? Can J Surg. 2016;59(4):254–61.
30. Mudatsakis N, Nikolaou M, Krithinakis K, Matalliotakis M, Politis N, Andreadakis E. Solitary cecal diverticulitis: an unusual cause of acute right iliac fossa pain-a case report and review of the literature. Case Rep Surg. 2014;2014:131452.
31. Gordon GHNS. Principles and practice of surgery for the colon, rectum and anus. 3rd ed. New York: Informa Healthcare USA; 2007. p. 1330.
32. Kachroo N, Sivakumar R, Hakim A, Semeraro D, Speake W. An unusual presentation of caecal diverticulitis. BMJ Case Rep. 2009;2009
33. Harbi H, Kardoun N, Fendri S, Dammak N, Toumi N, Guirat A, et al. Jejunal diverticulitis. Review and treatment algorithm. Presse Med. 2017;46(12 Pt 1):1139–43.
34. Hall J, Hardiman K, Lee S, Lightner A, Stocchi L, Paquette IM, et al. The American Society of Colon and Rectal Surgeons clinical practice guidelines for the treatment of left-sided colonic diverticulitis. Dis Colon Rectum. 2020;63(6):728–47.
35. Francis NK, Sylla P, Abou-Khalil M, Arolfo S, Berler D, Curtis NJ, et al. EAES and SAGES 2018 consensus conference on acute diverticulitis management: evidence-based recommendations for clinical practice. Surg Endosc. 2019;33(9):2726–41.
36. Tan JP, Barazanchi AW, Singh PP, Hill AG, Maccormick AD. Predictors of acute diverticulitis severity: a systematic review. Int J Surg. 2016;26:43–52. https://doi.org/10.1016/j.ijsu.2016.01.005. Epub 2016 Jan 9. PMID: 26777741
37. Daniels L, Ünlü Ç, de Korte N, van Dieren S, Stockmann HB, Vrouenraets BC, et al. Randomized clinical trial of observational versus antibiotic treatment for a first episode of CT-proven uncomplicated acute diverticulitis. Br J Surg. 2017;104(1):52–61.
38. Ambrosetti P, Robert JH, Witzig JA, Mirescu D, Mathey P, Borst F, et al. Acute left colonic diverticulitis: a prospective analysis of 226 consecutive cases. Surgery. 1994;115(5):546–50.
39. Gallo A, Ianiro G, Montalto M, Cammarota G. The role of biomarkers in diverticular disease. J Clin Gastroenterol. 2016;50(Suppl 1):S26–8.
40. Mäkelä JT, Klintrup K, Takala H, Rautio T. The role of C-reactive protein in prediction of the severity of acute diverticulitis in an emergency unit. Scand J Gastroenterol. 2015;50(5):536–41.
41. Hogan J, Sehgal R, Murphy D, O'Leary P, Coffey JC. Do inflammatory indices play a role in distinguishing between uncomplicated and complicated diverticulitis? Dig Surg. 2017;34(1):7–11.
42. Kechagias A, Rautio T, Mäkelä J. The early C-reactive protein trend does not have a role in monitoring acute diverticulitis progression. Chirurgia (Bucharest, Romania: 1990). 2016;111(1):43–7.
43. Nizri E, Spring S, Ben-Yehuda A, Khatib M, Klausner J, Greenberg R. C-reactive protein as a marker of complicated diverticulitis in patients on anti-inflammatory medications. Tech Coloproctol. 2014;18(2):145–9.
44. Bolkenstein HE, van de Wall BJ, Consten EC, van der Palen J, Broeders IA, Draaisma WA. Development and validation of a diagnostic prediction model distinguishing complicated from uncomplicated diverticulitis. Scand J Gastroenterol. 2018;53(10–11):1291–7.
45. Jeger V, Pop R, Forudastan F, Barras JP, Zuber M, Piso RJ. Is there a role for procalcitonin in differentiating uncomplicated and complicated diverticulitis in order to reduce antibiotic therapy? A prospective diagnostic cohort study. Swiss Med Wkly. 2017;147:w14555.
46. Jegers M, Kesteloot K, De Graeve D, Gilles W. A typology for provider payment systems in health care. Health Policy. 2002;60(3):255–73.
47. Sartelli M, Weber DG, Kluger Y, et al. 2020 update of the WSES guidelines for the management of acute colonic diverticulitis in the emergency setting. World J Emerg Surg. 2020;15(1):32. https://doi.org/10.1186/s13017-020-00313-4.
48. Alshamari M, Norrman E, Geijer M, Jansson K, Geijer H. Diagnostic accuracy of low-dose CT compared with abdominal radiography in non-traumatic acute abdominal pain: prospective study and systematic review. Eur Radiol. 2016;26(6):1766–74.
49. Laméris W, van Randen A, Bipat S, Bossuyt PM, Boermeester MA, Stoker J. Graded compression ultrasonography and computed tomography in acute colonic diverticulitis: meta-analysis of test accuracy. Eur Radiol. 2008;18(11):2498–511.
50. Birnbaum BA, Balthazar EJ. CT of appendicitis and diverticulitis. Radiol Clin North Am. 1994;32(5):885–98.
51. Hulnick DH, Megibow AJ, Balthazar EJ, Naidich DP, Bosniak MA. Computed tomography in the evaluation of diverticulitis. Radiology. 1984;152(2):491–5.
52. Wasvary H, Turfah F, Kadro O, Beauregard W. Same hospitalization resection for acute diverticulitis. Am Surg. 1999;65(7):632–5. discussion 6
53. Ambrosetti P. Acute diverticulitis of the left colon: value of the initial CT and timing of elective colectomy. J Gastrointest Surg. 2008;12(8):1318–20.
54. Ambrosetti P, Becker C, Terrier F. Colonic diverticulitis: impact of imaging on surgical management – a prospective study of 542 patients. Eur Radiol. 2002;12(5):1145–9.
55. Hall JF, Roberts PL, Ricciardi R, Read T, Scheirey C, Wald C, et al. Long-term follow-up after an initial episode of diverticulitis: what are the predictors of recurrence? Dis Colon Rectum. 2011;54(3):283–8.
56. Nielsen K, Richir MC, Stolk TT, van der Ploeg T, Moormann GR, Wiarda BM, et al. The limited role of

ultrasound in the diagnostic process of colonic diverticulitis. World J Surg. 2014;38(7):1814–8.
57. Dirks K, Calabrese E, Dietrich CF, Gilja OH, Hausken T, Higginson A, et al. EFSUMB position paper: recommendations for gastrointestinal ultrasound (GIUS) in Acute appendicitis and diverticulitis. Ultraschall in der Medizin (Stuttgart, Germany: 1980). 2019;40(2):163–75.
58. Kameda T, Kawai F, Taniguchi N, Kobori Y. Usefulness of transabdominal ultrasonography in excluding adnexal disease. J Med Ultrason (2001). 2016;43(1):63–70.
59. Heverhagen JT, Sitter H, Zielke A, Klose KJ. Prospective evaluation of the value of magnetic resonance imaging in suspected acute sigmoid diverticulitis. Dis Colon Rectum. 2008;51(12):1810–5.
60. Heverhagen JT, Zielke A, Ishaque N, Bohrer T, El-Sheik M, Klose KJ. Acute colonic diverticulitis: visualization in magnetic resonance imaging. Magn Reson Imaging. 2001;19(10):1275–7.
61. Öistämö E, Hjern F, Blomqvist L, Von Heijne A, Abraham-Nordling M. Cancer and diverticulitis of the sigmoid colon. Differentiation with computed tomography versus magnetic resonance imaging: preliminary experiences. Acta radiologica (Stockholm, Sweden: 1987). 2013;54(3):237–41.
62. McKee RF, Deignan RW, Krukowski ZH. Radiological investigation in acute diverticulitis. Br J Surg. 1993;80(5):560–5.

4 Endoscopic Evaluation of Diverticulitis

Kyle Staller and Ryan Flanagan

Introduction

Colonoscopy for diverticular disease has traditionally been reserved for evaluation of the colon for colorectal cancer (CRC) after an acute episode of diverticulitis. In this setting, colonoscopy 4–8 weeks after an episode leads to a diagnosis of CRC in approximately 1.5% of cases. Recently, limited data has shown that the risks of perforation during colonoscopy for acute diverticulitis may not be as high as previously thought. However, the benefits of early colonoscopy are usually limited to patients with a protracted course of diverticulitis despite antibiotic therapy. Colonoscopy after an episode of diverticulitis can also be helpful in differentiating acute diverticulitis from segmental colitis associated with diverticulosis (SCAD), which helps guide medical and surgical management.

Endoscopic Features of Acute Diverticulitis

Typical endoscopic features of acute diverticulitis have not been rigorously defined, due to the historical avoidance of colonoscopy during an acute episode for fear of perforation. The majority of inflamed diverticula are found incidentally on a colonoscopy performed for screening or another diagnostic indication. The rate of endoscopic evidence of diverticulitis in asymptomatic individuals has not been widely reported. One cross-sectional study of 2566 patients found that inflamed diverticula were identified in 0.8% of patients without prior clinical evidence of acute diverticulitis [1]. Inflamed diverticula may have an erythematous base, surrounding edema, granulation tissue in an orifice, or visible pus at the orifice (Fig. 4.1). Since diverticulitis is generally an extraluminal disease, a normal appearance on colonoscopy cannot rule out the presence of diverticulitis. Thus, computed tomography (CT) can better characterize the extraluminal portion of diverticula for inflammation, abscess, or perforation.

K. Staller (✉)
Division of Gastroenterology, Massachusetts General Hospital, Boston, MA, USA
e-mail: kstaller@mgh.harvard.edu

R. Flanagan
Division of Gastroenterology, Hepatology and Endoscopy, Brigham and Women's Hospital, Boston, MA, USA

M. Boutros et al. (eds.), *Diverticulitis*, https://doi.org/10.1007/978-3-032-21720-2_4

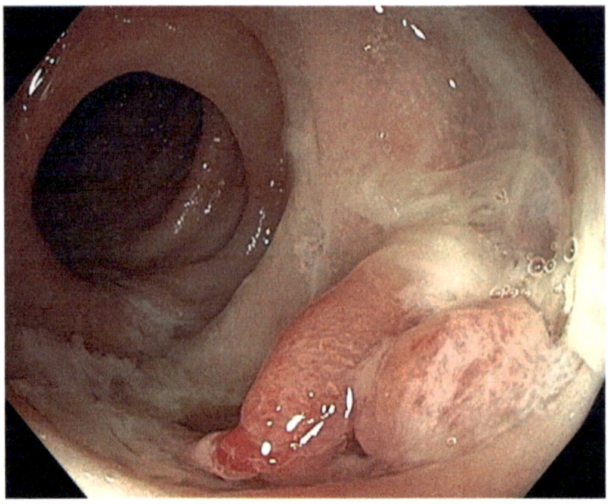

Fig. 4.1 Erythematous diverticula with visible pus at the orifice

Table 4.1 Components of the Diverticular Inflammation and Complication Assessment (DICA) score

Endoscopic feature	Points
Diverticulosis extension	
Left	2
Right	1
Number of diverticula	
Grade I (≤15)	0
Grade II (>15))	1
Presence of inflammation	
Edema/hyperemia	1
Erosions	2
SCAD	3
Presence of complications	
Rigidity of the colon	4
Stenosis	4
Pus	4
Bleeding	4

SCAD segmental colitis associated with diverticulitis
DICA score: 0: 0 points; 1: 1–3 points; 2: 4–7 points; 3: >7 points

Endoscopic Classification of Diverticulosis

Recent efforts in understanding the common endoscopic features of diverticular disease have focused on the ability to predict future complications, especially diverticulitis. The Diverticular Inflammation and Complication Assessment (DICA) score has been validated as a simple, reliable, and reproducible tool to help predict complications of diverticular disease [2–4]. Four main factors were chosen for inclusion in DICA: (1) diverticulosis extension (left vs. right), (2) number of diverticula, (3) presence of inflammation, and (4) presence of complications (F). Each of these factors on endoscopy contributes to the overall DICA score, in a weighted fashion, with DICA 1 being the lowest score and DICA 3 being the highest score. This score was developed by a panel of expert endoscopists based on experience and video footage of 30 endoscopies featuring diverticular disease. The score has been shown to positively correlate with erythrocyte sedimentation rate (ESR), C-reactive protein (CRP), and abdominal pain (Table 4.1).

After initial development and validation of the DICA score, further studies have assessed its reproducibility and ability to predict future episodes of diverticulitis. Reproducibility among 66 endoscopists was found to be moderate to good overall: 70.2% for DICA 1, 70.5% for DICA 2, and 81.3% for DICA 3. Among a subset of expert endoscopists, agreement was slightly higher with 78.8% for DICA 1, 80.2% for DICA 2, and 88.5% for DICA 3 [4]. In a study of 1651 patients, DICA was found to best predict the occurrence of diverticulitis and risk of surgery during follow-up compared with other potential risk factors, including age, presence of abdominal pain, CRP, and fecal calprotectin [3].

Limited Role for Colonoscopy During Acute Diverticulitis

Colonoscopy during acute diverticulitis is thought to carry a higher risk of perforation than endoscopy for other indications, though data supporting this theory has been limited.

Diverticulitis is thought to arise due to obstructed diverticula with associated mucosal damage, inflammation, and microperforations leading to bacterial translocation [5]. Although alternative hypotheses have more recently arisen, inflammation is thought to be the main driver in the pathogenesis [6]. Endoscopists generally believe the increased risk of perforation in the setting of acute diverticulitis arises from the presence of thin-walled, inflamed diverticula, which may rupture with air insufflation or mechanical stretch. The overall rate of perforation in colonoscopies (for all indications) has been reported extensively and appears to be approximately 0.08% based on the largest sample available [7]. Given that diverticulitis has been thought to be related to microperforations, there has been a logical assumption that the friable mucosa would be at higher risk of perforation during colonoscopy.

Two prospective trials have investigated the safety and utility of endoscopy during an acute episode of diverticulitis [8, 9]. These studies were designed to assess the safety of colonoscopy during an acute flare by performing colonoscopies on the day of discharge. The first noncontrolled study included 107 patients in two series. Of the 49 patients considered in the first series, 10 were excluded due to peri-diverticular air or fluid, and 39 patients underwent uncomplicated colonoscopies. In the second series, 58 patients were considered, and 4 patients were excluded due to peritoneal free air on CT. Of the remaining 54 patients who underwent colonoscopy, there was one patient with a perforation who had peri-diverticular air on imaging. Nine patients were found to have polyps, one of which was obstructing a diverticulum and the presumed source of diverticulitis. The two patients with diverticular obstructions were able to be treated endoscopically and there was perceived benefit given their protracted courses.

Based on this pilot study, a randomized controlled trial was done to further investigate the safety and potential advantages of early colonoscopy in diverticulitis [9]. This study included 86 patients without CT evidence of pericolic air or fluid. A total of 45 of these patients underwent colonoscopy approximately 5 days after clinical diagnosis (on the day of discharge), while 41 patients had colonoscopy at approximately 8 weeks. There were no perforations in either group and polyp incidence rates were similar between groups. A complete colonoscopy to the cecum was achieved in 82% of patients with early colonoscopy, compared to 93% in the delayed group (nonsignificant difference), though both rates were lower than would be expected in screening colonoscopies [10, 11]. Patients were more likely to undergo early colonoscopies compared with late colonoscopies (93% vs. 76%, $p = 0.033$), due to higher patient adherence. Notably, while early colonoscopy was not associated with higher complication risk, the study was likely underpowered given the rarity of perforations overall. Additionally, there were no patients who had a change in treatment or outcome as a result of early colonoscopy.

While early colonoscopy may have a lower risk than initially presumed, there are no data showing a benefit to early colonoscopy. Nevertheless, there are some situations where early colonoscopy may be a reasonable diagnostic or therapeutic consideration. If a patient has a lack of improvement on appropriate antimicrobial therapy or atypical imaging findings, repeat CT imaging is warranted to rule out perforation or abscess. If additional imaging remains unrevealing, an early colonoscopy may reveal an alternative diagnosis, such as inflammatory bowel disease, malignancy, or a frankly obstructed diverticulum, ultimately changing management. One study evaluated the utility of early colonoscopy in patients with a protracted course of diverticulitis, defined as longer than 7 days of appropriate antibiotic therapy with continued symptoms [12]. In this sample of 23 patients, 4 (17%) had an obstructed diverticulum, most commonly by an adenocarcinoma, and derived significant diagnostic benefit from early colonoscopy. None of the early colonoscopies performed in 201 patients without a protracted course led to significant diagnostic or therapeutic benefit. Notably, early colonoscopy should be avoided in cases where a CT shows peri-diverticular air or fluid, given that these findings suggest preexisting perforation, which may be exacerbated by colonoscopy [8, 13].

Indication for Colonoscopy After Acute Diverticulitis

Colonoscopy is typically recommended approximately 6–8 weeks after the initial diagnosis of acute diverticulitis to evaluate for malignancy, which could both precipitate diverticulitis or mimic diverticulitis [6, 14–18]. A 2014 systematic review and meta-analysis of eight studies found that the prevalence of malignancy in 1796 postdiverticulitis colonoscopies was approximately 15 per 1000 (95% confidence interval (CI), 10–21) [15]. The prevalence of advanced adenomas (≥1 cm, ≥25% villious features, or high-grade dysplasia) was slightly higher at 38 per 1000 colonoscopies (95% CI, 27–53). A more recent systematic review published in 2020 corroborated these findings. In this study, composed of 29,348 patients (30 studies) who had a colonoscopy following an episode of CT-proven acute diverticulitis, colonic malignancy occurred in 1.67% (95% CI, 1.24–2.14). The risk of malignancy in cases with uncomplicated diverticulitis was 1.22% (95% CI, 0.63–1.97) as compared with 6.14% (95% CI, 3.20–9.82) in cases with complicated diverticulitis, with a relative risk of 5.033 (95% CI, 3.194–7.930; $p < 0.001$). Most guidelines recommend a colonoscopy be performed if one has not been done in the past year, though no studies have assessed the sufficiency of a prior colonoscopy and time interval between procedures to exclude colorectal cancer (CRC) in this population [6].

Despite the evidence that colonoscopy after acute diverticulitis may reveal colon cancer or precancerous polyps [19], the recommendation that all patients undergo colonoscopy after acute diverticulitis is hardly unanimous [20]. Those arguing against universal screening in this setting point out that CRC rates are similar between general screening colonoscopies and colonoscopies performed after acute diverticulitis, particularly after cases of uncomplicated diverticulitis. The rate of colon cancer detection during screening colonoscopies has been found to be 0.5–1% in most studies [21–25], with the largest study reporting a rate of 0.9% [26]. This is similar to the rate of CRC after an episode of uncomplicated diverticulitis, which was reported to have a pooled estimate of 0.7% (95% CI 0.3–1.4%) [27]. Additionally, as the resolution of CT imaging has improved, some authors believe the sensitivity has improved to a degree sufficient to exclude CRC in the majority of cases [28]. However, the rate of CRC after an episode of complicated diverticulitis was estimated at 10.8% (95% CI 5.2–21.0%), highlighting the need for interval endoscopy in this patient population [27].

The American Gastroenterology Association (AGA) guidelines note that colonoscopies after diverticulitis may identify a small number of colorectal malignancies, though the procedure places a moderate burden on patients, and perforation rates in this setting have yet to be firmly established [6, 19]. The guidelines also appropriately state that many of the studies investigating colonoscopy after diverticulitis suffer from appreciable selection bias. Commonly, the studies investigating rates of CRC after diverticulitis have been retrospective, excluded patients with complicated diverticulitis, and overrepresented patients with atypical imaging or clinical course [6].

Recent epidemiologic data has suggested that there may be an increased long-term risk of colorectal malignancy after an episode of acute diverticulitis [29]. A longitudinal Danish cohort study of 445,456 people found the incidence of CRC in people with diverticulitis to be significantly higher than in people without diverticulitis (4.3% vs. 2.3%, $p < 0.001$). After adjusting for confounders, people with diverticulitis were still found to be approximately twice as likely to have CRC compared to controls (odds ratio (OR) 2.20, 95% CI 2.08 to 2.32). Furthermore, people with diverticulitis and no colonoscopy were at significantly higher risk of CRC compared to patients without diverticulitis and no colonoscopy (OR 2.72, 95% CI 2.64 to 2.94). Of the 1723 individuals with a history of both diverticulitis and CRC, 977 (57%) had the diagnosis of CRC within a year of the diagnosis of diverticulitis. Prior studies investigating the association between diverticulitis and CRC have been conflicting. In general, small single-center studies have found no association [30–32], while larger multicenter studies have found a significant association [33–35]. The latter finding may be related to the size of the larger studies, which allow the identification of significant associations even if the absolute risk of CRC after diverticulitis is relatively low.

Segmental Colitis Associated with Diverticulosis (SCAD)

Segmental colitis associated with diverticulosis (SCAD) is a distinct entity within diverticular disease that may present similarly to diverticulitis but has different endoscopic features and management [36–39]. SCAD is defined by inflammation of the colon in the interdiverticular mucosa, with sparing of the diverticula. It is a relatively common entity, with one study showing that about 1.5% of patients presenting for colonoscopy will have evidence of disease [40]. Among patients with diverticulosis, approximately 11% of patients will have evidence of SCAD on endoscopy. Clinically, the diagnosis of SCAD is suggested by chronic diarrhea, left lower quadrant abdominal pain, and occasionally hematochezia, especially among patients with known diverticulosis. However, the diagnosis of SCAD relies on particular endoscopic and histologic findings, given its nonspecific clinical symptoms.

On endoscopy, inflammation is present in the sigmoid and sometimes descending colon, but always spares the rectum. Additionally, the inflammation is confined to the colonic mucosa near diverticula, but always spares the diverticula themselves. Four distinct endoscopic patterns have been defined: type A (crescentic fold pattern), type B (mild to moderate ulcerative colitis-like pattern), type C (Crohn's disease colitis-like pattern), and type D (severe ulcerative colitis-like pattern) [40]. Type A is the most common, present in over 50% of patients with SCAD (Figs. 4.2 and 4.3).

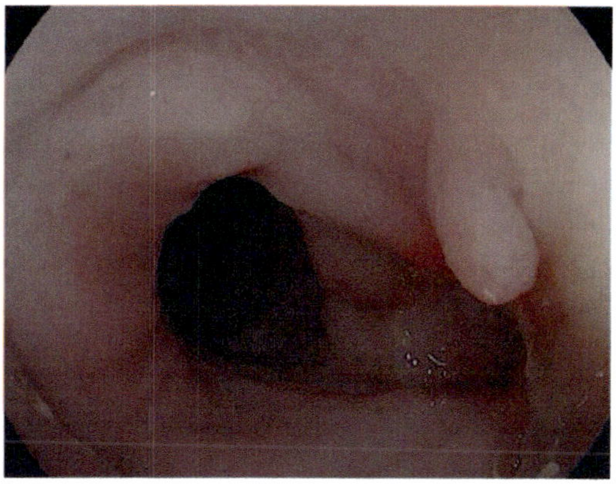

Fig. 4.2 Erythema on crescentic mucosal fold

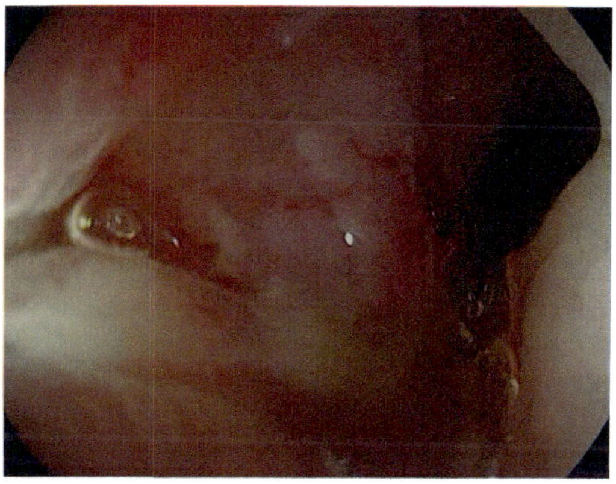

Fig. 4.3 Erythematous interdiverticular mucosa

The histology of SCAD is quite variable, but most often mimics that of the inflammatory bowel disease (IBD) that each type is named after [40, 41]. Type A often has lymphocyte and neutrophil infiltration and inflammation, but no significant disruption of glandular architecture. Type B and type D most often have histologic patterns similar to mild-to-moderate ulcerative colitis (B) or severe ulcerative colitis (D). Common findings in these types include diffuse mixed inflammation in the lamina propria, Pantaleth cell metaplasia, cryptitis, crypt distortion, and crypt abscesses. Type C commonly has transmural inflammation, granulomas, and fissures, without significant involvement of crypts. Given that the histological findings can be similar to findings in IBD, the differentiation between the two disease processes can be nuanced. However, rectal sparing on histology is always present in SCAD, while this is rare in ulcerative colitis. Additionally, there is almost never proximal extension in SCAD while this can occur in ulcerative colitis. By relying on the endoscopic, histologic, and clinical features of SCAD compared to IBD, a clinician can feel confident distinguishing between the two entities.

Conclusion

Colonoscopy during an acute episode of diverticulitis rarely changes management and is believed to carry a greater risk of perforation than screening colonoscopy. However, recent data has shown that the risk of perforation may be less than previously thought. A small number of patients with a protracted diverticulitis course or atypical imaging may benefit from colonoscopy after a short period of observation on appropriate antibiotic therapy. Colonoscopy is recommended 4–8 weeks after an acute episode of diverticulitis to screen for colorectal cancer, as the risk of malignancy appears to be greater in patients with diverticulitis, especially in complicated diverticulitis. Colonoscopy can also be useful in differentiating diverticulitis from SCAD in patients with ongoing symptoms after initial presentation. The DICA score offers an objective, validated tool to measure the severity of diverticular disease during endoscopy, which can predict the risk of a future episode of diverticulitis and need for surgery.

References

1. Ghorai S, Ulbright TM, Rex DK. Endoscopic findings of diverticular inflammation in colonoscopy patients without clinical acute diverticulitis: prevalence and endoscopic spectrum. Am J Gastroenterol. 2003;98(4):802–6.
2. Tursi A, Brandimarte G, Di Mario F, Andreoli A, Annunziata ML, Astegiano M, et al. Development and validation of an endoscopic classification of diverticular disease of the colon: the DICA classification. Dig Dis. 2015;33(1):68–76.
3. Tursi A, Brandimarte G, Di Mario F, Annunziata ML, Bafutto M, Bianco MA, et al. Predictive value of the Diverticular Inflammation and Complication Assessment (DICA) endoscopic classification on the outcome of diverticular disease of the colon: an international study. United European Gastroenterol J. 2016;4(4):604–13.
4. Tursi A, Brandimarte G, di Mario F, Nardone G, Scarpignato C, Picchio M, et al. The "DICA" endoscopic classification for diverticular disease of the colon shows a significant interobserver agreement among community endoscopists. J Gastrointestin Liver Dis. 2019;28(1):23–7.
5. Jacobs DO. Clinical practice. Diverticulitis. N Engl J Med. 2007;357(20):2057–66.
6. Strate LL, Peery AF, Neumann I. American Gastroenterological Association Institute Technical Review on the management of acute diverticulitis. Gastroenterology. 2015;149(7):1950–76 e12.
7. Arora G, Mannalithara A, Singh G, Gerson LB, Triadafilopoulos G. Risk of perforation from a colonoscopy in adults: a large population-based study. Gastrointest Endosc. 2009;69(3 Pt 2):654–64.
8. Sakhnini E, Lahat A, Melzer E, Apter S, Simon C, Natour M, et al. Early colonoscopy in patients with acute diverticulitis: results of a prospective pilot study. Endoscopy. 2004;36(6):504–7.
9. Lahat A, Yanai H, Menachem Y, Avidan B, Bar-Meir S. The feasibility and risk of early colonoscopy in acute diverticulitis: a prospective controlled study. Endoscopy. 2007;39(6):521–4.
10. Marshall JB, Barthel JS. The frequency of total colonoscopy and terminal ileal intubation in the 1990s. Gastrointest Endosc. 1993;39(4):518–20.
11. Waye JD, Bashkoff E. Total colonoscopy: is it always possible? Gastrointest Endosc. 1991;37(2):152–4.
12. Lahat A, Yanai H, Sakhnini E, Menachem Y, Bar-Meir S. Role of colonoscopy in patients with persistent acute diverticulitis. World J Gastroenterol. 2008;14(17):2763–6.
13. Tursi A, Papa V, Lopetuso LR, Vetrone LM, Gasbarrini A, Papa A. When to perform a colonoscopy in diverticular disease and why: a personalized approach. J Pers Med. 2022;12(10):1713. https://doi.org/10.3390/jpm12101713. PMID: 36294852; PMCID: PMC9605603
14. Sai VF, Velayos F, Neuhaus J, Westphalen AC. Colonoscopy after CT diagnosis of diverticulitis to exclude colon cancer: a systematic literature review. Radiology. 2012;263(2):383–90.
15. Daniels L, Unlu C, de Wijkerslooth TR, Dekker E, Boermeester MA. Routine colonoscopy after left-sided acute uncomplicated diverticulitis: a systematic review. Gastrointest Endosc. 2014;79(3):378–89. quiz 498–e5
16. Feingold D, Steele SR, Lee S, Kaiser A, Boushey R, Buie WD, et al. Practice parameters for the treatment of sigmoid diverticulitis. Dis Colon Rectum. 2014;57(3):284–94.
17. Koo CH, Chang JHE, Syn NL, Wee IJY, Mathew R. Systematic review and meta-analysis on colorectal cancer findings on colonic evaluation after CT-confirmed acute diverticulitis. Dis Colon Rectum. 2020;63(5):701–9. https://doi.org/10.1097/DCR.0000000000001664. PMID: 32271220
18. Meyer J, Orci LA, Combescure C, Balaphas A, Morel P, Buchs NC, Ris F. Risk of colorectal cancer in patients with acute diverticulitis: a systematic review and meta-analysis of observational studies. Clin Gastroenterol Hepatol. 2019;17(8):1448–1456.e17. https://doi.org/10.1016/j.cgh.2018.07.031. Epub 2018 Jul 26
19. Peery AF, Shaukat A, Strate LL. AGA clinical practice update on medical management of colonic diverticulitis: expert review. Gastroenterology.

2021;160(3):906–911.e1. https://doi.org/10.1053/j.gastro.2020.09.059. Epub 2020 Dec 3. PMID: 33279517; PMCID: PMC7878331
20. de Vries HS, Boerma D, Timmer R, van Ramshorst B, Dieleman LA, van Westreenen HL. Routine colonoscopy is not required in uncomplicated diverticulitis: a systematic review. Surg Endosc. 2014;28(7):2039–47.
21. Regula J, Rupinski M, Kraszewska E, Polkowski M, Pachlewski J, Orlowska J, et al. Colonoscopy in colorectal-cancer screening for detection of advanced neoplasia. N Engl J Med. 2006;355(18):1863–72.
22. Segnan N, Senore C, Andreoni B, Azzoni A, Bisanti L, Cardelli A, et al. Comparing attendance and detection rate of colonoscopy with sigmoidoscopy and FIT for colorectal cancer screening. Gastroenterology. 2007;132(7):2304–12.
23. Kahi CJ, Imperiale TF, Juliar BE, Rex DK. Effect of screening colonoscopy on colorectal cancer incidence and mortality. Clin Gastroenterol Hepatol. 2009;7(7):770–5. quiz 11
24. Boursi B, Halak A, Umansky M, Galzan L, Guzner-Gur H, Arber N. Colonoscopic screening of an average-risk population for colorectal neoplasia. Endoscopy. 2009;41(6):516–21.
25. Strul H, Kariv R, Leshno M, Halak A, Jakubowicz M, Santo M, et al. The prevalence rate and anatomic location of colorectal adenoma and cancer detected by colonoscopy in average-risk individuals aged 40–80 years. Am J Gastroenterol. 2006;101(2):255–62.
26. Pox CP, Altenhofen L, Brenner H, Theilmeier A, Von Stillfried D, Schmiegel W. Efficacy of a nationwide screening colonoscopy program for colorectal cancer. Gastroenterology. 2012;142(7):1460–7 e2.
27. Sharma PV, Eglinton T, Hider P, Frizelle F. Systematic review and meta-analysis of the role of routine colonic evaluation after radiologically confirmed acute diverticulitis. Ann Surg. 2014;259(2):263–72.
28. Bar-Meir S, Lahat A, Melzer E. Role of endoscopy in patients with diverticular disease. Dig Dis. 2012;30(1):60–3.
29. Mortensen LQ, Burcharth J, Andresen K, Pommergaard HC, Rosenberg J. An 18-year nationwide cohort study on the association between diverticulitis and colon cancer. Ann Surg. 2017;265(5):954–9.
30. Alexandersson BT, Hreinsson JP, Stefansson T, Jonasson JG, Bjornsson ES. The risk of colorectal cancer after an attack of uncomplicated diverticulitis. Scand J Gastroenterol. 2014;49(5):576–80.
31. Brar MS, Roxin G, Yaffe PB, Stanger J, MacLean AR, Buie WD. Colonoscopy following nonoperative management of uncomplicated diverticulitis may not be warranted. Dis Colon Rectum. 2013;56(11):1259–64.
32. Lam TJ, Meurs-Szojda MM, Gundlach L, Belien JA, Meijer GA, Mulder CJ, et al. There is no increased risk for colorectal cancer and adenomas in patients with diverticulitis: a retrospective longitudinal study. Color Dis. 2010;12(11):1122–6.
33. Lau KC, Spilsbury K, Farooque Y, Kariyawasam SB, Owen RG, Wallace MH, et al. Is colonoscopy still mandatory after a CT diagnosis of left-sided diverticulitis: can colorectal cancer be confidently excluded? Dis Colon Rectum. 2011;54(10):1265–70.
34. Meyer J, Thomopoulos T, Usel M, Gjika E, Bouchardy C, Morel P, et al. The incidence of colon cancer among patients diagnosed with left colonic or sigmoid acute diverticulitis is higher than in the general population. Surg Endosc. 2015;29(11):3331–7.
35. Stefansson T, Ekbom A, Sparen P, Pahlman L. Association between sigmoid diverticulitis and left-sided colon cancer: a nested, population-based, case control study. Scand J Gastroenterol. 2004;39(8):743–7.
36. Goldstein NS, Leon-Armin C, Mani A. Crohn's colitis-like changes in sigmoid diverticulitis specimens is usually an idiosyncratic inflammatory response to the diverticulosis rather than Crohn's colitis. Am J Surg Pathol. 2000;24(5):668–75.
37. Schembri J, Bonello J, Christodoulou DK, Katsanos KH, Ellul P. Segmental colitis associated with diverticulosis: is it the coexistence of colonic diverticulosis and inflammatory bowel disease? Ann Gastroenterol. 2017;30(3):257–61.
38. Rezapour M, Ali S, Stollman N. Diverticular disease: an update on pathogenesis and management. Gut Liver. 2018;12(2):125–32.
39. Freeman HJ. Segmental colitis associated diverticulosis syndrome. World J Gastroenterol. 2016;22(36):8067–9.
40. Tursi A, Elisei W, Brandimarte G, Giorgetti GM, Lecca PG, Di Cesare L, et al. The endoscopic spectrum of segmental colitis associated with diverticulosis. Color Dis. 2010;12(5):464–70.
41. Harpaz N, Sachar DB. Segmental colitis associated with diverticular disease and other IBD look-alikes. J Clin Gastroenterol. 2006;40(Suppl 3):S132–5.

5 Imaging Modalities for Diverticular Disease

Vincent Pelsser and Jean-François Toupin

Introduction

On all imaging modalities, diverticular sacs are visualized as rounded and oval saccular outpouchings extending beyond the bowel wall. They are seen primarily in the sigmoid and descending colon but may occur in any other segment of the bowel. The rectum is spared due to the fusion of the taenia resulting in a stronger rectal wall. Diverticula can be of various size, with the majority ranging from 5 to 10 mm. The internal content and density on imaging are also variable, as diverticula can be filled with gas, soft stools, dense calcified inspissated stools (fecalith), or oral contrast agent. In the sigmoid colon, diverticula are often associated with thickening of the adjacent circular muscles of the muscularis propria and shortening of the taenia coli, termed myochosis coli. This hypertrophy results in narrowing of the colon lumen with irregularly spaced indentations in segments affected by diverticulosis.

Multidetector computed tomography (CT) is the main imaging modality for diverticular disease (Fig. 5.1); however, it is not infrequent that it is diagnosed or suspected on other modalities.

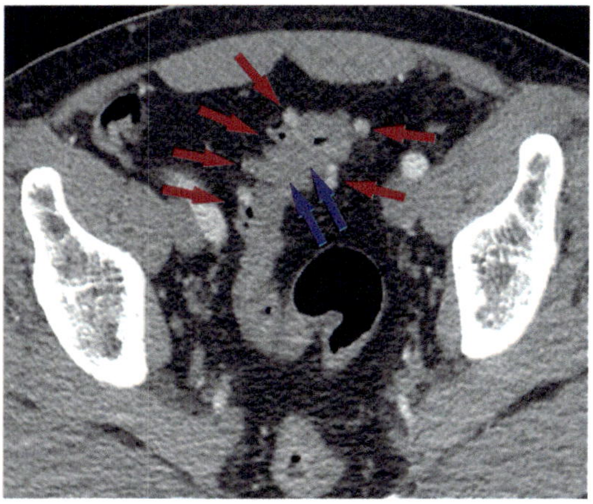

Fig. 5.1 Diverticulosis on CT. Diverticula appear as small outpouchings containing air or dense fecal materials extending into the pericolic fat (red arrows). The involved colonic wall shows circumferential thickening and shortening due to myochosis (blue arrows)

Imaging Modalities

Radiographs

Conventional abdominal radiograph can demonstrate numerous gas-filled sacs parallel to the colon in approximately 50% of individuals with significant diverticulosis (Fig. 5.2). It has a poor sensitivity for milder forms of the disease and diverticula may not be visualized when filled with stool or masked by overlapping gas-filled bowel loops. Literature has previously suggested a relationship between calcified pelvic phlebolith and diverticular disease as both may result from

V. Pelsser (✉)
Department of Radiology, Jewish General Hospital, Montreal, QC, Canada

J.-F. Toupin
Department of Diagnostic Radiology, McGill University Health Center, Montreal, QC, Canada

M. Boutros et al. (eds.), *Diverticulitis*, https://doi.org/10.1007/978-3-032-21720-2_5

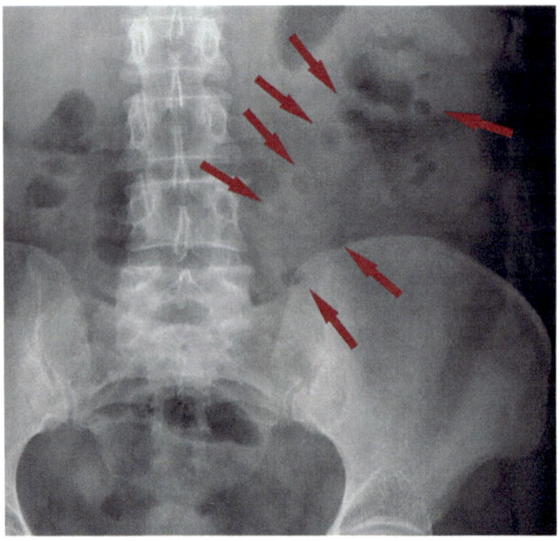

Fig. 5.2 Diverticulosis on radiograph. Numerous gas-filled sacs (red arrows) parallel to the proximal sigmoid colon in a patient with significant diverticular disease

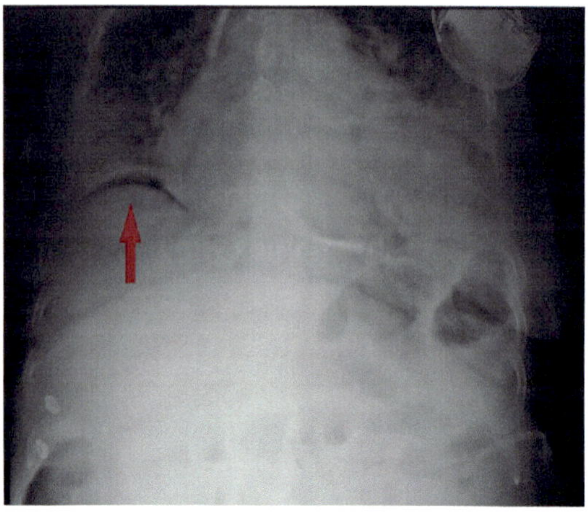

Fig. 5.3 Intraperitoneal free air on radiograph. The patient was diagnosed a week earlier with acute uncomplicated diverticulitis. He presented with acute worsening of the symptoms and hypotension. A crescent of free air (red arrow) is seen under the right hemidiaphragm, in keeping with pneumoperitoneum secondary to perforated diverticulitis

low-fiber diets; however, subsequent studies have shown no statistically significant relation other than with advanced age [1].

In the context of diverticulitis, conventional radiographs are rarely diagnostic except in severe, complicated cases. The diagnosis on abdominal plain films can be suggested in the presence of a localized ileus with an ill-defined pericolonic mass to indicate an abscess. Intraperitoneal free air may also suggest complicated perforated diverticulitis in the proper clinical context, and in hemodynamically normal patients, should prompt further imaging with CT to exclude other etiologies and better stage the disease (Fig. 5.3). In acute uncomplicated diverticulitis, most conventional radiographs are unremarkable and are therefore not used for diagnostic purposes in diverticular disease.

Fluoroscopic Contrast Enema

Barium contrast enema studies used to be the initial diagnostic test in suspected diverticulitis until it was replaced by CT in the 1990s. Diverticula can be demonstrated on both single and double-contrast enemas as barium-filled outpouchings, with double-contrast studies having a greater sensitivity than plain radiographs to detect diverticula due to greater colonic distension [2]. The shortening and thickening of the taenia coli (myochosis coli) may also be visualized on contrast enema, characterized by irregularly spaced indentations with narrowing of the lumen of the colon.

When viewed en face, diverticula appear either as well-defined, dense round foci (when filled with barium) or as dark rings (when filled with gas). Diverticula can be difficult to distinguish from polyps when viewed en face and both may show the appearance of a bowler hat. The bowler hat sign suggests the presence of a polyp when the tip of the hat points toward the center of the lumen of the colon [3]. When diverticula are inverted into the lumen, they cannot be differentiated from polyps and are often misdiagnosed [4]. On profile view, diverticula usually appear as barium-filled outpouchings with a discernible neck. The neck can be obstructed by adherent fecal matter and the diverticula can remain filled with gas or partially filled with barium. When partially filled, a streak of contrast within the neck or a dependent meniscus in the outpouching can be identified (Fig. 5.4).

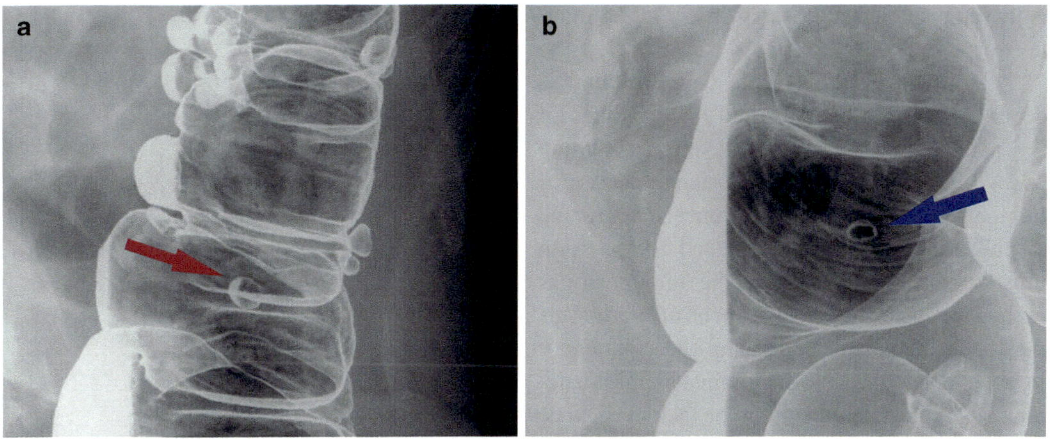

Fig. 5.4 Double-contrast barium enema. (**a**) Multiple barium-filled outpouchings along the descending colon. Note a round filling defect viewed en face (red arrow) with a meniscus of contrast indicating a diverticulum. (**b**) Round filling defect (blue arrow) confirmed to be a polyp by colonoscopy, showing a similar appearance to a diverticulum viewed en face

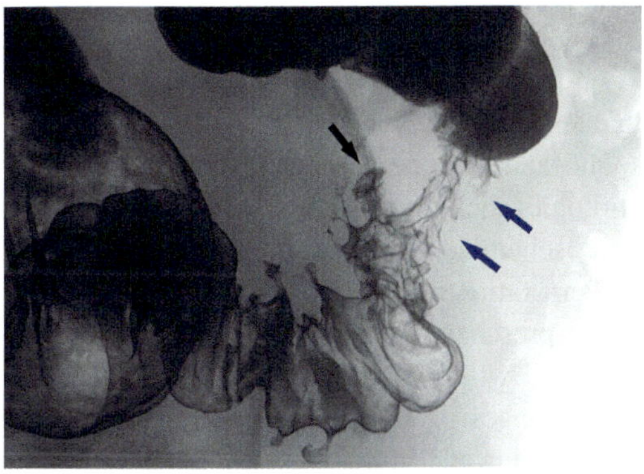

Fig. 5.5 Acute diverticulitis: double contrast barium enema. Luminal narrowing (blue arrows) on a short segment of the proximal colon adjacent to a prominent diverticulum (black arrow). Differential diagnosis includes an acute diverticulitis and colon carcinoma. Colonoscopy with biopsy confirmed an acute diverticulitis

In the context of diverticulitis, barium enema may show deformed diverticular sacs with focal narrowing of the lumen secondary to the inflammation. The inflammation itself is not visualized and the diagnosis can only be inferred from the clinical context as these signs are not specific for diverticulitis (Fig. 5.5). Diagnosis can be made more confidently in cases of complicated diverticulitis when contrast material is seen extravasating within the peritoneal cavity, or into an associated abscess, sinus tract, or fistula; however, this is observed in only 50% of perforations. Contrast enema studies are specific when complications are present but remain poorly sensitive as colovesical fistulas are only identified 20% of the time when present [5]. These complications can also be seen in the context of perforated colorectal carcinoma and with Crohn's disease and should be correlated with the medical history and other signs of disease in the sigmoid, in the rest of the colon and terminal ileum.

Ultrasound

The utilization of ultrasonography in the diagnosis of diverticulitis is highly variable and operator-dependent. While it is typically not the first imaging modality used for suspected diverticulitis, it can be performed reliably in centers with expertise [6]. Ultrasonography may also be the initial diagnostic modality of choice in pregnant women with suspected diverticulitis if MRI is not readily available. Diverticular disease is also not uncommonly imaged on ultrasound while assessing for other diseases such as appendicitis, cholecystitis, or pelvic pathology. However, CT has shown to be more accurate in diagnosing and staging diverticulitis, as well as identifying alternate pathologies, compared to ultrasound [7], and is therefore preferred as the primary initial diagnostic study [8].

Assessment of the bowels on ultrasound is dependent on the operator and body habitus of the patient and can be rather time-consuming given the length of the colon and presence of luminal gas [9]. To achieve proper sonographic visualization of the bowels, graded compression must be performed to reduce the amount of gas within the lumen. The assessment of the bowels may be technically difficult in an obese patient or in a patient with acute abdominal pain as adequate compression may not be achieved. The advantages of ultrasonography compared to other modalities are the relatively lower cost and the absence of ionizing radiation and contrast.

On high-resolution sonography, the different layers of the colonic wall can be identified by alternating bands of different echogenicity (Table 5.1). The internal appearance of the diverticula varies in echogenicity according to the content; it may be hypo or iso-echoic if filled with soft stool and hyperechoic in the presence of gas or fecalith. The myochosis coli may be visualized as a thick hypoechoic band within the adjacent wall, reflecting the enlarged muscularis propria.

In the context of acute diverticulitis, typical sonographic findings include the presence of a noncompressible, inflamed diverticula with hypoechoic segmental concentric bowel wall thickening, measuring more than 4 mm [10]. The surrounding mesenteric fat often appears hyperechoic due to the inflammatory changes (Fig. 5.6). Graded compression may be difficult to achieve due to focal pain at this location. In the absence of a definitive inflamed diverticulum, bowel wall thickening alone remains nonspecific on ultrasound and may be explained by multiple other etiologies including inflammatory disease, infection, ischemia, or neoplasm.

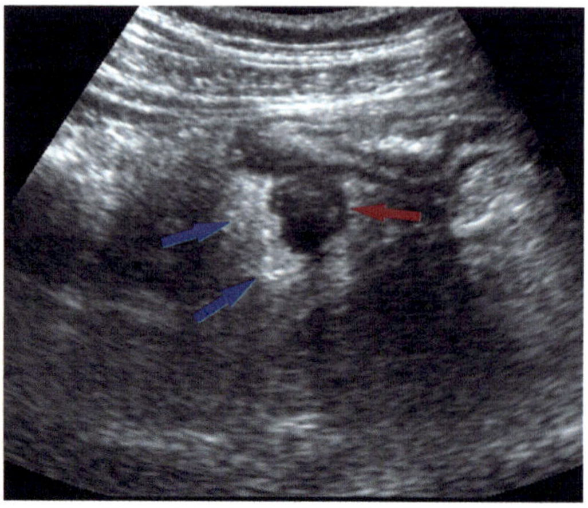

Fig. 5.6 Acute diverticulitis: ultrasonography. An inflamed diverticulum (red arrow) is identified in the sigmoid colon with hyperechogenicity of the surrounding fat (blue arrows) indicative of acute inflammatory changes. This corresponded to the patient's maximal point of tenderness, compatible with an acute diverticulitis. A CT was performed to confirm the diagnosis and exclude complications

Perforation may be identified sonographically in the presence of ill-definition of the diverticulum wall with extra-luminal fluid or phlegmonous changes. An abscess will appear as an organized, walled-off collection that may contain gas. Mesenteric venous pylephlebitis and fistulas are not adequately assessed on ultrasound. Clinical-sonographic assessment showed optimal sensitivity (92.7%) and specificity (90.9%) for diverticulitis. However, the sensitivity (50%) for complicated diverticulitis was low [11].

Table 5.1 The different layers of colonic wall on sonography

Layer	Echogenicity
Mucosa	Echogenic
Deep and muscularis mucosa	Hypoechoic
Submucosa	Echogenic
Muscularis propria	Hypoechoic
Serosa	Echogenic

Magnetic Resonance Imaging (MRI)

MRI can effectively diagnose diverticular disease and may be the initial diagnostic study in the context of pregnant women with suspected diverticulitis. It can adequately assess for diverticulitis with a reported sensitivity of 86–94% and specificity of 88–92% [12]. The only major advantage of MRI compared to CT is the lack of ionizing radiation, and the disadvantages include the susceptibility to motion artifacts from bowel peristalsis, a longer scan time, and higher cost. Given the greater efficiency and effectiveness of CT, MRI is not routinely used for diverticular disease. In addition, MRI is not widely available in all centers and Emergency Departments and should only be considered in pregnant patients to avoid ionizing radiation and in patients with contrast allergy or renal dysfunction who cannot be given IV contrast.

The MRI protocol varies according to institution but typically involves axial and coronal T1 and T2-weighted acquisition before and after gadolinium contrast administration. In the context of acute diverticulitis, bowel wall thickening and pericolic inflammation are best assessed on two sequences [13]. T1-weighted fat-suppressed gadolinium-enhanced spoiled gradient-echo sequence shows hyperintense enhancing bowel wall thickening and surrounding inflammatory changes on the background of dark suppressed mesenteric fat (Fig. 5.7). It also demonstrates possible enhancing complications such as sinus tracts, fistulas, or walls of abscesses [14]. T2-weighted fast spin echo (T2 FSE) is a rapidly acquired fluid-sensitive sequence that also shows hyperintense signals to indicate inflammatory changes surrounding diverticula and is less prone to motion artifacts due to the rapid acquisition [15].

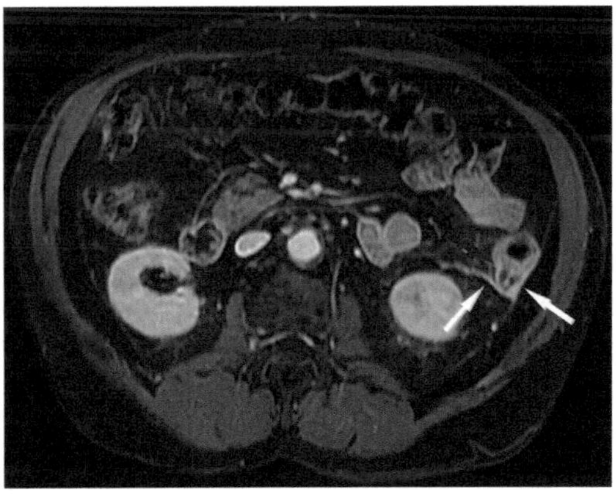

Fig. 5.7 Acute diverticulitis on MRI. MRI Axial image of a T1-weighted, contrast-enhanced, fat-saturated sequence. An enhancing inflamed diverticulum (red arrow) with adjacent mural thickening is visualized in the descending colon. There are mild enhancing pericolic inflammatory changes with reactive thickening of the anterior renal fascia and lateroconal fascia (white arrows)

Computed Tomography

Since the 1990s, multidetector computed tomography (CT) has become the primary imaging modality to assess diverticular disease with reported sensitivity and specificity up to 99% [16, 17]. In the context of suspected diverticulitis, a contrast-enhanced CT is currently the initial study recommended [18]. Oral or rectal contrast is not recommended routinely but may be used to assess for fistula when complications are suspected.

CT is now widespread and available in most institutions. It provides fast scanning time with good spatial resolution, allowing excellent visualization of diverticular disease and its complications. The main disadvantage is the presence of ionizing radiation, with a single-phase CT abdomen associated with an approximate effective dose of 10 mSv, the equivalent of 3 years of natural background radiation.

Diverticula on CT are well seen as outpouchings arising from the colon, with the density in soft tissue window varying from air (black), stool (gray), and dense calcified inspissated stools or oral contrast (white). The myochosis coli can also be identified by shortening and thickening of the adjacent wall in segments most affected by diverticulosis.

In the context of acute diverticulitis, the most common findings (Table 5.2) are pericolic fat stranding and segmental mural edema of the colon adjacent to diverticula. The amount of surrounding inflammatory changes in the pericolic fat can vary significantly. A mild uncomplicated diverticulitis may only show subtle increase in attenuation of the surrounding fat, while more severe cases will show extensive surrounding fat stranding with engorgement of the vasa recta. When the inflammation extends to the fascia, reactive thickening can be visualized. The principle inflamed diverticulum can sometimes be identified at the epicenter of the inflammatory changes, often appearing hyperdense compared to the others. More severe forms of diverticulitis can demonstrate pericolic gas bubbles from perforation and extensive inflammatory changes with areas of increased heterogeneous densities representing phlegmons (Fig. 5.8). Other findings in complicated diverticulitis will be discussed in the next section. Of note, virtual CT colonography is contraindicated in the settings of acute diverticulitis due to the risk of perforation by the distension of the colon with gas.

Table 5.2 Findings in acute diverticulitis on CT

Findings	Sensitivity (%)
Mural edema of the colon	96
Fat stranding	95
Fascial thickening	50
Free fluid	45
Inflamed diverticulum	43

Adapted from Kircher MF, Rhea JT, Kihiczak D, et al.: Frequency, sensitivity and specificity of individual signs of diverticulitis on thin-section helical CT with colonic contrast material: Experience with 312 cases. AJR 178:1313–1318, 2002

Complications

Perforation

Histopathological studies have demonstrated that there is bacterial translocation beyond the bowel wall in acute diverticulitis [19]. In most cases, this cannot be specifically identified on imaging other than by the surrounding fat stranding. Small pericolic gas bubbles are visible in approximately 30% of acute diverticulitis, reported as microperforation; however, it is not clear whether this finding is associated with a more aggressive form of diverticulitis [20].

Rarely, acute diverticulitis will lead to free perforation in the peritoneal cavity that will not be contained by the mesocolon or walled off into an abscess. This leads to extravasation of gas and fluid diffusely in the peritoneal cavity with subsequent peritonitis. CT will show the presence of free air distant to the site of diverticulitis and dense peritoneal free fluid (>20 HU) with diffuse enhancement and thickening of the peritoneal linings indicating peritonitis (Fig. 5.9). Free

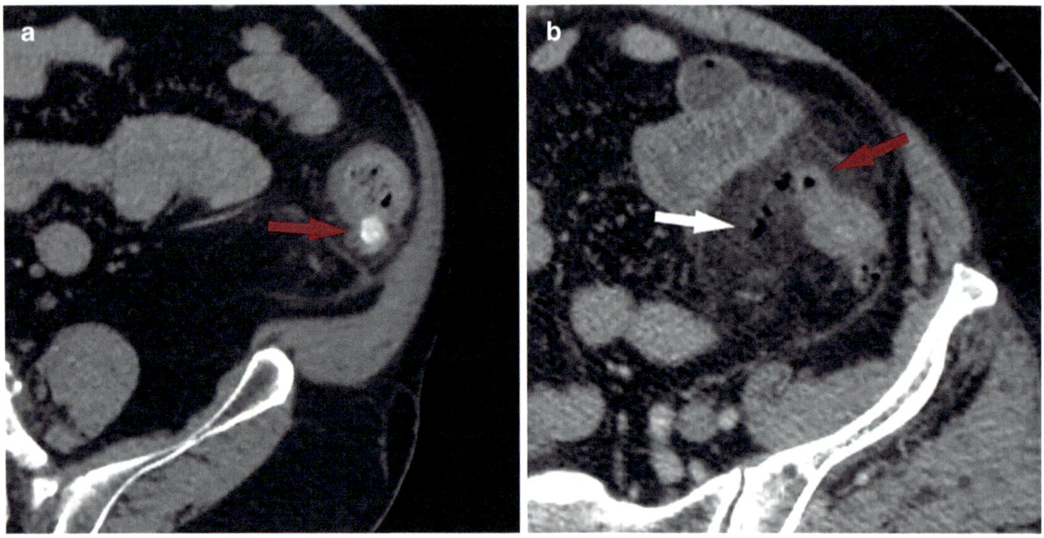

Fig. 5.8 Acute diverticulitis on CT. (**a**) An inflamed hyperdense diverticulum (red arrow) with adjacent mural thickening can be visualized in the distal descending colon. There are mild surrounding fat stranding and thickening of the fascia, compatible with a mild uncomplicated acute diverticulitis. (**b**) Acute diverticulitis (red arrow) with extensive fat stranding and pericolic gas bubbles (white arrow) indicating microperforation, associated with a worse prognosis

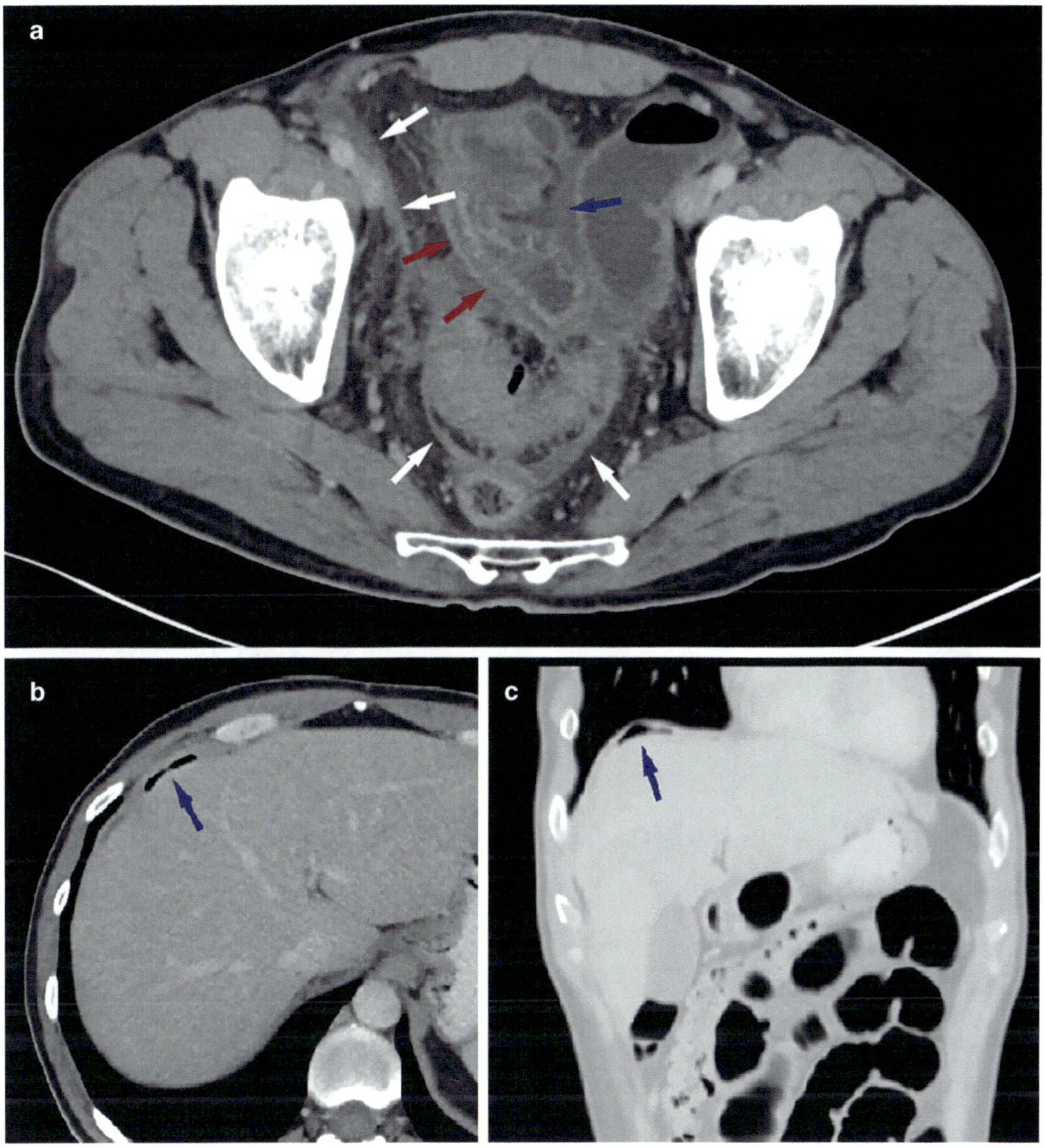

Fig. 5.9 Acute diverticulitis complicated by free perforation. (**a**) Diffuse mural thickening of the sigmoid colon (red arrows) with dense free fluid (blue arrow). Diffuse enhancement and thickening of peritoneum (white arrows), indicating peritonitis. (**b**, **c**). Intraperitoneal free gas (blue arrow) is also noted under the right hemidiaphragm, in keeping with free perforation. A perforated sigmoid diverticulum was identified at surgery

intraperitoneal gas in the settings of colonic diverticulitis is the most important finding on CT to indicate the need for surgery [21].

Abscess

An abscess refers to a walled-off collection and is the most common complication seen in acute diverticulitis. The appearance on imaging is an organized collection with enhancing walls, containing fluid with or without gas. Abscesses can develop locally within the colon wall at the site of diverticulitis, termed intramural abscesses. These are usually smaller abscesses (<3 cm) that are well contained. Pericolic abscesses adjacent to the inflamed colon are one of the most common complications seen in acute diverticulitis with contained perforation in the adjacent mesocolon [22, 23]. Distant abscesses within the peritoneal cavity can be seen when the mesocolon is unable to contain the perforation. These are most frequently seen in the pelvis at the rectouterine or rectovesical pouch, as the fluid accumulates in the lowest dependent aspect of the peritoneal cavity (Fig. 5.10). Rarely, abscesses can also

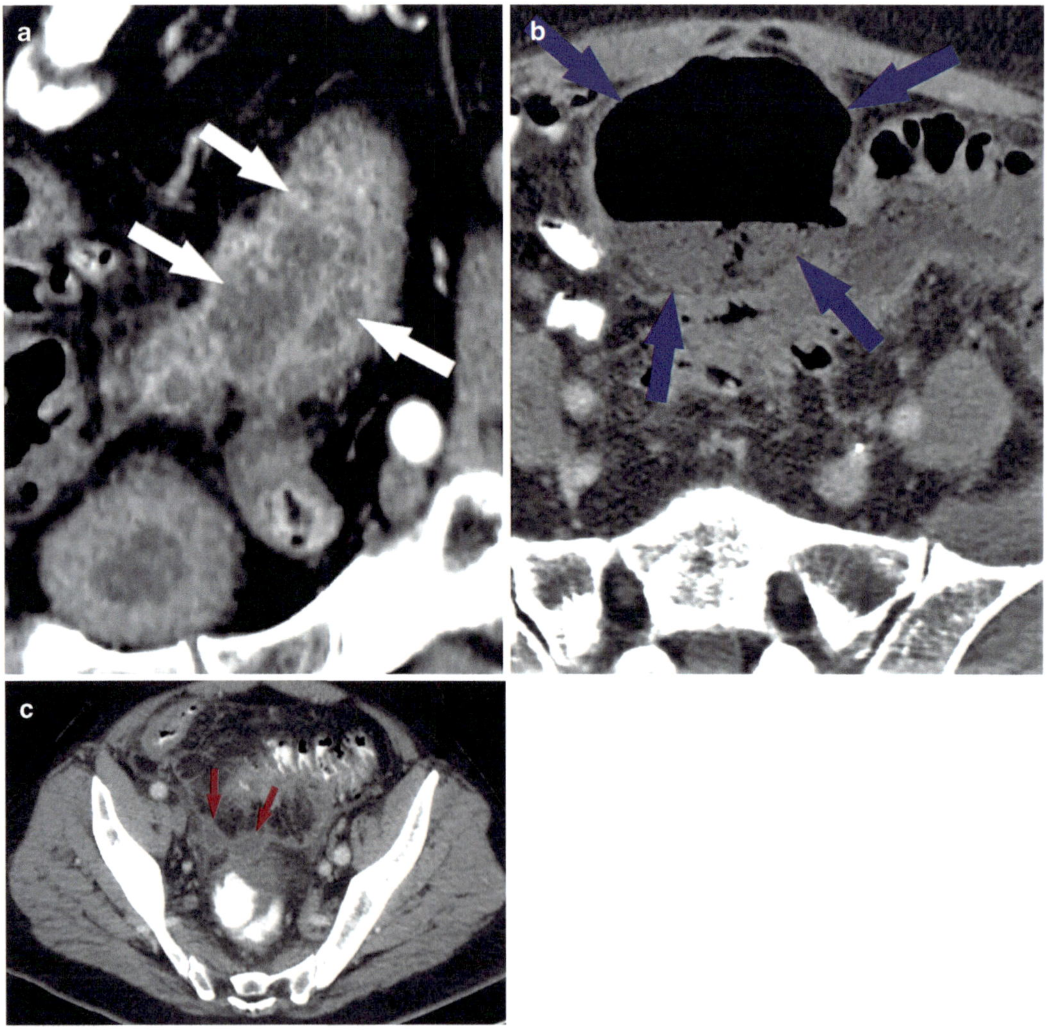

Fig. 5.10 Diverticulitis complicated by abscesses. (**a**) Intramural abscess. Rim-enhancing fluid collection embedded within the wall of the sigmoid colon (white arrows). (**b**) Pericolic abscess. Large organized fluid collection with air-fluid level adjacent to the sigmoid (blue arrows). (**c**) Pelvic abscess. Bilobed rim-enhancing fluid collection at the dependent of aspect of the peritoneal space (red arrows)

develop distantly in the retroperitoneal space, psoas muscle, groin, abdominal wall or subphrenic space.

When abscesses are larger than 5 cm in diameter, the risk of failed medical management alone increases and percutaneous drainage should be attempted if there is no contraindication. Abscesses between 3 and 4 cm may be drained in patients who do not respond to antibiotics [24]. Contraindications to percutaneous drainage include coagulopathy and lack of direct access. Access is most commonly percutaneous by transabdominal or transgluteal approach, depending on the location of the abscess. A transabdominal approach is favored in abscesses located anteriorly and adjacent to the descending colon or proximal sigmoid colon, and a transgluteal approach is often favored for deeper abscesses adjacent to the distal sigmoid colon. The safest approach is chosen by the radiologist after assessing the imaging to avoid unnecessary injury to adjacent structures. Alternatively, deep pelvic abscesses may also be accessed by a transrectal or transvaginal approach [25]. Complications related to percutaneous drainage are rare and include hemorrhage in approximately 2% of the cases [26].

Fistulas and Sinus Tracts

Fistulas occur in 2% of patients with complicated diverticular disease and are best identified with a contrast-enhanced CT [27]. An enhancing tract arising from a diverticula can be blind-ended (sinus tract) or communicate with an adjacent structure, indicating a fistula. More specifically, a fistula represents the communication between two epithelium-lined surfaces, most frequently between the bowels and another hollow organ (e.g., bladder, small bowel) and much less commonly to skin. If a fistula is suspected but remains uncertain clinically, it is helpful to perform a CT with oral or rectal contrast material and without intravenous contrast to assess for the presence of endoluminal contrast within any tracts or adjacent organs.

Colovesical fistulas represent approximately 65% of all encountered diverticulitis-related fistulas [28]. On CT, colovesical fistula can be diagnosed when the enhancing tract filled with contrast is identified between the colon and bladder (Fig. 5.11). Colovesical fistulas should also be suspected when the bladder is adherent to the colon with thickening of the walls, or when gas is

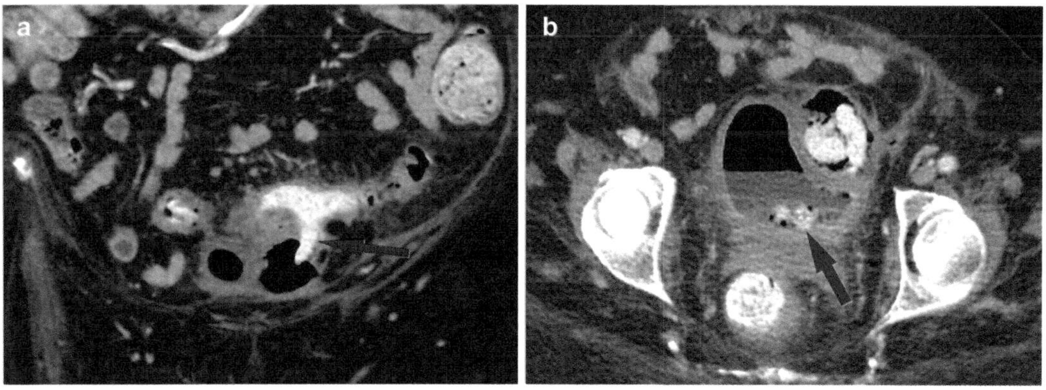

Fig. 5.11 Diverticulitis complicated by a colovesical fistula. (**a**) A tract filled with oral contrast (red arrow) is connecting the sigmoid colon to the superior aspect of the bladder. (**b**) The bladder demonstrates wall thickening and is adherent to the sigmoid colon. It contains gas and a small amount of oral contrast at its dependent aspect (blue arrow), in keeping with a colovesical fistula

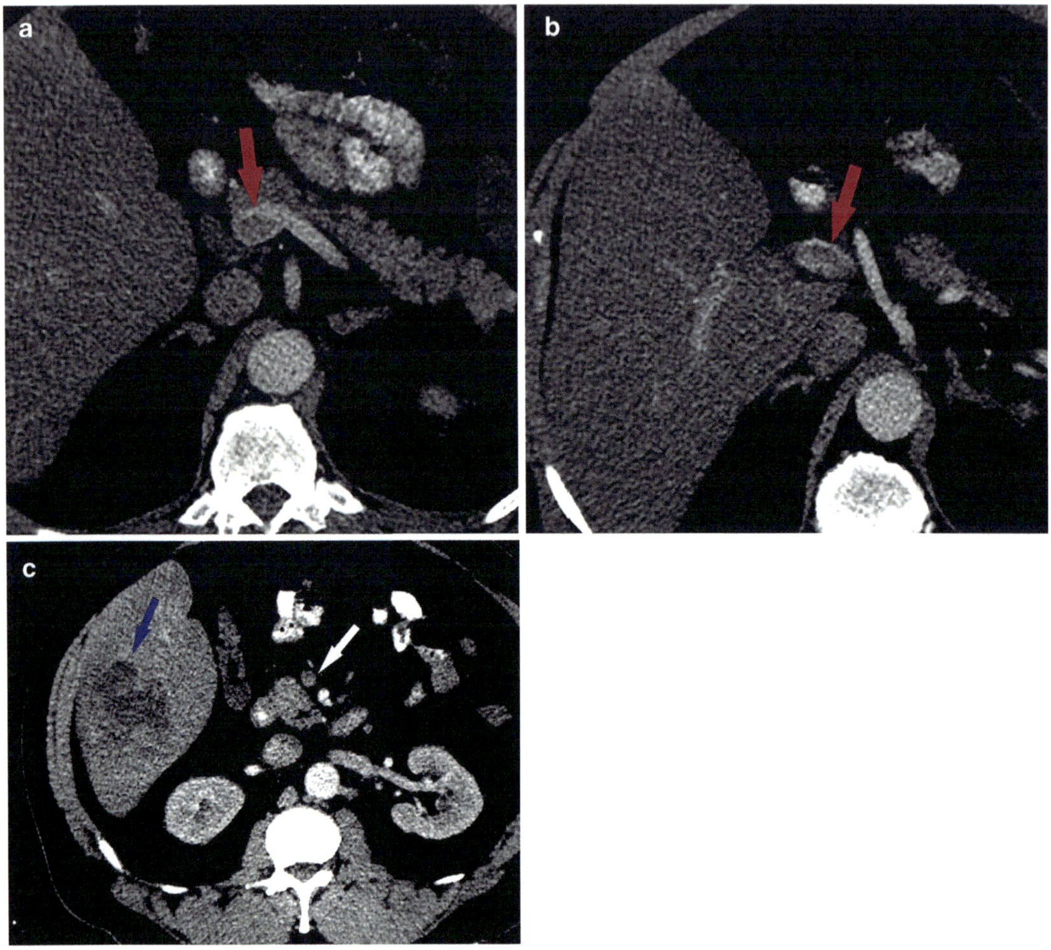

Fig. 5.12 Diverticulitis complicated by a liver abscess and septic thrombosis of the mesenteric and portal veins. (**a**, **b**) Patient presenting in septic shock with an acute sigmoid diverticulitis. The superior mesenteric vein is occluded (white arrow), and the septic thrombus extends into the portal vein causing a partial filling defect (red arrows). (**c**). An irregular hypodense hepatic lesion (blue arrow) in segment VI with subtle peripheral enhancement, compatible with an abscess

present in the bladder in the absence of recent catheterization [29].

Other less common types of diverticulitis-related fistulas include communication with the uterus, vagina, adnexae, small or large bowels, and skin. In severe chronic cases, complex multi-directional fistulas and sinus tracts can be seen.

Pylephlebitis and Liver Abscess

One of the most morbid complications of acute diverticulitis is the spread of infection into the mesenteric venous vessels, leading to septic thrombosis, termed pylephlebitis. The septic thrombosis can extend to the portal veins and lead to pyogenic liver abscess, a serious complication with an overall mortality of 32% [30, 31]. The diagnosis can be made with a contrast-enhanced CT showing thrombosis or air within the mesenteric and portal veins (Fig. 5.12).

Pyogenic liver abscess may not be present at the initial diagnosis, and short-term follow-up should be performed if pylephlebitis is diagnosed and signs of sepsis persist. Early signs of liver involvements include perfusion abnormalities within the parenchyma in the vicinity of the portal venous supply. It takes several days for a fully organized liver abscess to develop and prompt diagnosis is essential as it may require percutaneous drainage.

Bowel Obstruction

After colorectal cancer and volvulus, diverticulitis is the third most frequent cause of large bowel obstruction [32]. In the acute setting, the inflammation causing wall thickening may lead to luminal narrowing significant enough to cause an obstruction (Fig. 5.13). A large pericolic abscess may also cause compression and result in obstruction. In the chronic setting, stricture and fibrosis from recurrent diverticulitis can cause chronic luminal narrowing leading to obstruction. Rarely, small bowel can be trapped in the inflamed pericolonic inflammatory changes and lead to small bowel obstruction [33].

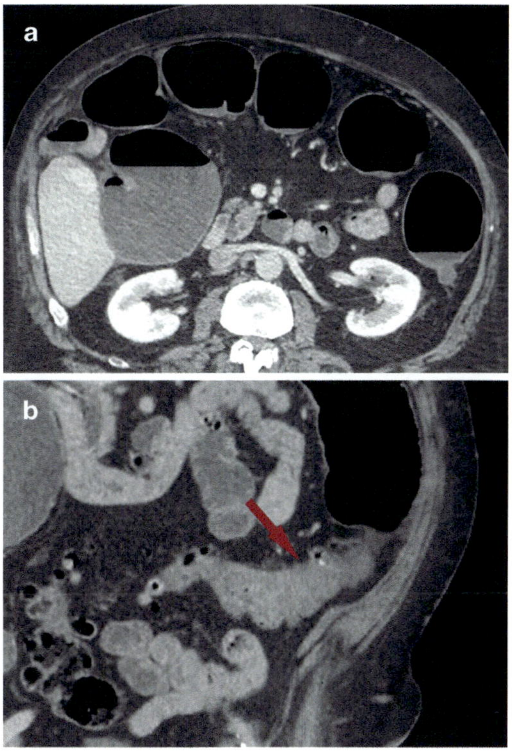

Fig. 5.13 Acute diverticulitis complicated by large bowel obstruction. (**a**) Dilated colonic loops with air-fluid levels indicating a large bowel obstruction. (**b**) Transition point in the proximal sigmoid colon (red arrow) secondary to a thickening segment with diverticula. The obstruction resolved with medical management and colonoscopy confirmed a diverticulitis

Other

Giant Diverticulum

Giant diverticulum is a rare entity with less than 200 cases documented in the literature [34]. It is defined as a large diverticulum measuring more than 4 cm in one dimension, and the majority are observed in the sigmoid colon (Fig. 5.14).

Three types of giant diverticulum have been described [35]. Type I (22%) are giant pseudodiverticula as the colonic muscularis propria ends abruptly at the neck of the pseudodiverticulum. The colonic mucosa is also often incomplete and interspersed with chronic granulation tissue. Type II is the most common (66%) and the wall is made of dense fibrous tissue with chronic inflammatory cells and foreign body giant cells. Type III (12%) are true diverticula that contain all colonic layers, and likely represent a communicating bowel duplication cyst. On imaging, the appearance is of a large diverticulum with perceptible walls, usually containing stool and gas.

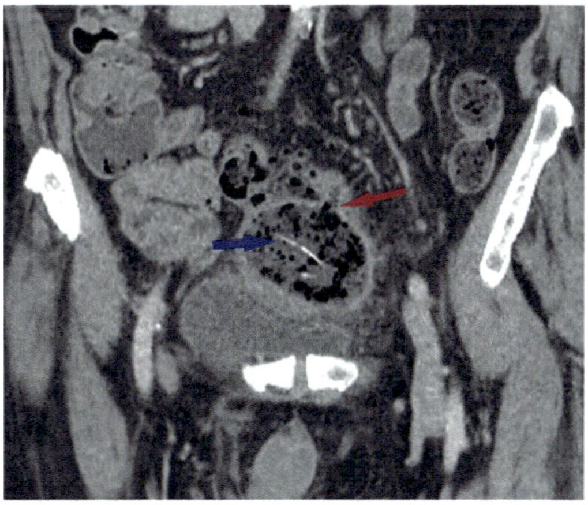

Fig. 5.14 Giant sigmoid diverticulum. Large diverticulum arising from the sigmoid colon (red arrow) containing partially calcified inspissated stools (blue arrow)

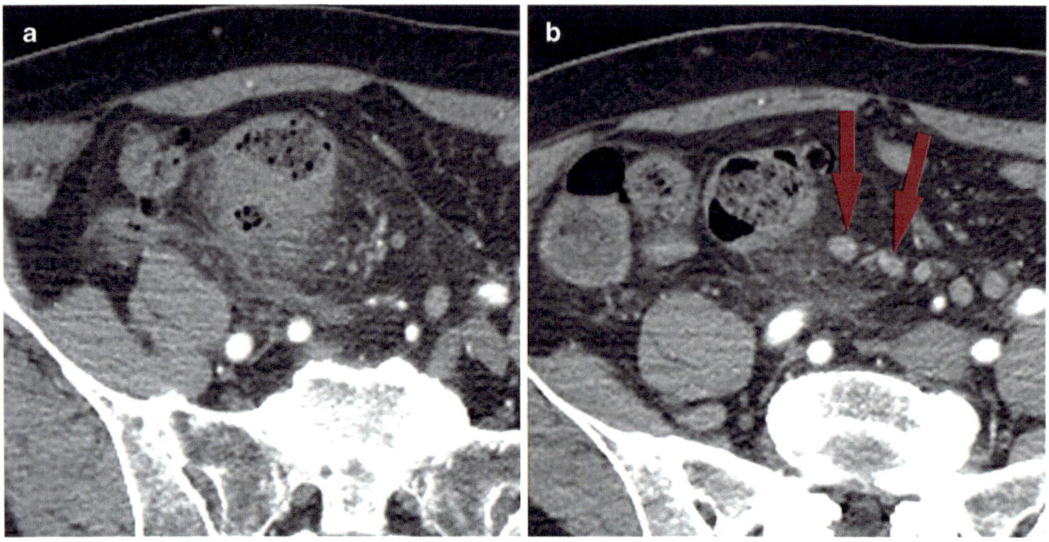

Fig. 5.15 Colon cancer mimicking a diverticulitis. (**a**) Asymmetric wall edema adjacent to a diverticulum in the distal sigmoid colon with surrounding inflammatory changes. (**b**) Suspicious prominent enhancing mesosigmoid lymph nodes are noted. Colonoscopy confirmed the presence of a perforating colon carcinoma

If administered, oral contrast can be seen pooling in the diverticulum. These can be complicated by diverticulitis and all the aforementioned diverticulitis complications.

Differential Diagnosis

Colon Cancer

Diverticulitis and colon carcinoma can be impossible to differentiate from each other on all imaging modalities, with diagnostic uncertainty on CT reported in up to 25% of cases [36]. Colonic neoplasm often arises in segments with significant diverticulosis and may mimic the appearance of acute diverticulitis, with similar findings of colon wall thickening and fat stranding adjacent to diverticula (Fig. 5.15).

Several findings on CT scan suggest the presence of an acute diverticulitis or a colon carcinoma. Findings that favor a diagnosis of acute diverticulitis include identification of an inflamed diverticulum, extensive pericolic fat stranding compared to the degree of colon wall thickening, and extraluminal gas and free fluid. Carcinoma of the colon should be suspected when there are prominent mesenteric lymph nodes, asymmetric wall thickening, or an endoluminal mass. In the context of a large bowel obstruction secondary to diverticulitis, the zone of transition should be gradual with preservation of mucosal folds, while a colon carcinoma often demonstrates an abrupt transition point with a narrowed lumen, giving the appearance of an apple core [37, 38]. In equivocal cases, follow-up varies by institution but generally consists of endoscopic assessment or CT colonography after the acute inflammation has subsided (usually 6 weeks).

Colitis

Colitis often causes colonic wall thickening in segments affected by diverticulosis. Most infectious and inflammatory colitides usually affect longer segments of the colon than those observed in acute diverticulitis and are less likely to be associated with focal pericolic fat stranding or extraluminal gas. Other CT findings may suggest an inflammatory bowel disease, including the presence of fatty submucosal infiltration, small bowel involvement, sacroiliitis, or primary sclerosing cholangitis. Segmental colitis associated with diverticulosis, also known as SCAD, is defined as inflammation of the interdiverticular colonic mucosa that typically spares the diverticula. This may be difficult to appreciate on CT scan but should be considered in a short-segment colitis centered on diverticula-containing colon.

Epiploic Appendagitis

Primary epiploic appendagitis is an uncommon self-limiting process caused by intraperitoneal focal fat infarction secondary to a torsed appendix epiploica of the colon. It appears as a small oval or round fat-containing mass with inflammatory changes adjacent to the mesenteric side of the colon and is most often seen in younger patients compared to sigmoid diverticulitis. A central hyperdense dot can often be seen representing the thrombosed vascular pedicle (Fig. 5.16) [39]. Epiploic appendagitis can usually be differentiated from acute diverticulitis as it is not associated with significant thickening of the colon and should not feature any evidence of complication. On follow-up imaging, it can resolve entirely or leave coarse calcifications at the site of the infarcted epiploic appendage [40].

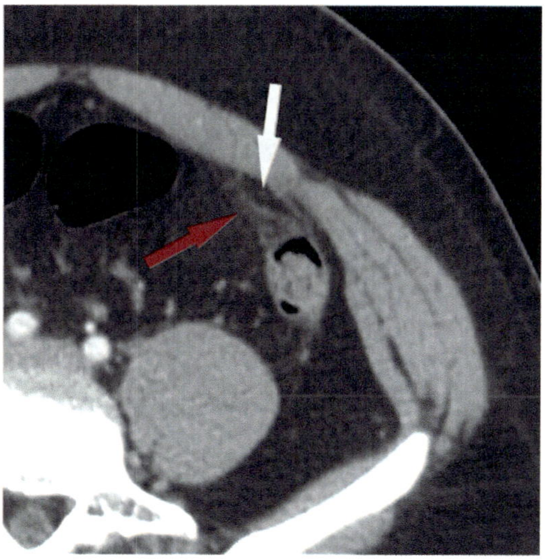

Fig. 5.16 Epiploic appendagitis. Inflammatory changes centered around a round focus of fat (red arrow) adjacent to the distal descending colon. A central hyperdense dot sign (white arrow) indicating a torsed vascular peduncle. The appendagitis is not in continuity with the colon and there is no significant mural thickening

Appendicitis

Cecal and ascending colon diverticulitis are uncommon but may present with a similar clinical picture to acute appendicitis (Fig. 5.17) [41]. On imaging, reactive thickening of the appendix can be visualized if the offending diverticulum is near the appendix, mimicking an acute appendicitis. Right-sided diverticulitis can be differentiated from appendicitis by the identification of an affected diverticulum. Furthermore, the inflammatory changes are typically not centered around the appendix itself.

Gynecologic Disease

Multiple gynecologic pathologies can mimic diverticulitis, including pelvic inflammatory disease, ovarian torsion, and endometriosis. A tubo-ovarian abscess in close proximity with a segment of the sigmoid colon affected by diverticulosis can appear similar to a diverticulitis complicated by a peri-sigmoid abscess. If there is suspected involvement of the pelvic organs on CT when assessing for acute diverticulitis and the diagnosis remains equivocal, further characterization can be achieved with an endovaginal ultrasound or MRI.

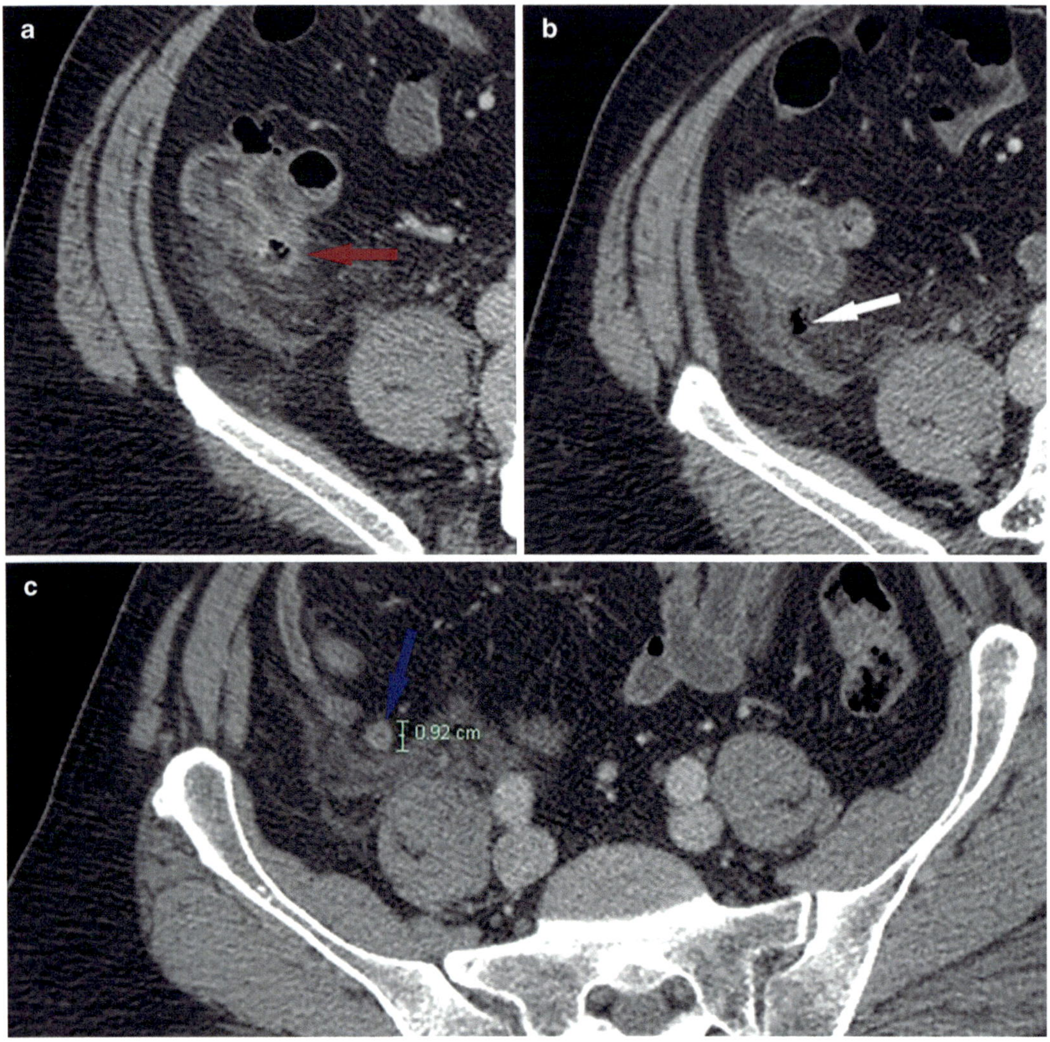

Fig. 5.17 Cecal diverticulitis with reactive thickening of the appendix. (**a**) An enhancing cecal diverticulitis (red arrow) with surrounding fat stranding. (**b**) Free gas bubbles adjacent to the diverticulitis (white arrow). (**c**) Reactive thickening of the appendix (blue arrow) measuring 9.2 mm with adjacent fat stranding mimicking an acute appendicitis

Conclusion

Contrast-enhanced CT is the primary imaging modality to assess diverticular disease, and is the initial study recommended when an acute diverticulitis is suspected. The high sensitivity and specificity for complications make it an essential diagnostic modality to guide treatment and potential therapeutic interventions. The main diagnostic challenge remains the differentiation from a colon cancer arising in a segment of diverticulosis, and short-term follow-up or endoscopic assessment should be considered if any suspicious features are present. If CT is contraindicated by pregnancy or other reasons, MRI and ultrasound provide a reasonable alternative with no ionizing radiation.

References

1. de Vries EH, Ginai AZ, Robben SG, Hop WC. Pelvic phleboliths: is there an association with diverticulitis? Br J Radiol. 1992;65:868–70.
2. Fox JA, Stollman NH. Diverticular disease of the colon. In: Feldman M, Friedman LS, Brandt LJ, editors. Sleisenger and Fordtran's gastrointestinal and liver disease: pathophysiology, diagnosis, management. 9th ed. Philadelphia: Elsevier; 2010. p. 2073–89.
3. Miller WT, Levine MS, Rubesin SE, Laufer I. Bowler-hat sign: a simple principle for differentiating polyps from diverticula. Radiology. 1989;173:615–7.
4. Paoluzi OA, Tosti C, Andrei F, Stroppa I, Pallone F. Look out before polypectomy in patients with diverticular disease – a case of a large, inverted diverticulum of the colon resembling a pedunculated polyp. Can J Gastroenterol. 2010;24:61–3.
5. Laufer I, Lavine MS, Laufer I: Double contrast gastrointestinal radiology, 2, Philadelphia,1992, WB Saunders.
6. Francis NK, Sylla P, Abou-Khalil M, et al. EAES and SAGES 2018 consensus conference on acute diverticulitis management: evidence-based recommendations for clinical practice. Surg Endosc. 2019;33:2726–41.
7. Laméris W, van Randen A, Bipat S, Bossuyt PMM, Boermeester MA, Stoker J. Graded compression ultrasonography and computed tomography in acute colonic diverticulitis: meta-analysis of test accuracy. Eur Radiol. 2008;18:2498–511.
8. Kaewlai R, Nazinitsky KJ. Acute colonic diverticulitis in a community-based hospital: CT evaluation in 138 patients. Emerg Radiol. 2007;13:171–9.
9. Smereczyński A, Kołaczyk K. Pitfalls in ultrasound imaging of the stomach and the intestines. J Ultrason. 2018;18:207–11.
10. Mazzei MA, Cioffi Squitieri N, Guerrini S, Stabile Ianora AA, Cagini L, Macarini L, Giganti M, Volterrani L. Sigmoid diverticulitis: US findings. Crit Ultrasound J. 2013;5(Suppl 1):S5.
11. Nazerian P, Gigli C, Donnarumma E, et al. Diagnostic accuracy of point-of-care ultrasound integrated into clinical examination for acute diverticulitis: a prospective multicenter study. Ultraschall Med. 2021;42(6):614–22. https://doi.org/10.1055/a--1161-0780. Epub 2020 Jul 20. English
12. Halpenny DF, McNeil G, Snow A, Geoghegan T, Torreggiani WC. Prospective evaluation of the value of magnetic resonance imaging in suspected acute sigmoid diverticulitis. Dis Colon Rectum. 2009;52:1030–1. author reply 1031.
13. Chung JJ, Semelka RC, Martin DR, Marcos HB. Colon diseases: MR evaluation using combined T2-weighted single-shot echo train spin-echo and gadolinium-enhanced spoiled gradient-echo sequences. J Magn Reson Imaging. 2000;12:297–305.
14. Buckley O, Geoghegan T, McAuley G, Persaud T, Khosa F, Torreggiani WC. Pictorial review: magnetic resonance imaging of colonic diverticulitis. Eur Radiol. 2007;17:221–7.
15. Jerjen F, Zaidi T, Chan S, et al. Magnetic resonance imaging for the diagnosis and management of acute colonic diverticulitis: a review of current and future use. J Med Radiat Sci. 2021;68(3):310–9. https://doi.org/10.1002/jmrs.458.
16. Ünlü Ç, van de Wall BJ, Gerhards MF, Wiezer M, Draaisma WA, Consten EC, Boermeester MA, Vrouenraets BC. Influence of age on clinical outcome of acute diverticulitis. J Gastrointest Surg. 2013;17:1651–6.
17. Rotert H, Nöldge G, Encke J, Richter GM, Düx M. The value of CT for the diagnosis of acute diverticulitis. Radiologe. 2003;43:51–8.
18. ACR Expert Panel on Gastrointestinal Imaging: ACR Appropriateness Criteria: Left Lower Quadrant Pain – Suspected Diverticulitis, 2018. https://acsearch.acr.org/docs/69356/Narrative/. Accessed 2 June 2019.
19. Khalil HA, Yoo J. Colorectal emergencies: perforated diverticulitis (operative and nonoperative management). J Gastrointest Surg. 2014;18:865–8.
20. García-Gómez MA, Belmonte-Montes C, Cosme-Reyes C, Aguirre Garcia MP. Prognostic value of the presence of pericolic air bubbles detected by computed tomography in acute diverticulitis. Cir Cir. 2017;85:471–7.
21. Shin S, Kim D, Kang UR, Yang C-S. Impact of CT imaging on predicting the surgical management of acute diverticulitis. Ann Surg Treat Res. 2018;94:322–9.
22. Gore RM, Miller FH, Pereles FS, Yaghmai V, Berlin JW. Helical CT in the evaluation of the acute abdomen. AJR Am J Roentgenol. 2000;174:901–13.
23. Pradel JA, Adell JF, Taourel P, Djafari M, Monnin-Delhom E, Bruel JM. Acute colonic diverticulitis: prospective comparative evaluation with US and CT. Radiology. 1997;205:503–12.
24. Young-Fadok TM. Diverticulitis. N Engl J Med. 2018;379:1635–42.
25. Maher MM, Gervais DA, Kalra MK, Lucey B, Sahani DV, Arellano R, Hahn PF, Mueller PR. The inaccessible or undrainable abscess: how to drain it. Radiographics. 2004;24:717–35.
26. Harisinghani MG, Gervais DA, Maher MM, Cho CH, Hahn PF, Varghese J, Mueller PR. Transgluteal approach for percutaneous drainage of deep pelvic abscesses: 154 cases. Radiology. 2003;228:701–5.
27. Strati T-M, Sapalidis K, Koimtzis GD, et al. Sigmoidocecal fistula: a rare case of complicated recurrent diverticulitis and a review of the literature. Am J Case Rep. 2018;19:1386–139226.
28. Woods RJ, Lavery IC, Fazio VW, Jagelman DG, Weakley FL. Internal fistulas in diverticular disease. Dis Colon Rectum. 1988;31:591–6.

29. Jarrett TW, Vaughan ED. Accuracy of computerized tomography in the diagnosis of colovesical fistula secondary to diverticular disease. J Urol. 1995;153:44–6.
30. Van De Wauwer C, Irvin TT. Pylephlebitis due to perforated diverticulitis. Acta Chir Belg. 2005;105:229–30.
31. Lee BK, Ryu HH. A case of pylephlebitis secondary to cecal diverticulitis. J Emerg Med. 2012;42:e81–5.
32. Taourel P, Kessler N, Lesnik A, Pujol J, Morcos L, Bruel JM. Helical CT of large bowel obstruction. Abdom Imaging. 2003;28:267–75.
33. Kim AY, Bennett GL, Bashist B, Perlman B, Megibow AJ. Small-bowel obstruction associated with sigmoid diverticulitis: CT evaluation in 16 patients. AJR Am J Roentgenol. 1998;170:1311–3.
34. Zeina A-R, Nachtigal A, Matter I, Benjaminov O, Abu-Gazala M, Mahamid A, Kessel B, Amitai M. Giant colon diverticulum: clinical and imaging findings in 17 patients with emphasis on CT criteria. Clin Imaging. 2013;37:704–10.
35. Thomas S, Peel RL, Evans LE, Haarer KA. Best cases from the AFIP: giant colonic diverticulum. Radiographics. 2006;26:1869–72.
36. Zaman S, Chapman W, Mohammed I, Gill K, Ward ST. Patients with computed tomography-proven acute diverticulitis require follow-up to exclude colorectal cancer. Intest Res. 2017;15:195–202.
37. Chintapalli KN, Chopra S, Ghiatas AA, Esola CC, Fields SF, Dodd GD. Diverticulitis versus colon cancer: differentiation with helical CT findings. Radiology. 1999;210:429–35.
38. Chintapalli KN, Esola CC, Chopra S, Ghiatas AA, Dodd GD. Pericolic mesenteric lymph nodes: an aid in distinguishing diverticulitis from cancer of the colon. AJR Am J Roentgenol. 1997;169:1253–5.
39. Almeida AT, Melão L, Viamonte B, Cunha R, Pereira JM. Epiploic appendagitis: an entity frequently unknown to clinicians--diagnostic imaging, pitfalls, and look-alikes. AJR Am J Roentgenol. 2009;193:1243–51.
40. Singh AK, Gervais DA, Hahn PF, Sagar P, Mueller PR, Novelline RA. Acute epiploic appendagitis and its mimics. Radiographics. 2005;25:1521–34.
41. Chiu T-C, Chou Y-H, Tiu C-M, Chiou H-J, Wang H-K, Lai Y-C, Chiou Y-Y. Right-sided colonic diverticulitis: clinical features, sonographic appearances, and management. J Med Ultrasound. 2017;25:33–9.

Classification Systems and Definitions of Diverticulitis

6

Scott C. Dolejs and Dimitrios Stefanidis

Introduction

Diverticulosis is a common finding in adults, and most commonly remains asymptomatic. However, in a small proportion of patients, diverticular disease can manifest as diverticulitis or diverticular bleeding. Within the spectrum of diverticulitis, there is a wide phenotypic variation, ranging from mild abdominal pain to an acute surgical abdomen with sepsis. In light of this wide disease presentation, several classification systems have been proposed to stratify and categorize diverticulitis severity. Classification systems may help predict patient outcomes, define treatment strategies, and can aid in the comparison of research studies on diverticulitis.

Hughes and Hinchey Classifications

The classification and reclassification of diverticulitis have been an ongoing exercise for over 50 years. Hughes et al. [1] first published a four-stage classification system in 1963 that has formed the basis for many of the subsequent classification systems. Fifteen years later, Hinchey et al. [2] published their classification of diverticulitis that was very similar to the work by Hughes. Despite being published 15 years later with minimal changes from the Hughes classification, the Hinchey classification has largely been considered the standard classification since that time. Both of these early classifications were predominantly based on surgical findings (Fig. 6.1). With the increasing use of CT scan, the Hinchey classification system has undergone at least three modifications; however, it still remains a clinical (rather than purely radiological) classification schema [1–3]. For the purposes of this chapter, the Wasvary modification of the Hinchey classification will be used as this is the most widely accepted modification (Fig. 6.2; Table 6.1) [2].

S. C. Dolejs
Franciscan Health Indianapolis, Indiana Colon and Rectal Specialists, Indianapolis, IN, USA

D. Stefanidis (✉)
Department of Surgery, Indiana University School of Medicine, Indiana University Health North Hospital, Carmel, IN, USA
e-mail: dimstefa@iu.edu

M. Boutros et al. (eds.), *Diverticulitis*, https://doi.org/10.1007/978-3-032-21720-2_6

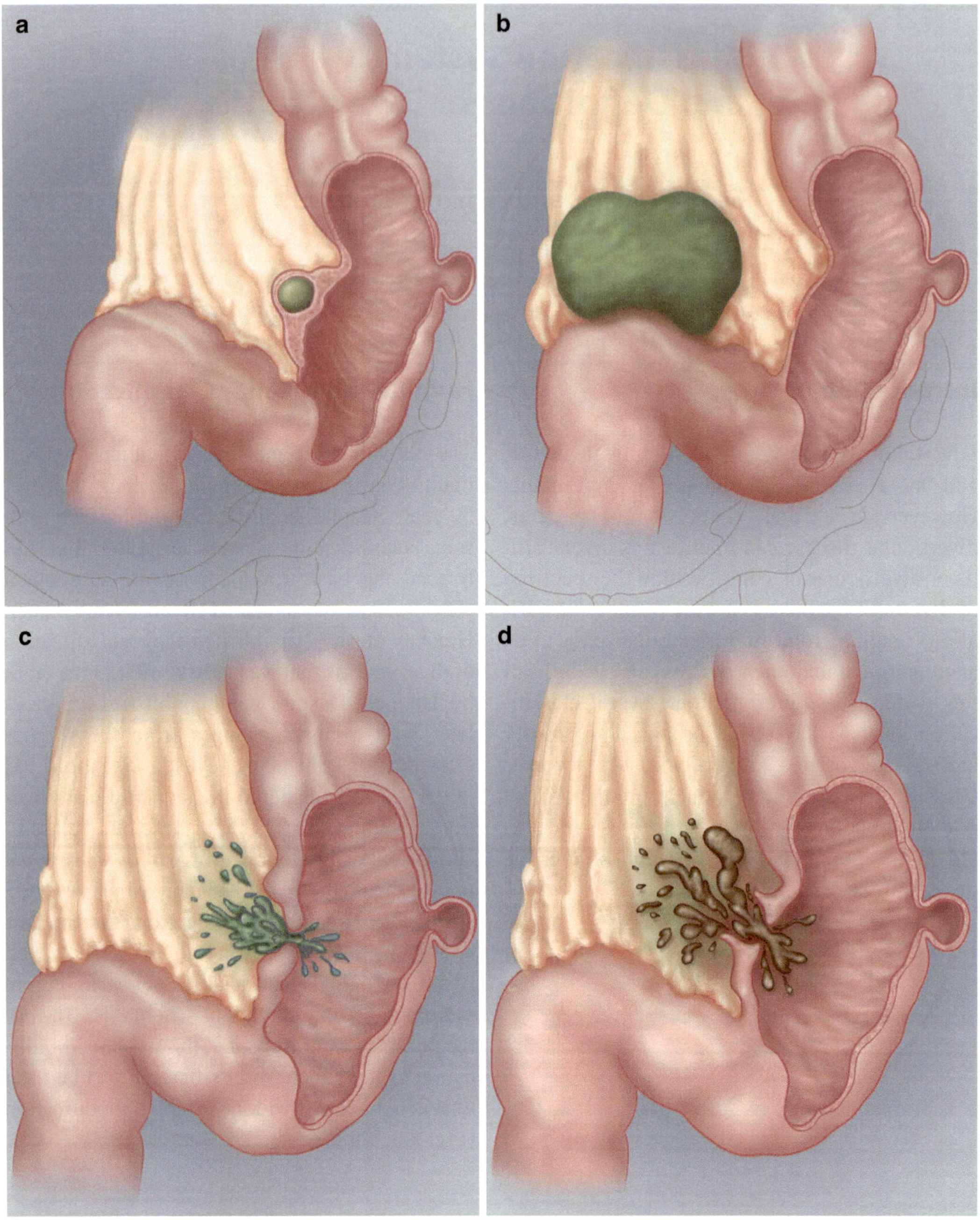

Fig. 6.1 (**a**–**d**) Figure of original Hinchey Classification. (**a**) Hinchey Class I with a pericolic abscess. (**b**) Hinchey Class II with a pelvic abscess. (**c**) Hinchey Class III with purulent fluid from perforation with purulent peritonitis. (**d**) Hinchey Class IV with fecal spillage resulting in feculent peritonitis

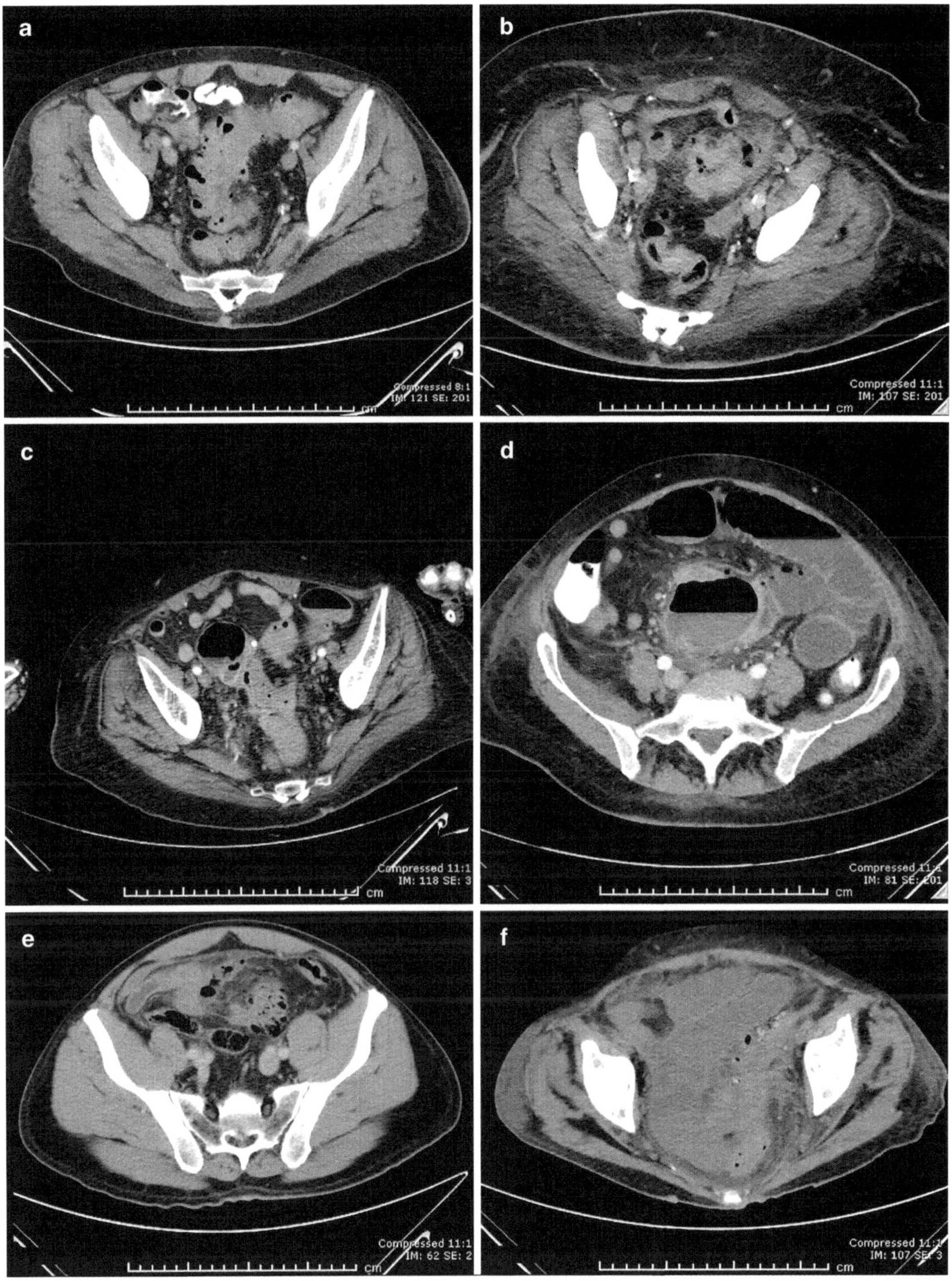

Fig. 6.2 (**a**–**f**) CT scans demonstrating the various Hinchey Classification. Of note, determining Hinchey Class III versus IV is difficult on CT scan. (**a**) Hinchey Class 0 with sigmoid colon thickening and mild inflammatory changes. (**b**) Hinchey Class Ia with sigmoid colon thickening and a pericolic phlegmon. (**c**) Hinchey Class Ib with a pericolic abscess. (**d**) Hinchey Class II with a pelvic abscess with a large air fluid collection. (**e**) Hinchey Class III with pneumoperitoneum and free fluid. (**f**) Hinchey Class IV with pneumoperitoneum, a large amount of free fluid which was found to be feculent peritonitis at the time of operation

Table 6.1 Hinchey classification system with Wasvary modification [2]

Classification	Definition
0	Mild clinical diverticulitis
Ia	Pericolic phlegmon
Ib	Pericolic or mesocolic abscess
II	Pelvic, distant abscess
III	Purulent peritonitis
IV	Feculent peritonitis

Modified Hinchey Classification

With this modified Hinchey classification schema, the full range of acute diverticulitis is accurately categorized.

Hinchey class 0 corresponds to mild clinical diverticulitis. If imaging is obtained, the colon will appear thickened with minimal surrounding fat stranding.

Hinchey class Ia is diverticulitis with a pericolonic phlegmon but no organized fluid collection. *Hinchey class Ib* represents a pericolic or mesocolic abscess. There has thus been a progression from unorganized inflammation into an organized collection.

Hinchey class II represents a pelvic, or distant abscess, suggesting the spread of bacteria further away from the site of inflammation or perforation.

Hinchey class III represents purulent peritonitis with an active communication between the colon and the peritoneum resulting in widespread bacterial spillage.

Hinchey class IV represents the next step in peritonitis wherein a hole has formed that is large enough to allow free flow of stool from the colon into the peritoneal cavity. The Hinchey classification has been the most studied classification system, is predictive of morbidity, mortality, and the need for operative intervention, and is the most widely utilized classification for diverticulitis worldwide [4–8].

Despite its widespread use, there are still significant gaps in the Hinchey classification system. With improvements in cross-sectional imaging, CT scans can reliably detect microperforations, defined as small amounts of pericolic air bubbles without the formation of a phlegmon or abscess, which the Hinchey classification does not address. Further, the Hinchey classification does not take into account the physiologic status of the patient, which may significantly impact outcomes. The Hinchey classification is additionally designed for an acute episode of diverticulitis. Thus, it fails to address chronic sequelae that may arise from diverticulitis, such as stricture or fistula.

Other Classifications

As a result of the gaps in the Hinchey classification, up to 10 additional classifications have been proposed to stage the severity of diverticulitis [6, 9]. Examples of radiographic classifications include the American Association for the Surgery of Trauma (AAST) grading system for acute colonic diverticulitis and the Ambrosetti Classification [6, 8, 10–18]. Examples of clinical and operative classification systems include the Mannheim Peritonitis Index (MPI), the Boostrom Classification, and the Cleveland Clinic Diverticular Disease Propensity Score (CCDDP) [6, 8, 10–18]. Examples of combined radiographic and clinical classifications systems include the Hinchey classification system, the Hansen-Stock Classification, and the Kruis classification [6, 8, 10–18]. These various classification systems are presented in Table 6.2.

The majority of these classifications find their roots in the Hinchey classification, or perhaps more accurately, the Hughes classification system. Despite their differences, most classifications do not address chronic diverticulitis and its complications. They generally classify acute diverticulitis as uncomplicated or complicated based on the presence or absence of an abscess, fistula, or free intraperitoneal contamination [6, 8, 10–16]. Complicated diverticulitis is frequently further subdivided into contained perforation (perforation with an abscess either pericolic or distant) and uncontained perforation (free intraperitoneal contamination with

Table 6.2 Various classification systems of diverticulitis

Classification	Definition
Radiographic classifications:	
AAST[a]	
I	Colonic inflammation
II	Microperforation or phlegmon
III	Localized abscess
IV	Distant abscess
V	Free perforation
Ambrosetti	
Moderate/mild	Localized sigmoid wall thickening (<5 mm) and/or pericolic fat stranding
Severe	Abscess, extraluminal air or contrast
Clinical and operative classifications:	
Mannheim Peritonitis Index	Combination of age, gender, organ failure, malignancy, symptoms>24 h, origin of peritonitis, diffuse peritonitis, purulent vs. feculent peritonitis
CR-POSSUM[b]	Score based on 6 physiologic and 4 operative variables. Not diverticular specific
Cleveland Clinic Diverticular Disease Propensity Score	Combination of operative urgency, BMI, MPI, and Hinchey classification
Boostrom	
Acute	Discrete episodes that resolve
Chronic	Persistent pain for 3 months
Atypical	Prolonged LLQ pain, but no radiographic evidence
Combined clinical and radiographic classifications:	
Hinchey	*See* Table 6.1
Hansen-Stock	
0	Diverticulosis
I	Uncomplicated diverticulitis
IIa	Phlegmon, peridiverticulitis
IIb	Abscess, sealed perforation
IIc	Free perforation
III	Chronic, recurrent
Sallinen	
1	Uncomplicated acute
2	Abscess <6 cm
3	Abscess >6 cm or distant intra- or retroperitoneal air. Peritonitis without organ dysfunction
4	Peritonitis with organ dysfunction
5	
Kruis	
0	Asymptomatic Diverticulosis
1	Acute uncomplicated diverticulitis
1a	Diverticulitis without peridiverticulitis
1b	Diverticulitis with phlegmonous peridiverticulitis
2	Acute complicated diverticulitis
2a	Microabscess
2b	Macroabscess
2c1	Purulent peritonitis
2c2	Feculent peritonitis
3	Chronic diverticular disease
3a	Symptomatic uncomplicated diverticular disease
3b	Relapsing diverticulitis without complications
3c	Relapsing diverticulitis with complications
4	Diverticular bleeding

[a]*AAST* American Association of Surgical Trauma
[b]*CR-POSSUM* ColoRectal Physiological and Operative Severity Score for the Enumeration of Mortality and Morbidity

either purulent or feculent peritonitis) [6, 8, 10–16]. As can be seen in Table 6.2, these classification schemes, in general, mirror the Hinchey classification system. This is not surprising as the classification by Hinchey remains clinically useful. In particular, determining whether there is complicated or uncomplicated disease, and if there is complicated disease, if the perforation is contained or not contained is useful as this dictates the therapeutic course approach [10–12, 19].

Classifications Based on Chronicity of Symptoms

Only the Boostrom [17], Kruis [11], and Hansen-Stock [18] classification systems include categories based on the chronicity of symptoms.

Type 0 refers to asymptomatic diverticulosis.

Type 1 refers to acute uncomplicated diverticular disease/diverticulitis and is further subdivided into type 1a and 1b; type 1a is defined as diverticulitis without peridiverticulitis (defined as diverticular symptoms with laboratory findings of inflammation, but without cross-sectional imaging or with only have colonic wall thickening on CT scan), while type 1b is defined as diverticulitis with phlegmonous peridiverticulitis on cross-sectional imaging.

Type 2 diverticulitis is acute, complicated diverticulitis and is subdivided into type 2a, 2b, 2c1, and 2c2, which closely follow Hinchey I–IV. Type 2a refers to a microabscess (defined as ≤1 cm), type 2b a macroabscess (defined as an abscess >1 cm), type 2c1 a perforation with purulent peritonitis, and type 2c2 a free perforation with feculent peritonitis.

Type 3 refers to chronic diverticular disease, defined as relapsing or persistent symptomatic diverticular disease. Type 3a is defined by persistent symptomatic uncomplicated diverticular disease, type 3b by relapsing diverticulitis without complications, and type 3c by relapsing diverticulitis with complications such as obstruction, fistula, or tumors.

Type 4 refers to diverticular bleeding.

The Kruis classification has the advantage of succinctly summarizing the varying phenotypes of diverticulitis, which may better correlate with management decisions. Despite the utility of this classification, there are some areas of possible improvement. For example, the abscess size cutoff of 1 cm is not a useful clinical cutoff based on several studies that have demonstrated that most abscesses <4 cm in size resolve without percutaneous intervention [13, 14]. Recent practice guidelines have thus not recommended percutaneous drainage until an abscess is greater than 3 or 4 cm depending on the guideline [13, 14]. Despite its potential usefulness, this classification has not been widely adopted in the literature or widely utilized outside of Germany.

While the literature is rife with single studies that have proposed a new classification system, there is a paucity of literature comparing the diagnostic accuracy and utility of these scoring systems. This limits the clinician's ability to select one classification system over another. There is only one retrospective cohort study by Sallinen et al. [8] that directly compares scoring systems. The authors included 631 patients and calculated the area under the curve (AUC) for several classification systems. They also created their own classification that is similar to the Hinchey classification, but with an additional stage for patients with generalized peritonitis and organ dysfunction [6]. The AUC for predicting 30-day mortality, need for operation, and ICU admission was 0.89–0.96 (very good predictive capability) for the Hinchey Classification, Hansen-Stock Classification, and Sallinen Classification, but was only 0.74–0.80 (good predictive capability) for the Ambrosetti Classification [6].

There is more literature that supports the efficacy of the various classification systems without directly comparing them. The Hinchey classification system has been the most widely studied [4, 5, 7, 8, 15–18, 20, 21]. The MPI has also been well studied; in six retrospective and one prospective studies, a higher MPI severity has been associated with higher mortality [8, 9, 15, 22–26]. In one large, retrospective, multicenter cohort study, the AAST diverticulitis grading system was found to be associated with complications, need for surgery, intensive care unit utilization, and 30-day readmission [27]. The AAST classification also has a category for a microperforation, making this a potentially appealing classification in an era of advanced computed tomography. In the AAST classification, microperforation is considered a lower grade of diverticulitis than even an abscess. This is also echoed in the recent American Society of Colon and Rectal Surgeons Clinical Practice Guidelines, wherein "small amounts of contained, extraluminal gas in the absence of a systemic inflammatory response" is not considered complicated disease [14].

There is not a single perfect classification system. Given the wide adoption of the modified Hinchey classification and its utilization in several clinical trials on diverticulitis, it is reasonable to use this system to classify acute diverticulitis [10–12, 19]. The AAST classification may be the best classification system as far as predictive power and representation of current practice in the setting of acute diverticulitis and is also reasonable to use. For chronic diverticulitis, the Kruis classification nicely summarizes the various phenotypes. However, given the lack of recognition of this classification system, it is likely more beneficial for a clinician to describe the phenotype of chronic disease rather than the Kruis classification.

Conclusion

In clinical practice, the actual classification system used is likely not as important as understanding the key decision points that are common in almost all the various classification systems and relate directly to clinical outcomes and management decisions (Fig. 6.3). We therefore suggest that the clinician encountering patients with this disease first determine if they are dealing with an acute or chronic episode of diverticulitis. If acute, they should determine if it is complicated (i.e., abscess, free perforation, or fistula) or uncomplicated (i.e., pericolonic inflammation or phlegmon). If complicated, they should determine if there is an abscess that may require percutaneous drainage or antibiotics versus a free perforation with peritonitis that will require urgent surgery. If chronic, it is

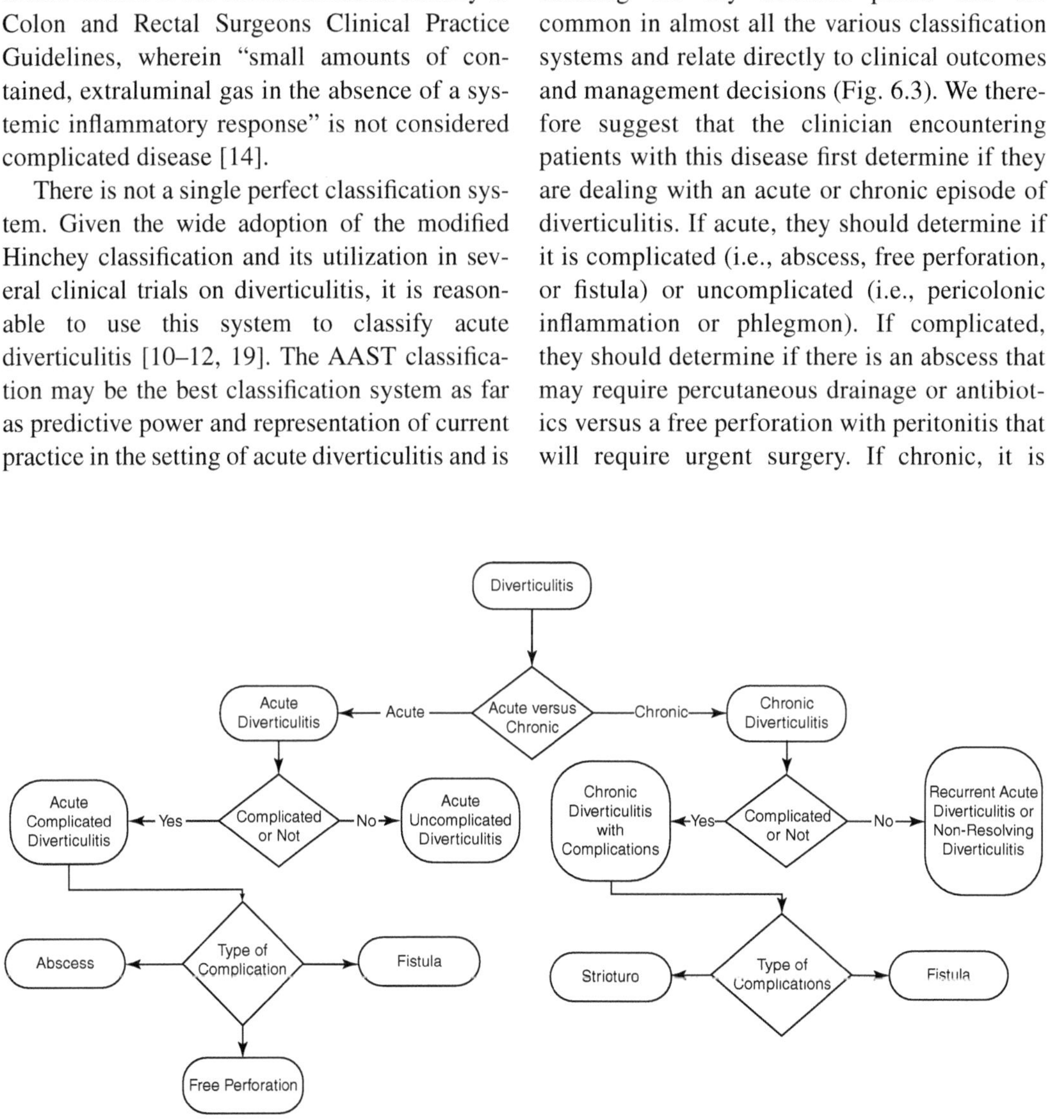

Fig. 6.3 Flowchart demonstrating a simplified workflow to characterize diverticulitis

important to determine the time course (persistent and unresolving versus individual recurrent attacks over a long timeframe) and if there are any complications of this chronic inflammatory process (fistula or obstruction). Separating patients into these simple categories should allow clinicians to follow appropriate therapeutic pathways to most efficaciously manage patients with this challenging disease.

References

1. Hughes ES, Cuthbertson AM, Carden AB. The surgical management of acute diverticulitis. Med J Aust. 1963;50(1):780–782.
2. Hinchey EJ, Schaal PG, Richards GK. Treatment of perforated diverticular disease of the colon. Adv Surg. 1978;12:85–109.
3. Sher ME, et al. Laparoscopic surgery for diverticulitis. Surg Endosc. 1997;11(3):264–7.
4. Constantinides VA, Tekkis PP, Senapati A. Comparison of POSSUM scoring systems and the surgical risk scale in patients undergoing surgery for complicated diverticular disease. Dis Colon Rectum. 2006;49(9):1322–31.
5. Kaiser AM, et al. The management of complicated diverticulitis and the role of computed tomography. Am J Gastroenterol. 2005;100(4):910–7.
6. Sallinen VJ, Leppäniemi AK, Mentula PJ. Staging of acute diverticulitis based on clinical, radiologic, and physiologic parameters. J Trauma Acute Care Surg. 2015 Mar;78(3):543–51. https://doi.org/10.1097/TA.0000000000000540. PMID: 25710425.
7. Antolovic D, et al. Surgical treatment of sigmoid diverticulitis—analysis of predictive risk factors for postoperative infections, surgical complications, and mortality. Int J Color Dis. 2009;24(5):577–84.
8. Vermeulen J, et al. Long-term survival after perforated diverticulitis. Color Dis. 2011;13(2):203–9.
9. Pasternak I, et al. Use of severity classification systems in the surgical decision-making process in emergency laparotomy for perforated diverticulitis. Int J Color Dis. 2010;25(4):463–70.
10. Galbraith N, et al. Laparoscopic lavage in the management of perforated diverticulitis: a contemporary meta-analysis. J Gastrointest Surg. 2017;21(9):1491–9.
11. Kruis W, Germer CT, Böhm S, Dumoulin FL, Frieling T, Hampe J, Keller J, Kreis ME, Meining A, Labenz J, Lock JF, Ritz JP, Schreyer A, Leifeld L; German Society of Gastroenterology, Digestive and Metabolic Diseases (DGVS) and the German Society of General and Visceral Surgery (DGAV) (AWMF-Register 021-20). German guideline diverticular diseaseerticulitis: Part I: Methods, pathogenesis, epidemiology, clinical characteristics (definitions), natural course, diagnosis and classification. United European Gastroenterol J. 2022 Nov;10(9):923–939. https://doi.org/10.1002/ueg2.12309. Epub 2022 Nov 21. PMID: 36411504; PMCID: PMC9731664.
12. Schultz JK, et al. Laparoscopic lavage vs primary resection for acute perforated diverticulitis: the SCANDIV randomized clinical trial. JAMA. 2015;314(13):1364–75.
13. Francis NK, et al. EAES and SAGES 2018 consensus conference on acute diverticulitis management: evidence-based recommendations for clinical practice. Surg Endosc. 2019;33(9):2726–41.
14. Hall J, et al. The American Society of Colon and Rectal Surgeons clinical practice guidelines for the treatment of left-sided colonic diverticulitis. Dis Colon Rectum. 2020;63(6):728–47.
15. Bielecki K, Kaminski P, Klukowski M. Large bowel perforation: morbidity and mortality. Tech Coloproctol. 2002;6(3):177–82.
16. Murphy SF, et al. Predictive factors for colonic resection in patients less than 49 years with symptomatic diverticular disease. Am J Surg. 2016;212(1):47–52.
17. Boostrom SY, Wolff BG, Cima RR, Merchea A, Dozois EJ, Larson DW. Uncomplicated diverticulitis, more complicated than we thought. J Gastrointest Surg. 2012 Sep;16(9):1744–9. https://doi.org/10.1007/s11605-012-1924-4. Epub 2012 Jun 13. PMID: 22696233.
18. Hansen O, Graupe F, Stock W. Prognostic factors in perforating diverticulitis of the large intestine. Chirurg. 1998;69:443–9.
19. Angenete E, et al. Laparoscopic lavage is feasible and safe for the treatment of perforated diverticulitis with purulent peritonitis: the first results from the randomized controlled trial DILALA. Ann Surg. 2016;263(1):117–22.
20. Setti Carraro PG, et al. Predictive value of a pathophysiological score in the surgical treatment of perforated diverticular disease. Chir Ital. 1999;51(1):31–6.
21. van de Wall BJ, et al. Does the presence of abscesses in diverticular disease prelude surgery? J Gastrointest Surg. 2013;17(3):540–7.
22. Gooszen AW, et al. Prospective study of primary anastomosis following sigmoid resection for suspected acute complicated diverticular disease. Br J Surg. 2001;88(5):693–7.
23. Pisanu A, Cois A, Uccheddu A. Surgical treatment of perforated diverticular disease: evaluation of factors predicting prognosis in the elderly. Int Surg. 2004;89(1):35–8.
24. Pisanu A, et al. Factors predicting in-hospital mortality of patients with diffuse peritonitis from perforated colonic diverticulitis. Ann Ital Chir. 2012;83(4):319–24.

25. Thaler K, et al. Utility of appropriate peritonitis grading in the surgical management of perforated sigmoid diverticulitis. Color Dis. 2000;2(6):359–63.
26. Wysocki A, Poźniczek M, Zub A. Selected prognostic factors in perforated left colon diverticula. Pol Przegl Chir. 2005;77(2):121–31.
27. Shafi S, et al. Multicenter validation of American Association for the Surgery of Trauma grading system for acute colonic diverticulitis and its use for emergency general surgery quality improvement program. J Trauma Acute Care Surg. 2016;80(3):405–10; discussion 410–1.

Treatment of Uncomplicated Diverticulitis: Separating Myth from Science

7

Sebastiano Biondo and Thomas Golda

Introduction

Acute diverticulitis (AD) is an inflammatory condition affecting colonic diverticula, often associated with pericolonic inflammation [1], and can be categorized into uncomplicated and complicated diverticulitis. Colonic diverticula may occur in all segments of the colon but mostly in the sigmoid colon, with the second most common site in the right colon [2].

As the majority of individuals with diverticulosis remain asymptomatic throughout life, the true incidence and prevalence of diverticular disease of the colon has still not been accurately established. It is widely accepted that the global incidence of both uncomplicated and complicated AD is increasing. However, the natural history of diverticulosis with recurrent episodes, complications, and symptom progression is poorly understood.

In 1975, Parks proposed a rate of symptomatic diverticulitis ranging from 10% to 25% [3] and traditional teaching suggests that approximately 5%–25% of patients with colonic diverticulosis will develop an episode of AD, being 85% of those episodes uncomplicated [4, 5]. Current data from the American Gastroenterology Association (AGA) suggest that 4% of patients with diverticulosis develop diverticulitis and 15% of these will have complicated disease [6]. In the United Kingdom National Health Service acute admissions with diverticulitis increased by 16% in males and 12% in females over a 10-year period [7]. In the United States, AD is the third most common inpatient gastrointestinal diagnosis with approximately 300,000 hospitalizations, resulting in 1.5 million days of inpatient care [8, 9]. Additionally, AD is one of the most common gastrointestinal diagnoses in outpatient clinics and emergency departments [10] with 1.5–1.9 million outpatient visits each year [9, 11].

There has been increased interest in treating patients with AD conservatively. Treatment goals in AD include reduction of symptoms and inflammation along with prevention of complications and recurrence [11, 12]. Unfortunately, prevention of AD recurrence remains undefined [13] and even after surgical resection, AD recurrence can occur in 2.6%–10% [11, 14].

Clinicians try to clarify which patient needs to be hospitalized [15] and if antibiotics can be avoided [16]. Moreover, outcomes of recurrent AD are particularly relevant for planning long-term management [17].

S. Biondo (✉) · T. Golda
Colorectal Unit, Bellvitge University Hospital, University of Barcelona, Barcelona, Spain
e-mail: sbiondo@ub.edu; tgolda@bellvitgehospital.cat

M. Boutros et al. (eds.), *Diverticulitis*, https://doi.org/10.1007/978-3-032-21720-2_7

Focused on uncomplicated diverticulitis, this chapter summarizes the existing evidence and characteristics defining an acute uncomplicated episode of diverticulitis. This chapter discusses controversies and different options in the medical management of uncomplicated diverticulitis considering hospital admission vs. outpatient treatment, the need for antibiotic therapy and dietary restrictions. The debate on colonoscopic follow-up after an episode of uncomplicated diverticulitis and signs leading to a repetition of cross-sectional imaging is reviewed. This chapter summarizes findings and ambiguities on recurrence after an uncomplicated episode of diverticulitis and the risk factors for recurrence.

Definition of Acute Uncomplicated Diverticulitis

The term diverticulitis describes a peridiverticular inflammation of the bowel wall and in most cases the surrounding tissue. The pathophysiologic mechanism underlying diverticulitis is not well understood. The long-held statement that diverticulitis is caused by microperforation or translocation of intestinal bacteria through the mucosa of the diverticulum on the basis of a weak barrier resulting in colonic wall inflammation and bacterial infection has been challenged by the concept that diverticulitis may be a primary inflammatory process [11, 18] and the true etiology is unclear [19].

In general, uncomplicated (simple) acute diverticulitis is differentiated from complicated acute diverticulitis. Acute uncomplicated diverticulitis is defined as inflammation in a diverticula-bearing bowel segment and the surrounding tissue without signs of perforation (extraluminal air) or abscess formation [20]. Typical complications of acute diverticulitis occur if the inflammatory process extends beyond the colonic wall. However, peridiverticulitis alone is not considered complicated disease [21].

Uncomplicated diverticulitis does not include the clinical findings of free perforation with systemic inflammatory response, fistula, abscess, stricture, or obstruction, as all of these findings define complicated diverticulitis [22]. Nevertheless, as stated in the most recent guidelines of the European Society of Coloproctology, the cut-off between uncomplicated and complicated acute diverticulitis is poorly defined and depends on the degree of inflammation [20]. In the same manner, the most recent guidelines of the American Society of Colon and Rectal Surgeons (ASCRS) state that microperforation with small amounts of contained, extraluminal gas, in the absence of a systemic inflammatory response, is not necessarily considered complicated diverticulitis [23].

This classification does not predict severity or the need for surgery. Uncomplicated (simple) diverticulitis does not necessarily mean that surgical intervention will not be indicated (e.g., a microperforation in an immunosuppressed patient may extend to a diffuse peritonitis), and complicated diverticulitis may not require surgery as antibiotic treatment may be sufficient for a small abscess without the necessity of radiological drainage.

If an AD does not resolve completely, chronic diverticulitis can emerge, defined as wall thickening or chronic mucosal inflammation in the absence of stenosis. Diverticulitis is typically associated with symptoms and signs of peridiverticular inflammation characterized by clinical, radiological, and laboratory findings. These findings led to the development of various classifications differentiating between uncomplicated and complicated as well as acute and chronic diverticulitis. Traditionally, most used is the Hinchey classification, originally developed to classify intraoperative findings in patients with perforated diverticulitis including only patients with abscess or free perforation (See Chap. 6) [20, 21, 24–26].

Treatment of Acute Uncomplicated Diverticulitis

Antibiotics

Before effective broad-spectrum antibiotics were available, diverticulitis was a severe disease associated with high morbidity and mortality [27]. However, with modern antibiotic therapy, most cases of AD resolve with medical treatment [4]. In recent years, the traditional treatment paradigm of AD including antibiotics and hospital admission has been questioned. Few studies have evaluated the use, dosage, and administration of antibiotics in patients with uncomplicated AD, and this practice is based largely on expert opinion. Several prospective randomized and open-label trials have found no benefit of intravenous versus oral antibiotics in this setting [28, 29]. Likewise, a short 4-day course may be equivalent to a 7-day course [30, 31]. Trials comparing specific antibiotics for the treatment of diverticulitis are limited. In general, broad-spectrum antibiotics with gram-negative and anaerobic coverage are prescribed. Commonly used antibiotics for stable patients include the combination of a fluoroquinolone or trimethoprim-sulfamethoxazole with metronidazole, or amoxicillin plus clavulanic acid or moxifloxacin as single agents or a short-course therapy with ertapenem [30]. The combination of ciprofloxacin and metronidazole is probably the most prescribed oral treatment [32].

Until 2010, antibiotics were considered mandatory in the treatment of AD. This practice was based on the theory that diverticulitis resulted due to obstruction of a diverticulum leading to mucosal abrasions, microperforation and bacterial translocation [1]. However, this concept has been largely questioned, as some authors have suggested that AD may be primarily an inflammatory disease, with increased expression of proinflammatory mediators [33, 34] rather than infectious [35]. Conversely, there is increasing concern regarding antibiotic resistance and antibiotic-related complications, namely, *Clostridium difficile* colitis, both of which have further fueled an interest in non-antibiotic therapy for uncomplicated AD [34].

Two recent prospective randomized controlled trials (RCTs) [27, 36], retrospective studies [37], and systematic reviews with more than 2000 patients [38–43] have shown no benefit for the routine use of antibiotics in the treatment of uncomplicated AD, suggesting that its use should be reserved for the treatment of complicated disease or in selected cases of uncomplicated AD. In addition, a systematic review found that antibiotics may be indicated in patients with comorbidities [44].

The first RCT (AVOD) included 623 patients with computed tomography (CT)-proven uncomplicated AD, and compared antibiotic treatment [at least a 7-day course of intravenous (IV)/oral] with antibiotic treatment (IV fluids only). This study concluded that antibiotic treatment neither accelerated recovery nor reduced complications [36]. Ten patients (3.2%) allocated to the nonantibiotic arm required antibiotic treatment because of increasing C-reactive protein levels, fever, or abdominal pain. After a long-term follow-up (median 11 years), the authors found no significant differences between the two groups in terms of recurrences (both 31.3%), complications, surgery for diverticulitis, or reported quality of life [45].

One recent multicenter RCT (the Diverticulitis Antibiotics or close Observation trial; DIABOLO) that included 528 patients compared observation without antibiotics versus antibiotic treatment (IV for at least 48 h and then orally) for a first episode of AD (Hinchey 1a–b [abscess size up to 5 cm]) [27]. No significant differences were found in the median time to recovery [14 days (6–35 days) vs. 12 days (7–30 days), $p = 0.151$], complicated diverticulitis ($p = 0.377$), recurrent diverticulitis ($p = 0.494$), sigmoid resection ($p = 0.323$), readmission ($p = 0.148$), or adverse events ($p = 0.221$). However, the antibiotic group had a higher rate of antibiotic-related adverse events (0.4% versus 8.3%; $p = 0.006$) and mortality ($p = 0.432$). The long-term outcomes of the DIABOLO trial after a 2-year follow-up were recently published, and reported no differences in disease recurrence, complicated diverticulitis, or sigmoid resections [46]. A more recent RCT, the DINAMO study published in 2021 [47], included 480 patients who were randomly assigned to nonantibiotics group ($n = 242$) or antibiotic group ($n = 238$). Hospitalization rates were 14/238 (5.8%) in the antibiotics group and 8/242 (3.3%) in the nonantibiotics group [mean difference 2.58%, 95% confidence interval (CI)

6.32 to −1.17], confirming noninferiority margin. Revisits were 16/238 (6.7%) in the antibiotics group and 17/242 (7%) in the nonantibiotics group (mean difference −0.3, 95% CI 4.22 to −4.83). Poor pain control at 2 days follow-up was 13/230 (5.7%) int the antibiotics group and 5/221 (2.3%) (mean difference 3.39, 95% CI 6.96 to −0.18) in the antibiotics group. The authors concluded that non-antibiotic outpatient treatment of mild AD is safe and effective and is not inferior to current standard treatment.

A Cochrane review on antibiotic use has also found that the best available data do not support use of antibiotics in uncomplicated AD [48] and a meta-analysis found that antibiotic use increases the length of hospital stay but is not associated with a reduction in overall or individual complication rates [39].

Several studies indicate that C-reactive protein (CRP) levels are correlated to the severity of disease and recurrence rates; certain discrimination between the stages of the disease seems difficult [49, 50]. One retrospective study showed high CRP levels (>170 mg/L) at admission as a predictive factor for the failure risk of nonantibiotic treatment in patients with Hinchey Ia diverticulitis [51].

The most recent Clinical Practice Guidelines for the Treatment of Left-Sided Colonic diverticulitis of the ASCRS state that selected otherwise healthy patients with uncomplicated diverticulitis can be safely treated without antibiotics. The use of antibiotics continues to be appropriate for higher-risk patients with significant comorbidities, signs of systemic infection, or immunosuppression [23].

The recently published guidelines of the European Society of Coloproctology state with high level of evidence that patients with acute uncomplicated diverticulitis do not routinely require antibiotics. Antibiotic treatment should be reserved for immunocompromised patients and those with sepsis. These guidelines state that patients with radiological signs of complicated diverticulitis should normally be treated with antibiotics [20].

The recent European Association for Endoscopic Surgery (EAES) and the Society of American Gastrointestinal and Endoscopic Surgeons (SAGES) consensus conference of 2018 state that a trial of nonantibiotic therapy can be considered with appropriate follow-up in selected immunocompetent individuals presenting with uncomplicated acute diverticulitis. Members voting, however, did not reach consensus on this recommendation nor its likelihood to change practice [52].

The AGA guidelines from 2015 recommend that antibiotics should be used selectively [6]. A more updated guideline was published in 2021 [53]. Antibiotics may decrease the risk of recurrence and diverticular complications in comparison with no antibiotics. The effect of antibiotics on the development of sepsis and the need for surgery or colostomy is uncertain [54].

The recently updated guidelines of the World Society of Emergency Surgery (WSES) recommend not prescribing antibiotic therapy in immunocompetent patients [55].

In summary, the existing data [38, 56] have demonstrated that antibiotic treatment for AD (modified Hinchey stage Ia and Ib) neither accelerates recovery nor prevents complications. Thus, antibiotics should be reserved for the treatment of complicated diverticulitis, uncomplicated diverticulitis in the presence of significant comorbidities or immunosuppression, and diverticulitis in the presence of sepsis.

Admission

The treatment of uncomplicated AD has notably evolved since the initial report of the practice parameters of the ASCRS in 1995 with IV antibiotics, IV fluids, and bowel rest [57]. Nevertheless, three aspects are critical for an adequate outpatient or inpatient management of an episode of uncomplicated AD: precise diagnosis, tolerance of oral medication, and clinical assessment of the patient [23].

Computed tomography, introduced over the past decade as a standard diagnostic tool in AD, now precisely and reliably distinguishes complicated AD (with perforation, abscess or phlegmon) from uncomplicated AD [58]. This has changed the thinking about the fear of missing an alternative pathology or difficulty in establishing a diagnosis, but also the management of uncomplicated AD [4]. The diagnosis of uncomplicated AD by CT is now standard and the modified Hinchey classification by Wasvary (Hinchey I divided into Ia when inflammation is restricted to a pericolic phlegmon and Ib when a pericolic abscess is identified) [21] has been used in several multicenter studies including the DIABOLO trial [27] and the AVOD trial [36]. The most recent Guidelines for the Treatment of Left-Sided Colonic diverticulitis of the ASCRS state that CT, even without IV, oral, and endoluminal contrast is highly sensitive and specific and therefore the exploration of choice to confirm the suspicion of AD [23]. Secondly, established guidelines advocating antibiotics were questioned for uncomplicated AD, as discussed earlier, in the same way that hospitalization for uncomplicated AD in selected patients was challenged [28, 29].

Generally, clinical improvement in patients affected by uncomplicated AD is observed within 3–4 days. In hospitalized patients, following the change from IV to oral treatment and discharge, a 7–10 day course of oral antibiotics is usually completed [59–61]. However, various studies have questioned this standard of hospitalization.

A recent meta-analysis identified 19 studies investigating outpatient treatment versus hospitalization for uncomplicated diverticulitis of the left colon [15]. These studies requested CT-confirmed diagnosis of AD, and only one study asked for a CT or ultrasound [62]. Of these 19 studies including 2303 ambulatory-treated patients, there is one randomized multicenter study (the DIVER trial) [63]. A more recent meta-analysis included 21 studies and 1781 patients who had outpatient management of AD including (11 prospective, 9 retrospective and only 1 randomized trial). The authors showed that outpatient management is safe, and the overall failure rate in an outpatient setting was 4.3% (95% CI 2.6%–6.3%). In patients who failed outpatient treatment, the majority had prolonged antibiotic therapy and only few had percutaneous drainage for an abscess (0.13%) or surgical intervention for perforation (0.06%). However, the authors cautioned that the results should be interpreted with some caution because of the low quality of available data [64].

Several international guidelines and various meta-analysis emphasize that ambulatory treatment is only applicable in patients who tolerate oral diet, have an adequate social network, and do not suffer from associated severe comorbidities or immunosuppression [62, 65]. All these criteria ensure that the patient is able to fulfill the prescribed oral antibiotic treatment, understands the situation and warning signs, does not suffer an increased vulnerability to infectious complications, and knows when to ask for help in case of being unable to fend for oneself. Various studies did not exclude patients fulfilling the aforementioned criteria, but used these as a reference group accepting a high risk of selection bias [66–72].

In the DIVER trial, the treatment in both management groups failed in a total of 7 of 132 patients. Of these, 4 patients (6.1%) from the hospitalization group and 3 patients (4.5%) from the outpatient group required re-admittance to the hospital. No differences were found between both groups with respect to the primary objective, readmission to hospital ($p = 0.619$). Reported readmission rates from all other studies ranged between 0% and 14.3% for patients with outpatient treatment. In comparison, the incidence of readmission for the hospitalized group ranged from 0% to 33% [63].

The aforementioned meta-analysis performed a pooled analysis of the incidence of readmission on all 2303 outpatient treatments, finding a readmission rate of 7% (95% CI 6%–9%). After outpatient treatment, the rate of re-admission and drainage of a diverticular abscess was 0.2% (2 of 1082 patients) and the rate of urgent surgery was 0.2% (2 of 1288 patients) [15]. In the DIVER study, no percutaneous drainage or urgent surgery was necessary. There was no related mortality within 60 days of the diagnosis.

Readmission was necessary in the majority of cases for persisting abdominal pain or vomiting and, thus, inability to take oral medication. Several systematic reviews show that even if readmission is needed for parenteral treatment or pain control, the risk that the clinical picture has worsened and requires aggressive measures is low [73, 74]. These findings demonstrate the safety of outpatient treatment for a selected group of patients with uncomplicated AD.

Clinical control in the outpatients´ management varies essentially between the different studies from one visit in outpatient clinics 4–7 days after diagnosis [75] or a daily visit at home by a medical team or an outpatient-hospitalization of sorts, including parenteral antibiotic treatment at home [71]. The daily follow-up telephone call within the DIVER trial to control temperature, general conditions, pain, and to adjust diet and painkillers was abandoned in the routine practice after completion of the DIVER study. There is just one appointment in the outpatients´ clinic scheduled at 10–15 days after diagnosis. Nevertheless, the threshold to repeat the diagnostic workup with clinical exploration, blood analysis, and CT scan should be low for the patient re-presenting in the Emergency Department with worsening of the clinical condition or increase of pain. However, there are no studies or recommendations on the diagnostic workup if treatment failure is suspected. A great number of studies have assessed the risk of treatment failure for complicated diverticulitis with abscesses, but not for uncomplicated diverticulitis.

The DIVER trial also assessed the quality of life at day 14 and day 60 after diagnosis. We observed an improvement in the quality of life without differences between the hospitalized and ambulatory patients [63].

Finally, it has been shown that outpatient treatment significantly reduces the costs of treating uncomplicated AD. Five studies refer to the costs of the two treatments [63, 66, 69, 76, 77]. The cost reduction of ambulatory treatment ranges between 42% and 82%. In the DIVER trial, the costs were three times lower for ambulatory treatment versus hospitalization (with an average hospital stay of 3 days) with a savings of €1124.70 for each patient treated on an outpatient basis.

All guidelines and consensus conferences on diverticulitis of the main national and international associations of colorectal surgery and gastroenterology published in the last 5 years recommend outpatient treatment for uncomplicated diverticulitis in selected patients [20].

The recently published guidelines of the Japan Gastroenterological Association [78] and the Clinical Practice Guidelines of the ASCRS do not even dedicate a individual paragraph to the outpatient treatment of uncomplicated diverticulitis, but the ASCRS goes even further with the statement that, "antibiotic treatment alone for abscesses smaller than 3cm is typically successful and, in stable patients, treatment can usually be administered in the outpatient setting" [23]. This acceptance of ambulatory treatment in uncomplicated diverticulitis is reflected in a decline in hospital admissions from 58.0% in 2006 to 47.1% in 2013 in the US, although diverticulitis-related emergency department visits rose from 89.8 to 113.9 visits per 100,000 population between 2006 and 2013 [79].

Diet

Upon diagnosis of acute, uncomplicated diverticulitis, short-term food deprivation or low dietary fiber intake for bowel rest is traditionally used in clinical practice as it is thought that a less active bowel reduces colonic irritation and re-inflammation [80]. This low-residue diet regimen is usually administered in the inpatient setting but may also be provided as outpatient care. Although there is a lack of studies supporting that bowel rest is required for resolution of an acute episode in uncomplicated cases, traditional practice and some guidelines advise a low fiber diet [61, 81, 82]. However, the Dutch guideline of 2012 abandoned this advice [83].

Evidence, however, is scarce with a lack of high-quality interventional research and risk of bias [84], demonstrated that a liberalized diet in uncomplicated diverticulitis shortens the time of hospitalization but equal to a restricted diet for the outcomes of recovery, gastrointestinal symptoms, and complications; moreover, a liberalized diet tends to have lower health care use and costs. A prospective study found a complication rate of 8.1% leaving patients with an unrestrictive diet in a first episode of acute uncomplicated diverticulitis [85], which is similar to literature data on restrictive diets [15, 86]. These data were confirmed in a retrospective study and an RCT, showing no differences in complications but a shorter hospital stay in the groups of less restricted diets [29, 87]. Moreover, there are data suggesting that bowel rest in acute diseases of the colon is ineffective in reducing inflammation, risk of infection, and other complications [88].

Based on the aforementioned studies and a systematic literature review, a liberalized diet is recommended for patients with uncomplicated diverticulitis (i.e., allowing consumption of solid food). There seems to be no evident difference between liberalized and restricted diets for treatment failures, recurrence or patient symptoms; conversely, liberalized diets may decrease length of hospital stay and prevent restriction of essential nutrient intake [84].

As with outpatient treatment of uncomplicated AD, the majority of patients would probably prefer food autonomy, having a low risk of harm and likely benefits to patients and the health care system.

Interval Colonoscopy

The majority of the previous guidelines recommended routine colonoscopy some weeks after an episode of acute diverticulitis [89]. The rationale was that early detection of colorectal cancer in misdiagnosed patients with bleeding, changed bowel habits, or ongoing pain, could reduce the chance of dissemination.

The AVOD trial, which evaluated the use of antibiotics in the treatment of uncomplicated diverticulitis, reported a 0% detection rate for cancer among 545 patients who received a follow-up colonoscopy 6–8 weeks after their disease presentation [36]. Beyond that, there are no RCTs to investigate the usefulness of an interval colonoscopy (by comparing cancer-specific survival). Various retrospective studies have investigated detection rates for colorectal cancer with colonoscopy after acute diverticulitis. Conducting meta-analysis has been difficult due to inconsistent definitions of uncomplicated and complicated diverticulitis, missing CT verification of diverticulitis, heterogeneity of the studies, lack of a valid reference population, and most importantly missing information about ongoing symptoms in the included patients [90, 91]. However, various systematic reviews report a pooled estimate for cancer detection among patients with uncomplicated diverticulitis of 0.5% (95% CI 0.2%–1.2%) [82] to 1.5% (95% CI 1.0%–2.3%) [91, 92] and for nonmalignant polyps a pooled estimate of 16.5% (95% CI, 11.2%–23.8%) [90]. A more recent meta-analysis found a higher cancer rate of 2% [93]. These findings are comparable to a cancer rate of 0.78% among 68,324 asymptomatic patients undergoing screening colonoscopy and 19% (15%–23%) for nonmalignant colorectal polyps, respectively [93, 94]. Comparing these data suggests that the risk of colorectal malignancy after an episode of CT-proven acute uncomplicated diverticulitis is not significantly different from that of the general asymptomatic population. Patients with uncomplicated diverticulitis have a low risk of malignancy and can be prioritized similarly to the asymptomatic population. In comparison, patients with a CT-proven complicated diverticulitis have a pooled estimate of 10.8% (95% CI, 5.2%–21.0%) of cancer detection [90]. Therefore, routine colonoscopy in conservatively treated complicated diverticulitis is generally accepted [92–94].

There is discrepancy between the different guidelines about colonoscopic follow-up after an episode of CT-proven acute uncomplicated diverticulitis. All guidelines comment on the low-mid quality evidence. A majority of national guidelines recommended routine colonoscopy after an episode of acute diverticulitis to rule out malignancy [89]. Two guidelines, the Dutch [83] and WSES [94, 95], recommend not performing routine colonoscopy after an episode of acute uncomplicated diverticulitis. The recent guidelines of the European Society of Coloproctology state that endoscopic follow-up after a single episode of CT-verified uncomplicated diverticulitis remains controversial and may be unnecessary [20]. The most recent Clinical Practice Guidelines of the ASCRS give only a strong recommendation for a follow-up colonoscopy after an episode of complicated diverticulitis, but only comment that patients may not require further colonoscopic workup beyond the cancer-screening colonoscopy after an episode of uncomplicated acute diverticulitis [23].

Data relative to the time point of follow-up colonoscopy are relatively scarce. The ASCRS and the American College of Gastroenterology guidelines recommend follow-up colonoscopy at 4–6 weeks after resolution of the acute attack [96]. Lahat et al. [97] showed in a single-center trial that 17% of 23 patients with persistent symptoms of AD (more than 1 week during standard treatment or recurrence within 2 months) benefited from early colonoscopic workup, as colonoscopy revealed a different underlying disease. None of the 201 patients with a regular nonpersisting course demonstrated any benefit of an early colonoscopy, keeping in mind the potential risk of converting a sealed into a free perforation during colonoscopy.

Recurrence After Episode of Acute Uncomplicated Diverticulitis

More than 40 years ago, Parks et al. [3] studied the natural course of diverticular disease and reported a 26% recurrence rate for conservatively treated AD with 46% occurring in the first year after the initial attack. Resection after two or more episodes of uncomplicated AD was advised [98]. At present, recurrence is not uniformly defined, not clearly separated from persistent diverticulitis, and may include treatment failure [99]. A diagnosis of recurrent AD most commonly should imply that the patient has completely recovered from the first episode. Recurrent episodes of AD are most consistently defined by an interval of 12 weeks, as in the recently published DIRECT trial, without symptoms between the two attacks and with CT confirmation [100]. In series without CT scan confirmation, recurrence rates range from 13% to 47%, depending on the definition [101–103]. Furthermore, the distinction between recurrent diverticulitis and persistent symptoms (smoldering diverticulitis) or treatment failure varies substantially among studies [104]. The current belief is that AD recurrence is relatively infrequent, and recurrent disease is rarely severe [105, 106].

The results of different studies confirm that a nonsurgical strategy for the treatment of uncomplicated AD is safe in the long term. They also contradict the former opinion that diverticulitis is a progressive disease [100, 107].

A recent large cohort study based on 65,162 patients, the largest to date, has defined the admission rate for recurrent AD in England. The risk of admission for recurrent AD was 11.5% over a minimum follow-up period of 4 years [108]. A similar retrospective cohort study from Canada involving 14,124 patients with a 5-year follow-up demonstrated an admission rate for recurrent AD of 9.0% with a low overall risk of emergency surgery of less than 2% [109]. Our own follow-up study analyzing 560 patients in a single institution at the University Hospital Bellvitge revealed an overall recurrence of 14.8% over 5 years with a severe recurrence rate of 3.4% [110]. A study from Kaiser Permanente that included 2366 hospitalized patients with AD and treated nonoperatively with nearly 9 years of follow-up reported recurrence in 13.3% of patients, and only 3.9% had a second recurrence. No patient with a second recurrence required surgical intervention, and repeated recurrences plateaued after 4 episodes. The authors observed that, although the risk for a second recurrence increased to 29% among those with a first recurrence, the overall recurrence rate was low and therefore does not warrant elective colectomy [103].

A recent review on AD and recurrence included 396,676 patients in 35 studies (only two randomized trials) and found an overall recurrence rate of 12.7% (range 1.6%–60.5%) at a median follow-up of 50 months [104].

After an episode of uncomplicated AD, the recurrence rate is even lower, and recurrences carry a very low rate of peritonitis requiring emergency surgery. Therefore, the available data do not support any more routine policy of sigmoidectomy as a prophylactic procedure to prevent further complications [111]. In addition, an important aspect to take into consideration is the risk of complications after sigmoidectomy for uncomplicated diverticulitis. It is probably equal or outweighs the risk of developing a complication related to the disease itself. Moreover, surgery does not completely protect against recurrence [105].

Decisions regarding elective surgery for recurrent AD should therefore be made on an individual basis and in consultation with the patient to prevent the morbidity and mortality associated with future attacks and emergency surgery, balanced against the risks of elective resection. Per the ASCRS guidelines, surgery for recurrent diverticulitis may be indicated when carcinoma cannot be excluded, quality of life is impacted, patients are immunosuppressed, have collagen-vascular diseases, or chronic renal failure.

Risk Factors for Recurrence After Treatment of Acute Diverticulitis

There are a large variety of risk factors for recurrence. Various factors influencing the probability and rate of recurrent episodes of AD were studied in a recent detailed review [105]. Factors studied included patient-level factors (gender, age, body mass index/obesity, ethnic origin, family history, ASA status, smoking, immunosuppression), disease-level factors (previous recurrences, abscess formation and free air, Hinchey stage, inflammatory extension), and treatment-level factors (duration and route of antibiotics, inpatient versus outpatient management). Table 7.1 reports the relationship of potential factors of AD recurrence.

Gender

Thirteen retrospective studies including 438,903 individuals analyzed the impact of gender on the recurrence of AD [104, 108]. Four studies presented a slightly increased risk in females and one study presented a protective tendency in males [112]. Nine studies showed no effect of gender on the risk of recurrence [103, 104, 113, 114]. In summary, female gender appears to be associated with recurrence, although the strength of association is poorly understood.

Table 7.1 Relationship of potential factors of acute diverticulitis recurrence

variables	
Gender	Relates likely to recurrence
Age	No stringent likelihood of young age to recurrent AD
Body mass index/obesity	Inconclusive results
Ethnic origin	Inconclusive results
Family history genetic predisposition	Genetic influence on recurrence
ASA score	Inconclusive results
Smoking	Inconclusive results
Immunosuppression	Opposite results do not support prophylactic surgery
Short/ long IV antibiotics	No difference on recurrence
Abscess formation	Recurrence more likely after diverticular abscess ≥1 abscess relates to recurrence Free air relates to recurrence Inconclusive data on abscess drainage and recurrence
Severity of index episode	After severe index episode recurrence not very likely Severe recurrence typical after severe first episode
Inflammatory extension	Inflammation >5 cm relates likely to recurrence
Outpatient treatment/ hospitalization	No correlation to recurrence
Number of recurrences	First episode is mostly the worst. Recurrence increases with episodes
Time to recurrence	Recurrence typically within first year

AD acute diverticulitis, *ASA* American Society of Anesthesiologists, *IV* intravenous

Age

The concept that younger patients with diverticulitis following a more severe course requiring surgery at an earlier stage [114] has been very controversial in recent years [115, 116]. Twenty-three studies including 452,085 patients investigated the association of age and recurrence. Two were prospective studies, one study contained both prospective and retrospective data, and 19 were retrospective studies [104, 108].

One prospective cohort study [107] and our own prospective single-center cohort study [115] found no significant influence of age on recurrence (age ≤45 years: 24%; age 45–70 years: 17%; age >70: 20%). Similarly, the distribution of complicated recurrences was similar among the different age groups. A study on retrospectively and prospectively collected data found an association of age younger than 40 years with a higher risk of recurrence on multivariate analysis [117].

Among the retrospective studies, 11 had results indicating a relationship between age and recurrence risk. Age younger than 50 years has been shown to be significantly associated with increased recurrence risk [104, 108]. However, there was no effect of age on the recurrence risk in the additional nine included studies [102, 110, 114, 118–121].

In another recent meta-analysis of 23,078 patients from eight studies, patients under the age of 50 years were more likely to have a recurrent attack [114]. However, the recurrence rates were highly variable (13.3%–36%) depending on the population under study and the length of follow-up. Additionally, all studies focused primarily on recurrences diagnosed and managed in a hospital setting, whereas there are no estimates of recurrent diverticulitis managed in the primary care setting [122].

In the past, sigmoidectomy was advocated in young patients (younger than 50 years at the first episode) [118]. However, younger patients seem to have a similar absolute risk of recurrence, albeit a higher lifetime risk [123, 124]. Younger patients may also be more willing to undergo surgery due to the lower relative surgical risk and their longer life expectancy with consequent increased potential for future episodes. However, most studies have not documented a greater likelihood of perforation or increased morbidity among young patients who develop recurrent disease. Considering all the existing data, there is no evidence that younger patients should be treated differently from older patients [35, 101, 115, 121, 124].

Overall, many of the retrospective studies lack an imaging-proven diagnosis, thereby possibly causing confusion with different diseases with comparable symptoms such as irritable bowel syndrome, inflammatory bowel disease, symptomatic uncomplicated diverticular disease, and constipation. Another confounding variable seems to be the huge variability in the duration of follow-up [125].

In our own retrospective study on age and recurrence of AD with 507 patients susceptible for recurrence, we analyzed three different age groups: Group 1: age 45 years or younger, Group 2: 45–70 years of age, and Group 3: 70 years or more. We did not find any statistical differences in the risk for AD recurrence between the three age groups, a more aggressive course of AD, or worse outcomes after a second episode of AD. The majority of patients did not require an emergency surgery after one or more episodes of AD recurrence [115].

In a more recent own study on 560 patients with a 14.8% recurrence rate within a mean of 6.5 years, multivariate analysis did not show age as a significantly influencing factor on recurrence. In this study, we again found a low risk (0.7%) for an emergency surgery due to recurrence after an uncomplicated first AD episode [110].

In summary, there seems to be no stringent likelihood of young age being associating with recurrent diverticulitis and there are many confounding factors (missing radiological confirmation of recurrent episode of AD, variability of follow-up time). Recent literature no longer supports age as a risk factor for recurrence of AD and this finding is reflected in newer guidelines. The ASCRS and the European Society of Coloproctology stipulate that young age does not increase the rate of recurrence [20, 23].

Body Mass Index/Obesity

Four studies including 66,060 individuals investigated the impact of body mass index (BMI) (≥30) on recurrence [104, 108]. A prospective and a retrospective study found no association between BMI and recurrence. Conversely, two retrospective studies found an increased risk of recurrence in obese patients [107, 126, 127]. Results from the available studies are inconclusive.

Ethnic Origin

Ethnic origin was analyzed in two studies for its influence on diverticulitis recurrence but with conflicting conclusions [104].

Family History

Family history and genetic predisposition of diverticulitis have been investigated in very few studies. One epidemiological study with 672 patients found an influence on recurrence, suggesting a genetic or an environmental component influencing the disease. However, this study did not include the number of patients with a positive family history [12]. A two-center cohort study in Canada that included 433 patients showed a family history with more than one relative diagnosed with diverticulitis with a higher recurrence rate (HR, 2.93; 95% CI, 1.96–4.39) and a higher rate of complicated recurrences (HR, 8.30; 95% CI, 3.64–18.9) [128].

American Society of Anesthesiologists Status

The correlation between the American Society of Gastroenterologists (ASA) score, which can be used as an aggregate marker of comorbidities, and diverticulitis recurrence has shown conflicting results. A higher comorbidity status was associated with increased risk of recurrence in one study but was not significant in another study and was actually associated with lower recurrence risk among certain patient groups. This reduced risk may be caused by early death due to severe comorbidity, decreasing the opportunity for patients to develop a recurrent episode [104, 114]. In summary, the relationship between ASA score and recurrence is unclear.

Smoking

A large English population-based cohort study with 65,162 National Health Service hospital admissions identified smoking as a risk factor for recurrent AD [108]. Two previous studies investigating smoking and diverticular disease are conflicting [129, 130]. These two epidemiological studies, however, were investigating the role of smoking in the development of symptomatic diverticular disease rather than as a risk factor for recurrent AD. In summary, results on smoking habits are conflicting and more data are needed.

Immunosuppression

There are conflicting results for immunosuppression leading to increased recurrence risk.

Immunosuppressed patients, such as those with solid organ transplants, collagen vascular diseases, steroid use, malnutrition, and chronic renal failure, were found to have a five-fold greater risk of complicated recurrence and perforation compared with non-immunosuppressed patients (36% vs. 7%) in one retrospective study [127].

We studied 931 patients with 1204 episodes of colonic diverticulitis over 14 years at our institution and identified 136 patients (14.6%) with a recurrence [131]. Excluding all patients who underwent an operation on, or soon after, the index admission, we analyzed 107 immunocompromised and 550 immunocompetent patients over a mean follow-up of over 6 years. No differences were observed between the two groups for recurrence (21.5% for the immunocompromised group and 20.5% in the immunocompetent group, $p = 0.82$). Immunosuppressed patients with a severe first episode experienced a significantly higher recurrence rate, and more severe recurrences, than their immunocompetent counterparts, but they did not require more emergency surgeries. Additionally, recurrence was more likely to occur in the first 6 months after the first diverticulitis episode in immunosuppressed patients. Among patients who underwent emergency surgery as treatment for the first episode, mortality was more than doubled in immunosuppressed patients: 33.3% vs. 15.9% ($p = 0.004$) [131]. Therefore, immunosuppressed patients seem to present with a more aggressive first episode of diverticulitis, with a higher need for emergency surgery and a higher mortality rate. However, after successful nonoperative management of AD, our data supports that immunosuppressed patients should not be advised to have an elective sigmoidectomy at a greater frequency than the immunocompetent patient.

These data are supported by a recent study on the surgical outcomes from the American College of Surgeons National Surgical Quality Improvement Program (ACS-NSQIP) database that included 4271 immunocompromised patients. This study analyzed the impact of immunosuppression on mortality and major morbidity after elective or emergent colectomy for diverticulitis and showed a higher mortality for emergent colectomy in immunosuppressed patients (16% versus 4%, $p < 0.001$). In the elective setting, there was a comparable mortality between the groups; however, there was an increased risk for major morbidity among immunosuppressed patients (25% versus 12%, $p < 0.001$) [132]. In summary, at present, no strong recommendation for elective surgery is possible in immunocompromised patients as data are inconclusive.

Duration of Intravenous Antibiotics

One study with 50 patients compared a 7-day fixed course of IV antibiotics to a shorter antibiotic course, with therapy only administered up until the patient has improved clinically. This study demonstrated the safety of short-duration IV antibiotics, with additional cost savings in hospitalization of 1244 € per patient [30]. One study compared short (5 days IV and 5 days oral) antibiotic (metronidazole and ceftriaxone) therapy with long therapy (5–10 days IV) after an index episode of Hinchey Ia AD. This study found no difference in recurrence rates; however, the effect was not compared with placebo [133]. Likewise, another study found that a short 4-day course may be equivalent to a 7-day course [30, 31]. In summary, data do not show differences for recurrence after short or long-term antibiotic treatment.

Abscess Formation and Free Air

The impact of a first episode of AD with abscess formation or free air on AD recurrence was reviewed in 15 studies with 433,614 individuals [104, 108], and appears to have a positive association with the likelihood of recurrence. Another recent review with 1051 patients from 22 studies also found an overall elevated recurrence rate of 28% among patients with abscess-complicated AD. The recurrence rate was even higher (39%) among patients awaiting elective surgery compared to patients without planned surgery (18%). Only 28% of this cohort with AD and abscess did not have a recurrence or need for surgery over the follow-up period [134]. A Canadian single-center study confirmed this finding as all of the nine included patients with a complicated recurrence underwent resection [135].

In our own single-center observational study, we found an increased recurrence risk when the index admission presented with more than one abscess (multivariate HR 5.29, 95% CI 2.11–13.3), but no difference in recurrence risk among patients without or with only one abscess [110].

In two studies, an abscess diameter of 5 cm was shown to be related to an increased recurrence risk, but another study could not find an association between abscess size or localization and recurrence on multivariate analysis. However, a significant association was reported between retroperitoneal abscesses at the primary episode (Hinchey II) and recurrence [104].

Among cases of AD that required CT-guided abscess drainage, recurrence rates were variable at between 25.2% and 74% [136–138]. Nevertheless, there are conflicting data on whether percutaneous drainage increases or decreases the risk of AD recurrence [108]. A recent multicenter study from Holland (447 patients with diverticular abscess, 15 of whom were percutaneously drained), did not find a significant difference in recurrence (28.0% for abscess drainage vs. 25.2% without drainage) [136]. However, the decision to undergo percutaneous drainage may be indicative of a larger abscess size, abscess location, patient comorbidity, or severity of disease; as such, this question is highly confounded and would best be answered in an RCT. The recurrence risk significantly increased after perforated diverticulitis with CT-verified free intra-abdominal air (Hinchey III) treated nonsurgically, compared with mild diverticulitis [118]. In summary, there is an association between AD recurrence and the presence of abscess formation on the index episode; however, the impact of abscess drainage is unclear. Abscess characteristics, including number, size and location, may also influence recurrence risk.

The most recent practice parameters of the ASCRS recommend consideration of elective resection after successful nonoperative treatment of a diverticular abscess. Conversely, the recent guidelines of the European Society of Coloproctology state that resection is not routinely recommended [20, 23].

Severity of First Episode of Acute Diverticulitis

A severe first episode of AD seems to correlate with a similar severity at the following episode. Likewise, uncomplicated primary diverticulitis lowers the risk for a secondary complicated episode, and complicated diverticulitis most commonly occurs during the first episode rather than during recurrent episodes [139]. After an episode of uncomplicated AD, the short-term risk of abscess or perforation is very low (2%) [140].

A recent population-based study in England including 3226 complicated AD (2924 without and 302 with drainage) patients and a recent review found that complicated AD (without drainage) was significantly associated with recurrence as high as 25.5% [108, 141]. Conversely, in our own study analyzing 560 patients with a first episode of AD, the recurrence risk after severe diverticulitis (Hinchey Ib-IV) did not differ statistically from that of recurrence after mild diverticulitis. However, within the first year, the rate of severe recurrence after a severe episode of diverticulitis was 9.6%, significantly higher than after uncomplicated AD. Among patients with primary severe AD, 54.5% presented with a severe recurrent episode. After primary mild diverticulitis, 88.5% experienced a similar mild recurrence and only 11.5% suffered a severe recurrence [110]. In summary, most commonly, a severe episode of AD occurs as a first episode, but a severe first episode of AD increases the likelihood of a recurrent severe episode. Uncomplicated primary AD lowers the risk for a recurrent complicated episode.

Inflammatory Extension

Two studies with 943 patients evaluated the impact of inflammatory extension within the colon on AD recurrence [12, 139]. Intestinal inflammation involving more than 5 cm measured by CT scan during the primary episode was associated with an increased risk of recurrence (multivariate HR 1.7, 95% CI 1.3–2.3) [12]. Inflammatory extension in patients with a primary and recurrent diverticulitis did not significantly differ [139]. In summary, an inflamed segment >5 cm may lead to an increased risk of AD recurrence.

Treatment of First Episode of Acute Diverticulitis as Outpatient or Hospitalized

Three studies including 240 patients with outpatient treatment reported a follow-up of approximately 1 year. These studies reported an AD recurrence rate of 13.0% in the outpatient group versus 12.1% in the hospitalization group [75, 141–143]. Recurrence was not analyzed in recent reviews on outpatient treatment. In summary, ambulatory treatment does not influence disease recurrence.

Number of Recurrences

Studies have found that the risk of AD recurrence increases with the number of AD episodes. Large cohort studies have reported a recurrence rate of 8.7%–9.0% after a first episode, 23.2%–36.0% after two episodes, 35.8%–65.4% after three episodes, 41.1% after four episodes, and 45.6% after five episodes [144, 145]. After a first episode of AD, the risk of recurrence is approximately 20% at 10 years. The risk of re-recurrence after the second episode is 55% at 10 years and after the third episode is 40% after 3 years [112]. A multicenter Italian study with a mean follow-up of 10.7 years confirmed that the risk of recurrence was greatest among patients with at least 3 previous episodes [117].

A prospective study on AD recurrence with 150 patients divided into two groups (patients with 1 or 2 previous diverticulitis episodes versus patients with more than 2 previous episodes) found no increase in major complications of diverticulitis at subsequent recurrences after more than 2 episodes [100]. Other studies have shown that complications mostly occur during the primary manifestation of diverticulitis [100, 146, 147]. In summary, patients with recurrent AD are at greater risk of future recurrences but are not at increased risk of developing diverticulitis complications.

Time to Recurrence

Recurrence rates within the first year after a first episode of AD were highest compared to after the first year, and with a frequency of 10.0%–82.0% [106, 108, 120]. Two studies showed a reduction in the proportion of recurrences at 2 years after disease remission. Our own study showed a reduction in the recurrence rate from 66% during the first year to 16% [132], while another study demonstrated a reduction in recurrence from 64% to 36% [118]. In summary, recurrence risk is higher within the first year after remission.

It is important to consider that the recurrence rate for diverticulitis after sigmoid colectomy is not negligible, and ranges from 2.6% to 10.0% [59, 117, 148]. Furthermore, prophylactic colectomy does not always result in symptom improvement, which can sometimes worsen after surgery [149, 150]. Moreover, up to 10.0% of operated patients are at risk of experiencing a major surgical complication [151, 152]. Consequently, various international guidelines have abandoned recommending elective surgery after two episodes of AD [89].

Similarities seem to exist in the pathophysiology between diverticulitis, irritable bowel syndrome, and inflammatory bowel disease [111, 153]. Although the mechanisms of inflammation are unknown, recurrent or smoldering diverticulitis displays histological and chemical similarities (higher levels of histamine, TNF-α and matrix metalloproteinases) [154, 155] to inflammatory bowel disease and irritable bowel syndrome [156]. Persistent low-grade inflammation following an episode of AD, even in the presence of uncomplicated AD, may also explain its recurrence. After a 24-month follow-up period, one study found endoscopic inflammation still detected in 27.6% of patients and active histological inflammation in 36.6%. This was shown to be a predictor of diverticulitis recurrence (p = 0.0004) [156]. Thus, inflammation persistence may play a role as a risk factor for disease recurrence. In addition, uncomplicated diverticulitis may not just be a benign self-limiting disease. Up to 30% of patients without further episodes have ongoing abdominal symptoms ("smouldering" diverticulitis). However, some authors believe that this is a different and not comparable entity [153, 157].

The gravity of inflammation (measured by the CRP level) may be associated with a higher probability of recurrence, as shown in one series [107]. The risk of recurrence at 6 months was 22% for patients with CRP >240 mg/L during their initial episode; thus, the CRP level at primary episode may be a useful predictor for short-term recurrence [107].

Conclusion

Looking to the future, understanding the pathogenic mechanisms for AD development, recurrence and its possible contributions such as mucosal inflammation, alterations of the gut microbiota, or diet and lifestyle factors, remains obscure. Proven explanations for the claimed mechanisms and their respective roles will enable an evidence-based therapeutic approach for patients and disease-severity-adjusted therapy together with primary and secondary prevention of AD.

References

1. Jacobs DO. Diverticulitis. N Engl J Med. 2007;357:2057–66.
2. Golder M, Ster IC, Babu P, Sharma A, Bayat M, Farah A. Demographic determinants of risk, colon distribution and density scores of diverticular disease. World J Gastroenterol. 2011;17(8):1009–17.
3. Parks TG. Natural history of diverticular disease of the colon. Clin Gastroenterol [Internet]. 1975;4(1):53–69. Available from: http://www.ncbi.nlm.nih.gov/pubmed/1109820.
4. Morris AM, Regenbogen SE, Hardiman KM, Hendren S. Sigmoid diverticulitis: a systematic review. JAMA – J Am Med Assoc. 2014;311(3):287–97.
5. Tursi A, Picchio M, Elisei W, Di Mario F, Scarpignato C, Brandimarte G. Management of patients with diverticulosis and diverticular disease: consensus statements from the 2nd international symposium on diverticular disease. J Clin Gastroenterol [Internet]. 2016;50(Suppl 1):S101–7. Available from: http://www.ncbi.nlm.nih.gov/pubmed/27622350.
6. Stollman N, Smalley W, Hirano I, AGA Institute Clinical Guidelines Committee. American Gastroenterological Association Institute guideline on the management of acute diverticulitis. Gastroenterology [Internet]. 2015;149(7):1944–9. Available from: http://www.ncbi.nlm.nih.gov/pubmed/26453777.
7. Kang JY, Hoare J, Tinto A, Subramanian S, Ellis C, Majeed A, et al. Diverticular disease of the colon—on the rise: a study of hospital admissions in England between 1989/1990 and 1999/2000. Aliment Pharmacol Ther [Internet]. 2003;17(9):1189–95. Available from: http://www.ncbi.nlm.nih.gov/pubmed/12752356.
8. Kozak LJ, DeFrances CJ, Hall MJ. National hospital discharge survey: 2004 annual summary with detailed diagnosis and procedure data. Vital Health Stat 13 [Internet]. 2006;(162):1–209. Available from: http://www.ncbi.nlm.nih.gov/pubmed/17091747.
9. Peery AF, Crockett SD, Murphy CC, Jennifer L, Dellon ES, Williams JL, et al. Diseases in the United States: update 2018. Gastroenterology. 2019;156(1):254–72.
10. Peery AF, Dellon ES, Lund J, Crockett SD, McGowan CE, Bulsiewicz WJ, et al. Burden of gastrointestinal disease in the United States: 2012 update. Gastroenterology [Internet]. 2012;143(5):1179–1187.e3. Available from: https://linkinghub.elsevier.com/retrieve/pii/S0016508512011572.
11. Shaheen NJ, Hansen RA, Morgan DR, Gangarosa LM, Ringel Y, Thiny MT, et al. The burden of gastrointestinal and liver diseases, 2006. Am J Gastroenterol [Internet]. 2006;101(9):2128–38. Available from: http://www.ncbi.nlm.nih.gov/pubmed/16848807.
12. Hall JF, Roberts PL, Ricciardi R, Read T, Scheirey C, Wald C, et al. Long-term follow-up after an initial episode of diverticulitis: what are the predictors of recurrence? Dis Colon Rectum [Internet]. 2011;54(3):283–8. Available from: http://www.ncbi.nlm.nih.gov/pubmed/21304297.
13. Nally DM, Kavanagh DO. Current controversies in the management of diverticulitis: a review. Dig Surg [Internet]. 2019;36(3):195–205. Available from: http://www.ncbi.nlm.nih.gov/pubmed/29672283.
14. Thaler K, Baig MK, Berho M, Weiss EG, Nogueras JJ, Arnaud JP, et al. Determinants of recurrence after sigmoid resection for uncomplicated diverticulitis. Dis Colon Rectum [Internet]. 2003;46(3):385–8. Available from: http://www.ncbi.nlm.nih.gov/pubmed/12626916.
15. van Dijk ST, Bos K, de Boer MGJ, Draaisma WA, van Enst WA, Felt RJF, Klarenbeek BR, Otte JA, Puylaert JBCM, van Geloven MAB AAW. A systematic review and meta-analysis of outpatient treatment for acute diverticulitis. Int J Color Dis. 2018;33(5):505–12.

16. Peery AF, Stollman N. Antibiotics for acute uncomplicated diverticulitis: time for a paradigm change? Gastroenterology [Internet]. 2015;149(7):1650–1. Available from: https://doi.org/10.1053/j.gastro.2015.10.022.
17. Biondo S, Lopez Borao J, Millan M, Kreisler E, Jaurrieta E. Current status of the treatment of acute colonic diverticulitis: a systematic review. Colorectal Dis [Internet]. 2012;14(1):e1–11. Available from: http://www.ncbi.nlm.nih.gov/pubmed/21848896.
18. Cuomo R, Cargiolli M, Cassarano S, Carabotti M, Annibale B. Treatment of diverticular disease, targeting symptoms or underlying mechanisms. Curr Opin Pharmacol [Internet]. 2018;43:124–31. Available from: http://www.ncbi.nlm.nih.gov/pubmed/30291995.
19. Strate LL, Morris AM. Epidemiology, pathophysiology, and treatment of diverticulitis. Gastroenterology [Internet]. 2019;156(5):1282–1298.e1. Available from: https://linkinghub.elsevier.com/retrieve/pii/S0016508519300460.
20. Schultz JK, Azhar N, Binda GA, Barbara G, Biondo S, Boermester MA, et al. European Society of Coloproctology: guidelines for the management of diverticular disease of the colon. Colorectal Dis. 2020;22 Suppl 2:5–28.
21. Wasvary H, Turfah F, Kadro O, Beauregard W. Same hospitalization resection for acute diverticulitis. Am Surg. 1999;65:632–6.
22. Hall J, Hammerich K, Roberts P. New paradigms in the management of diverticular disease. Curr Probl Surg. 2010;47(9):680–735.
23. Hall J, Hardiman K, Lee S, Lightner A, Stocchi L, Paquette IM, et al. The American Society of Colon and Rectal Surgeons clinical practice guidelines for the treatment of left-sided colonic diverticulitis. Dis Colon Rectum. 2020;6:728–47.
24. Hinchey EJ, Schaal PG, Richards GK. Treatment of perforated diverticular disease of the colon. [Internet]. Adv Surg. 1978;12:85–109. Available from: http://www.ncbi.nlm.nih.gov/pubmed/735943.
25. Kaiser AM, Jiang JK, Lake JP, Ault G, Artinyan A, Gonzalez-Ruiz C, et al. The management of complicated diverticulitis and the role of computed tomography. Am J Gastroenterol. 2005;100(4):910–7.
26. Bharucha AE, Parthasarathy G, Ditah I, Fletcher JG, Ewelukwa O, Pendlimari R, et al. HHS Public Access. 2016;2015(11):1589–96.
27. Daniels L, Ünlü Ç, de Korte N, van Dieren S, Stockmann HB, Vrouenraets BC, et al. Randomized clinical trial of observational versus antibiotic treatment for a first episode of CT-proven uncomplicated acute diverticulitis. Br J Surg [Internet]. 2017;104(1):52–61. Available from: http://www.ncbi.nlm.nih.gov/pubmed/27686365.
28. Hjern F, Josephson T, Altman D, Holmström B, Mellgren A, Pollack J, et al. Conservative treatment of acute colonic diverticulitis: are antibiotics always mandatory? Scand J Gastroenterol [Internet]. 2007;42(1):41–7. Available from: http://www.ncbi.nlm.nih.gov/pubmed/17190761.
29. Ridgway PF, Latif A, Shabbir J, Ofriokuma F, Hurley MJ, Evoy D, et al. Randomized controlled trial of oral vs intravenous therapy for the clinically diagnosed acute uncomplicated diverticulitis. Colorectal Dis [Internet]. 2009;11(9):941–6. Available from: http://www.ncbi.nlm.nih.gov/pubmed/19016815.
30. Schug-Pass C, Geers P, Hügel O, Lippert H, Köckerling F. Prospective randomized trial comparing short-term antibiotic therapy versus standard therapy for acute uncomplicated sigmoid diverticulitis. Int J Colorectal Dis [Internet]. 2010;25(6):751–9. Available from: http://www.ncbi.nlm.nih.gov/pubmed/20140619.
31. Smolarz CM, Hohertz B, Seupaul RA. Are antibiotics required for the treatment of uncomplicated diverticulitis? Ann Emerg Med [Internet]. 2014;63(1):52–3. Available from: http://www.ncbi.nlm.nih.gov/pubmed/23992942.
32. Scarpignato C, Barbara G, Lanas A, Strate LL. Management of colonic diverticular disease in the third millennium: highlights from a symposium held during the United European Gastroenterology Week 2017. Therap Adv Gastroenterol [Internet]. 2018;11:1756284818771305. Available from: http://www.ncbi.nlm.nih.gov/pubmed/29844795.
33. Tursi A, Elisei W, Brandimarte G, Giorgetti GM, Inchingolo CD, Nenna R, et al. Musosal tumour necrosis factor α in diverticular disease of the colon is overexpressed with disease severity. Colorectal Dis [Internet]. 2012;14(5):e258–63. Available from: http://www.ncbi.nlm.nih.gov/pubmed/22469482.
34. Floch MH. A hypothesis: is diverticulitis a type of inflammatory bowel disease? J Clin Gastroenterol [Internet]. 2006;40(Suppl 3):S121–5. Available from: http://www.ncbi.nlm.nih.gov/pubmed/16885694.
35. Ritz J-P, Lehmann KS, Stroux A, Buhr HJ, Holmer C. Sigmoid diverticulitis in young patients—a more aggressive disease than in older patients? J Gastrointest Surg [Internet]. 2011;15(4):667–74. Available from: http://www.ncbi.nlm.nih.gov/pubmed/21318443.
36. Chabok A, Påhlman L, Hjern F, Haapaniemi S, Smedh K. Randomized clinical trial of antibiotics in acute uncomplicated diverticulitis. Br J Surg. 2012;99(4):532–9.
37. Gaber CE, Kinlaw AC, Edwards JK, Lund JL, Stürmer T, Peacock Hinton S, Pate V, Bartelt LA, Sandler RS, Peery AF. Comparative effectiveness and harms of antibiotics for outpatient diverticulitis: two nationwide cohort studies. Ann Intern Med. 2021;174(6):737–46. https://doi.org/10.7326/M20-6315. Epub 2021 Feb 23. PMID: 33617725; PMCID: PMC9035276.
38. Desai M, Fathallah J, Nutalapati V, Saligram S. Antibiotics versus no antibiotics for acute uncomplicated diverticulitis: a systematic review and meta-analysis. Dis Colon Rectum [Internet]. 2019;62(8):1005–12. Available from: http://www.ncbi.nlm.nih.gov/pubmed/30664553.
39. Mocanu V, Dang JT, Switzer N, Tavakoli I, Tian C, de Gara C, et al. The role of antibiotics in

acute uncomplicated diverticulitis: a systematic review and meta-analysis. Am J Surg [Internet]. 2018;216(3):604–9. Available from: https://doi.org/10.1016/j.amjsurg.2018.01.039.
40. Seta T, Iwagami H, Agatsuma N, Noma A, Ikenouchi M, Kubo K, Akamatsu T, Uenoyama Y, Ito D, Yamashita Y, Nakayama T. Efficacy of antimicrobial therapy in patients with uncomplicated acute colonic diverticulitis: an updated systematic review and meta-analysis. Eur J Gastroenterol Hepatol. 2023;35(10):1097–106. https://doi.org/10.1097/MEG.0000000000002622. Epub 2023 Jul 28. PMID: 37577799.
41. Poh CW, Goh CK, Tan DJH, Chong CS. Antibiotics vs observational therapy in acute uncomplicated diverticulitis, a systemic review and meta-analysis. Int J Color Dis. 2023;38(1):97. https://doi.org/10.1007/s00384-023-04389-7. PMID: 37059809.
42. Correa Bonito A, Cerdán Santacruz C, Di Martino M, Blanco Terés L, Gancedo Quintana Á, Martín-Pérez E, Biondo S, García Septiem J. Treatment for acute uncomplicated diverticulitis without antibiotherapy: systematic review and meta-analysis of randomized clinical trials. Int J Surg. 2023;109(5):1412–9. https://doi.org/10.1097/JS9.0000000000000307. PMID: 37026842; PMCID: PMC10389615.
43. Zhao Y, Gao Y, Chen W, Hao Q, Ho C, Kennedy MK, Guyatt GH. Antibiotics for treatment of mild left-sided acute uncomplicated diverticulitis: meta-analysis of randomized trials. Br J Surg. 2023;110(3):373–4. https://doi.org/10.1093/bjs/znac433. PMID: 36791230.
44. Emile SH, Elfeki H, Sakr A, Shalaby M. Management of acute uncomplicated diverticulitis without antibiotics: a systematic review, meta-analysis, and meta-regression of predictors of treatment failure. Tech Coloproctol. 2018;22(7):499–509. https://doi.org/10.1007/s10151-018-1817-y. Epub 2018 Jul 6. PMID: 29980885.
45. Isacson D, Smedh K, Nikberg M, Chabok A. Long-term follow-up of the AVOD randomized trial of antibiotic avoidance in uncomplicated diverticulitis. Br J Surg. 2019;106(11):1542–8.
46. van Dijk ST, Daniels L, Ünlü Ç, de Korte N, van Dieren S, Stockmann HB, et al. Long-term effects of omitting antibiotics in uncomplicated acute diverticulitis. Am J Gastroenterol [Internet]. 2018;113(7):1045–52. Available from: http://www.ncbi.nlm.nih.gov/pubmed/29700480.
47. Mora-López L, Ruiz-Edo N, Estrada-Ferrer O, Piñana-Campón ML, Labró-Ciurans M, Escuder-Perez J, Sales-Mallafré R, Rebasa-Cladera P, Navarro-Soto S, Serra-Aracil X, DINAMO-Study Group. Efficacy and safety of nonantibiotic outpatient treatment in mild acute diverticulitis (DINAMO-study): a multicentre, randomised, open-label, noninferiority trial. Ann Surg. 2021;274(5):e435–42. https://doi.org/10.1097/SLA.0000000000005031. PMID: 34183510.
48. Shabanzadeh DM, Wille-Jørgensen P. Antibiotics for uncomplicated diverticulitis. Cochrane Database Syst Rev. 2012;11:CD009092.
49. Mäkelä JT, Klintrup K, Takala H, Rautio T. The role of C-reactive protein in prediction of the severity of acute diverticulitis in an emergency unit. Scand J Gastroenterol. 2015;50(5):536–41.
50. Jamal Talabani A, Endreseth BH, Lydersen S, Edna TH. Clinical diagnostic accuracy of acute colonic diverticulitis in patients admitted with acute abdominal pain, a receiver operating characteristic curve analysis. Int J Colorectal Dis [Internet]. 2017;32(1):41–7. Available from: https://doi.org/10.1007/s00384-016-2644-0.
51. Bolkenstein H, Draaisma W, van de Wall B, Consten E, Broeders I. Treatment of acute uncomplicated diverticulitis without antibiotics: risk factors for treatment failure. Int J Color Dis. 2018;33(7):863–9.
52. Francis NK, Sylla P, Abou-Khalil M, Arolfo S, Berler D, Curtis NJ, et al. EAES and SAGES 2018 consensus conference on acute diverticulitis management: evidence-based recommendations for clinical practice. Surg Endosc. 2019;33(9):2726–41.
53. Peery AF, Shaukat A, Strate LL. AGA clinical practice update on medical management of colonic diverticulitis: expert review. Gastroenterology. 2021;160(3):906–911.e1. https://doi.org/10.1053/j.gastro.2020.09.059. Epub 2020 Dec 3. PMID: 33279517; PMCID: PMC7878331.
54. Strate LL, Peery AF, Neumann I. American Gastroenterological Association Institute technical review on the management of acute diverticulitis. Gastroenterology [Internet]. 2015;149(7):1950–76.e12. Available from: https://doi.org/10.1053/j.gastro.2015.10.001.
55. Sartelli M, Weber DG, Kluger Y, Ansaloni L, Coccolini F, Abu-Zidan F, et al. 2020 update of the WSES guidelines for the management of acute colonic diverticulitis in the emergency setting. World J Emerg Surg. 2020;15(1):1–18.
56. van Dijk ST, Chabok A, Dijkgraaf MG, Boermeester MA, Smedh K. Observational versus antibiotic treatment for uncomplicated diverticulitis: an individual-patient data meta-analysis. Br J Surg. 2020;107(8):1062–9.
57. Roberts P, Abel M, Rosen L, Cirocco W, Fleshman J, Leff E, et al. Practice parameters for sigmoid diverticulitis. The Standards Task Force American Society of Colon and Rectal Surgeons. Dis Colon Rectum [Internet]. 1995;38(2):125–32. Available from: http://www.ncbi.nlm.nih.gov/pubmed/7851165.
58. Ambrosetti P, Becker C, Terrier F. Colonic diverticulitis: impact of imaging on surgical management—a prospective study of 542 patients. Eur Radiol [Internet]. 2002;12(5):1145–9. Available from: http://www.ncbi.nlm.nih.gov/pubmed/11976860.
59. Stollman N, Raskin JB. Diverticular disease of the colon. Lancet (London, England) [Internet]. 2004;363(9409):631–9. Available from: http://www.ncbi.nlm.nih.gov/pubmed/14987890.

60. Tursi A. Diverticulosis today: unfashionable and still under-researched. Therap Adv Gastroenterol [Internet]. 2016;9(2):213–28. Available from: http://www.ncbi.nlm.nih.gov/pubmed/26929783.
61. Köhler L, Sauerland S, Neugebauer E. Diagnosis and treatment of diverticular disease: results of a consensus development conference. The Scientific Committee of the European Association for Endoscopic Surgery. Surg Endosc [Internet]. 1999;13(4):430–6. Available from: http://www.ncbi.nlm.nih.gov/pubmed/10094765.
62. Estrada Ferrer O, Ruiz Edo N, Hidalgo Grau L-A, Abadal Prades M, Del Bas Rubia M, Garcia Torralbo EM, et al. Selective non-antibiotic treatment in sigmoid diverticulitis: is it time to change the traditional approach? Tech Coloproctol [Internet]. 2016;20(5):309–15. Available from: http://www.ncbi.nlm.nih.gov/pubmed/27053254.
63. Biondo S, Golda T, Kreisler E, Espin E, Vallribera F, Oteiza F, et al. Outpatient versus hospitalization management for uncomplicated diverticulitis: a prospective, multicenter randomized clinical trial (DIVER Trial). Ann Surg [Internet]. 2014 [cited 2015 May 24];259(1):38–44. Available from: http://www.ncbi.nlm.nih.gov/pubmed/23732265.
64. Cirocchi R, Randolph JJ, Binda GA, Gioia S, Henry BM, Tomaszewski KA, Allegritti M, Arezzo A, Marzaioli R, Ruscelli P. Is the outpatient management of acute diverticulitis safe and effective? A systematic review and meta-analysis. Tech Coloproctol. 2019;23(2):87–100. https://doi.org/10.1007/s10151-018-1919-6. Epub 2019 Jan 25. PMID: 30684110.
65. Cirocchi R, Randolph JJ, Binda GA, Gioia S, Henry BM, Tomaszewski KA, et al. Is the outpatient management of acute diverticulitis safe and effective? A systematic review and meta-analysis. Tech Coloproctol [Internet]. 2019;23(2):87–100. Available from: http://link.springer.com/10.1007/s10151-018-1919-6.
66. Moya P, Arroyo A, Pérez-Legaz J, Serrano P, Candela F, Soriano-Irigaray L, et al. Applicability, safety and efficiency of outpatient treatment in uncomplicated diverticulitis. Tech Coloproctol. 2012;16(4):301–7.
67. Ünlü Ç, Gunadi PM, Gerhards MF, Boermeester M a, Vrouenraets BC. Outpatient treatment for acute uncomplicated diverticulitis. Eur J Gastroenterol Hepatol [Internet]. 2013;25:1038–43. Available from: http://www.ncbi.nlm.nih.gov/pubmed/23636075.
68. Sirany A-ME, Gaertner WB, Madoff RD, Kwaan MR. Diverticulitis diagnosed in the emergency room: is it safe to discharge home? J Am Coll Surg [Internet]. 2017;225(1):21–5. Available from: http://www.ncbi.nlm.nih.gov/pubmed/28450063.
69. Lorente L, Cots F, Alonso S, Pascual M, Salvans S, Courtier R, et al. Outpatient treatment of uncomplicated acute diverticulitis: impact on healthcare costs. Cir Esp [Internet]. 2013;91(8):504–9. Available from: http://www.ncbi.nlm.nih.gov/pubmed/23764519.
70. Joliat G-R, Emery J, Demartines N, Hübner M, Yersin B, Hahnloser D. Antibiotic treatment for uncomplicated and mild complicated diverticulitis: outpatient treatment for everyone. Int J Colorectal Dis [Internet]. 2017;32(9):1313–9. Available from: http://www.ncbi.nlm.nih.gov/pubmed/28664347.
71. Mora López L, Flores Clotet R, Serra Aracil X, Montes Ortega N, Navarro Soto S. The use of the modified Neff classification in the management of acute diverticulitis. Rev Esp Enferm Dig [Internet]. 2017;109(5):328–34. Available from: http://www.ncbi.nlm.nih.gov/pubmed/28376628.
72. Mali JP, Mentula PJ, Leppäniemi AK, Sallinen VJ. Symptomatic treatment for uncomplicated acute diverticulitis: a prospective cohort study. Dis Colon Rectum [Internet]. 2016;59(6):529–34. Available from: http://www.ncbi.nlm.nih.gov/pubmed/27145310.
73. van Dijk ST, Rottier SJ, van Geloven AAW, Boermeester MA. Conservative treatment of acute colonic diverticulitis. Curr Infect Dis Rep. 2017;19(11):44.
74. Balasubramanian I, Fleming C, Mohan HM, Schmidt K, Haglind E, Winter DC. Out-patient management of mild or uncomplicated diverticulitis: a systematic review. Dig Surg [Internet]. 2017;34(2):151–60. Available from: http://www.ncbi.nlm.nih.gov/pubmed/27701164.
75. Alonso S, Pera M, Parés D, Pascual M, Gil MJ, Courtier R, et al. Outpatient treatment of patients with uncomplicated acute diverticulitis. Colorectal Dis [Internet]. 2010;12(10 Online):e278–82. Available from: http://www.ncbi.nlm.nih.gov/pubmed/19906059.
76. Martín Gil J, Serralta De Colsa D, García Marín A, Vaquero Rodríguez A, Rey Valcárcel C, Pérez Díaz MD, et al. Safety and efficiency of ambulatory treatment of acute diverticulitis. Gastroenterol Hepatol [Internet]. 2009;32(2):83–7. Available from: http://www.ncbi.nlm.nih.gov/pubmed/19231679.
77. Rodríguez-Cerrillo M, Poza-Montoro A, Fernandez-Diaz E, Romero AI. Patients with uncomplicated diverticulitis and comorbidity can be treated at home. Eur J Intern Med [Internet]. 2010;21(6):553–4. Available from: http://www.ncbi.nlm.nih.gov/pubmed/21111943.
78. Nagata N, Ishii N, Manabe N, Tomizawa K, Urita Y, Funabiki T, et al. Guidelines for colonic diverticular bleeding and colonic diverticulitis: Japan Gastroenterological Association. Digestion [Internet]. 2019;99(Suppl 1):1–26. Available from: http://www.ncbi.nlm.nih.gov/pubmed/30625484.
79. Bollom A, Austrie J, Hirsch W, Nee J, Friedlander D, Ellingson K, et al. Emergency department burden of diverticulitis in the USA, 2006–2013. Dig Dis Sci. 2017;62(10):2694–703.
80. de Korte N, Klarenbeek BR, Kuyvenhoven JP, Roumen RMH, Cuesta MA, Stockmann HBAC. Management of diverticulitis: results of a

survey among gastroenterologists and surgeons. Color Dis. 2011;13(12):411–7.
81. Wilkins T, Embry K, George R. Diagnosis and management of acute diverticulitis. Am Fam Physician [Internet]. 2013;87(9):612–20. Available from: http://www.ncbi.nlm.nih.gov/pubmed/23668524.
82. Pietrzak A, Bartnik W, Szczepkowski M, Krokowicz P, Dziki A, Reguła J, et al. Polish interdisciplinary consensus on diagnostics and treatment of colonic diverticulosis (2015). Pol Przegl Chir [Internet]. 2015;87(4):203–20. Available from: http://www.ncbi.nlm.nih.gov/pubmed/26146121.
83. Andeweg CS, Mulder IM, Felt-Bersma RJF, Verbon A, van der Wilt GJ, van Goor H, et al. Guidelines of diagnostics and treatment of acute left-sided colonic diverticulitis. Dig Surg [Internet]. 2013;30(4–6):278–92. Available from: http://www.ncbi.nlm.nih.gov/pubmed/23969324.
84. Dahl C, Crichton M, Jenkins J, Nucera R, Mahoney S, Marx W, et al. Evidence for dietary fibre modification in the recovery and prevention of reoccurrence of acute, uncomplicated diverticulitis: a systematic literature review. Nutrients. 2018;10(2):1–19.
85. Stam MAW, Draaisma WA, van de Wall BJM, Bolkenstein HE, Consten ECJ, Broeders IAMJ. An unrestricted diet for uncomplicated diverticulitis is safe: results of a prospective diverticulitis diet study. Color Dis. 2017;19(4):372–7.
86. World Gastroenterology Organization (WGO) practice guideline 2007. Diverticular disease. http://www.worldgastroenterologyorg/assets/en/pdf/guidelines/07_diverticular_diseasepdf2007. Accessed Apr 2008.
87. Van De Wall BJM, Draaisma WA, Van Iersel JJ, Van Der Kaaij R, Consten ECJ, Broeders IAMJ. Dietary restrictions for acute diverticulitis: evidence-based or expert opinion? Int J Color Dis. 2013;28(9):1287–93.
88. Mattei P, Rombeau JL. Review of the pathophysiology and management of postoperative ileus. World J Surg. 2006;30(8):1382–91.
89. Galetin T, Galetin A, Vestweber K-HH, Rink AD. Systematic review and comparison of national and international guidelines on diverticular disease. Int J Colorectal Dis [Internet]. 2018;33(3):261–72. Available from: http://www.ncbi.nlm.nih.gov/pubmed/29349481
90. Sharma PV, Eglinton T, Hider P, Frizelle F. Systematic review and meta-analysis of the role of routine colonic evaluation after radiologically confirmed acute diverticulitis. Ann Surg. 2014;259(2):263–72.
91. Rottier SJ, van Dijk ST, van Geloven AAW, Schreurs WH, Draaisma WA, van Enst WA, et al. Meta-analysis of the role of colonoscopy after an episode of left-sided acute diverticulitis. Br J Surg. 2019;106(8):988–97.
92. Daniels L, Ünlü Ç, De Wijkerslooth TR, Dekker E, Boermeester MA. Routine colonoscopy after left-sided acute uncomplicated diverticulitis: a systematic review. Gastrointest Endosc. 2014;79(3):378–89.
93. Cao AMY, Lam VW, Rickard MJFX. Endoscopic findings after CT proven acute diverticulitis: a systematic review and meta-analysis. ANZ J Surg. 2023;93(5):1150–8. https://doi.org/10.1111/ans.18190. Epub 2022 Dec 18. PMID: 36529882.
94. Niv Y, Hazazi R, Levi Z, Fraser G. Screening colonoscopy for colorectal cancer in asymptomatic people: a meta-analysis. Dig Dis Sci. 2008;53(12):3049–54.
95. Sartelli M, Catena F, Ansaloni L, Coccolini F, Griffiths EA, Abu-Zidan FM, et al. WSES Guidelines for the management of acute left sided colonic diverticulitis in the emergency setting. World J Emerg Surg [Internet]. 2016;11:37. Available from: http://www.ncbi.nlm.nih.gov/pubmed/27478494.
96. Hannan E, Harding T, Duggan W, Brosnan C, Maguire D. Routine endoscopy after acute sigmoid diverticulitis: would a sigmoidoscopy be sufficient? Cureus. 2021;13(9):e17648. https://doi.org/10.7759/cureus.17648. PMID: 34646695; PMCID: PMC8486147.
97. Lahat A, Yanai H, Sakhnini E, Menachem Y, Bar-Meir S. Role of colonoscopy in patients with persistent acute diverticulitis. World J Gastroenterol. 2008;14(17):2763–6.
98. Parks TG. Natural history of diverticular disease of the colon. A review of 521 cases. Br Med J [Internet]. 1969;4(5684):639–42. Available from: http://www.ncbi.nlm.nih.gov/pubmed/5359917.
99. Garfinkle R, Boutros M. Recurrent versus persistent diverticulitis: an important distinction. Dis Colon Rectum. 2016;59(10):e437.
100. Chapman JR, Dozois EJ, Wolff BG, Gullerud RE, Larson DR. Diverticulitis: a progressive disease? Do multiple recurrences predict less favorable outcomes? Ann Surg [Internet]. 2006;243(6):876–30; discussion 880–3. Available from: http://www.ncbi.nlm.nih.gov/pubmed/16772791.
101. Biondo S, Parés D, Martí Ragué J, Kreisler E, Fraccalvieri D, Jaurrieta E. Acute colonic diverticulitis in patients under 50 years of age. Br J Surg [Internet]. 2002;89(9):1137–41. Available from: http://www.ncbi.nlm.nih.gov/pubmed/12190679.
102. Mueller MH, Glatzle J, Kasparek MS, Becker HD, Jehle EC, Zittel TT, et al. Long-term outcome of conservative treatment in patients with diverticulitis of the sigmoid colon. Eur J Gastroenterol Hepatol [Internet]. 2005;17(6):649–54. Available from: http://www.ncbi.nlm.nih.gov/pubmed/15879727.
103. Broderick-Villa G, Burchette RJ, Collins JC, Abbas MA, Haigh PI. Hospitalization for acute diverticulitis does not mandate routine elective colectomy. Arch Surg [Internet]. 2005;140(6):576–81; discussion 581–3. Available from: http://www.ncbi.nlm.nih.gov/pubmed/15967905.
104. Hupfeld L, Burcharth J, Pommergaard HC, Rosenberg J. Risk factors for recurrence after acute colonic diverticulitis: a systematic review. Int J Color Dis. 2017;32(5):611–22.

105. Buchs NC. Natural history of uncomplicated sigmoid diverticulitis. World J Gastrointest Surg. 2015;7(11):313.
106. Eglinton T, Nguyen T, Raniga S, Dixon L, Dobbs B, Frizelle FA. Patterns of recurrence in patients with acute diverticulitis. Br J Surg [Internet]. 2010;97(6):952–7. Available from: http://www.ncbi.nlm.nih.gov/pubmed/20474006.
107. Buchs NC, Konrad-Mugnier B, Jannot A-S, Poletti P-A, Ambrosetti P, Gervaz P. Assessment of recurrence and complications following uncomplicated diverticulitis. Br J Surg [Internet]. 2013;100(7):976–9; discussion 979. Available from: http://www.ncbi.nlm.nih.gov/pubmed/23592303.
108. El-Sayed C, Radley S, Mytton J, Evison F, Ward ST. Risk of recurrent disease and surgery following an admission for acute diverticulitis. Dis Colon Rectum. 2018;61(3):283–9.
109. Li D, de Mestral C, Baxter NN, McLeod RS, Moineddin R, Wilton AS, et al. Risk of readmission and emergency surgery following nonoperative management of colonic diverticulitis: a population-based analysis. Ann Surg [Internet]. 2014;260(3):423–30; discussion 430–1. Available from: http://www.ncbi.nlm.nih.gov/pubmed/25115418.
110. Trenti L, Kreisler E, Galvez A, Golda T, Frago R, Biondo S. Long-term evolution of acute colonic diverticulitis after successful medical treatment. World J Surg [Internet]. 2015 [cited 2015 Jun 11];39(1):266–74. Available from: http://link.springer.com/10.1007/s00268-014-2773-y.
111. Morris AM, Regenbogen SE, Hardiman KM, Hendren S. Sigmoid diverticulitis: a systematic review. JAMA [Internet]. 2014;311(3):287–97. Available from: http://www.ncbi.nlm.nih.gov/pubmed/24430321.
112. Bharucha AE, Parthasarathy G, Ditah I, Fletcher JG, Ewelukwa O, Pendlimari R, et al. Temporal trends in the incidence and natural history of diverticulitis: a population-based study. Am J Gastroenterol [Internet]. 2015;110(11):1589–96. Available from: http://www.ncbi.nlm.nih.gov/pubmed/26416187.
113. Parente F, Bargiggia S, Prada A, Bortoli A, Giacosa A, Germanà B, et al. Intermittent treatment with mesalazine in the prevention of diverticulitis recurrence: a randomised multicentre pilot double-blind placebo-controlled study of 24-month duration. Int J Colorectal Dis [Internet]. 2013;28(10):1423–31. Available from: http://www.ncbi.nlm.nih.gov/pubmed/23754545.
114. van de Wall BJM, Draaisma WA, Consten ECJ, van der Kaaij RT, Wiezer MJ, Broeders IAMJ. Does the presence of abscesses in diverticular disease prelude surgery? J Gastrointest Surg [Internet]. 2013;17(3):540–7. Available from: http://www.ncbi.nlm.nih.gov/pubmed/23242845.
115. Lopez-Borao J, Kreisler E, Millan M, Trenti L, Jaurrieta E, Rodriguez-Moranta F, et al. Impact of age on recurrence and severity of left colonic diverticulitis. Color Dis. 2012;14(7):e407–12.
116. Katz LH, Guy DD, Lahat A, Gafter-Gvili A, Bar-Meir S. Diverticulitis in the young is not more aggressive than in the elderly, but it tends to recur more often: systematic review and meta-analysis. J Gastroenterol Hepatol. 2013;28(8):1274–81.
117. Binda GA, Arezzo A, Serventi A, Bonelli L, Italian Study Group on Complicated Diverticulosis (GISDIC), Facchini M, et al. Multicentre observational study of the natural history of left-sided acute diverticulitis. Br J Surg [Internet]. 2012;99(2):276–85. Available from: http://www.ncbi.nlm.nih.gov/pubmed/22105809.
118. Ünlü Ç, van de Wall BJ, Gerhards MF, Wiezer M, Draaisma WA, Consten EC, et al. Influence of age on clinical outcome of acute diverticulitis. J Gastrointest Surg [Internet]. 2013;17(9):1651–6. Available from: http://www.ncbi.nlm.nih.gov/pubmed/23733363.
119. Sallinen V, Mali J, Leppäniemi A, Mentula P. Assessment of risk for recurrent diverticulitis: a proposal of risk score for complicated recurrence. Medicine (Baltimore) [Internet]. 2015;94(8):e557. Available from: http://www.ncbi.nlm.nih.gov/pubmed/25715253.
120. Reisman Y, Ziv Y, Kravrovitc D, Negri M, Wolloch Y, Halevy A. Diverticulitis: the effect of age and location on the course of disease. Int J Colorectal Dis [Internet]. 1999;14(4–5):250–4. Available from: http://www.ncbi.nlm.nih.gov/pubmed/10647635.
121. Hjern F, Josephson T, Altman D, Holmström B, Johansson C. Outcome of younger patients with acute diverticulitis. Br J Surg [Internet]. 2008;95(6):758–64. Available from: http://www.ncbi.nlm.nih.gov/pubmed/18412297.
122. Humes DJ, Spiller RC. Review article: the pathogenesis and management of acute colonic diverticulitis. Aliment Pharmacol Ther. 2014;39(4):359–70.
123. Faria GR, Almeida AB, Moreira H, Pinto-de-Sousa J, Correia-da-Silva P, Pimenta AP. Acute diverticulitis in younger patients: any rationale for a different approach? World J Gastroenterol [Internet]. 2011;17(2):207–12. Available from: http://www.ncbi.nlm.nih.gov/pubmed/21245993.
124. Lahat A, Menachem Y, Avidan B, Yanai H, Sakhnini E, Bardan E, et al. Diverticulitis in the young patient—is it different ? World J Gastroenterol [Internet]. 2006;12(18):2932–5. Available from: http://www.ncbi.nlm.nih.gov/pubmed/16718822.
125. van Dijk ST, Rottier SJ, van Geloven AAWW, Boermeester MA. Conservative treatment of acute colonic diverticulitis. Curr Infect Dis Rep [Internet]. 2017;19(11):44. Available from: http://www.ncbi.nlm.nih.gov/pubmed/28942590.
126. Bose KP, Khorshidi I, Southern WN, Brandt LJ. The impact of ethnicity and obesity on the course of colonic diverticulitis. J Clin Gastroenterol [Internet]. 2013;47(2):160–4. Available from: http://www.ncbi.nlm.nih.gov/pubmed/22810106.
127. Klarenbeek BR, Samuels M, van der Wal MA, van der Peet DL, Meijerink WJ, Cuesta MA. Indications for elective sigmoid resection in diverticular dis-

ease. Ann Surg [Internet]. 2010;251(4):670–4. Available from: http://www.ncbi.nlm.nih.gov/pubmed/20224374.
128. Almalki T, Garfinkle R, Kmiotek E, Pelsser V, Bonaffini P, Reinhold C, et al. Family history is associated with recurrent diverticulitis after an episode of diverticulitis managed nonoperatively. Dis Colon Rectum. 2020;63(7):944–54.
129. Rosemar A, Angerås U, Rosengren A. Body mass index and diverticular disease: a 28-year follow-up study in men. Dis Colon Rectum [Internet]. 2008;51(4):450–5. Available from: http://www.ncbi.nlm.nih.gov/pubmed/18157570.
130. Aldoori VH, Giovannucci EL, Rimm EB, Wing AL, Trichopoulos DV, Willett WC. A prospective study of alcohol, smoking, caffeine, and the risk of symptomatic diverticular disease in men. Ann Epidemiol. 1995;5(3):221–8. https://doi.org/10.1016/1047-2797(94)00109-7.
131. Biondo S, Borao JL, Kreisler E, Golda T, Millan M, Frago R, et al. Recurrence and virulence of colonic diverticulitis in immunocompromised patients. Am J Surg [Internet]. 2012;204(2):172–9. Available from: http://www.ncbi.nlm.nih.gov/pubmed/22444713.
132. Al-Khamis A, Abou Khalil J, Demian M, Morin N, Vasilevsky C-A, Gordon PH, et al. Sigmoid colectomy for acute diverticulitis in immunosuppressed vs immunocompetent patients: outcomes from the ACS-NSQIP Database. Dis Colon Rectum [Internet]. 2016;59(2):101–9. Available from: http://www.ncbi.nlm.nih.gov/pubmed/26734967.
133. Scarpa CR, Buchs NC, Poncet A, Konrad-Mugnier B, Gervaz P, Morel P, et al. Short-term intravenous antibiotic treatment in uncomplicated diverticulitis does not increase the risk of recurrence compared to long-term treatment. Ann Coloproctol [Internet]. 2015;31(2):52–6. Available from: http://www.ncbi.nlm.nih.gov/pubmed/25960972.
134. Lamb MN, Kaiser AM. Elective resection versus observation after nonoperative management of complicated diverticulitis with abscess: a systematic review and meta-analysis. Dis Colon Rectum [Internet]. 2014;57(12):1430–40. Available from: http://www.ncbi.nlm.nih.gov/pubmed/25380010.
135. Garfinkle R, Kugler A, Pelsser V, Vasilevsky C-A, Morin N, Gordon P, et al. Diverticular abscess managed with long-term definitive nonoperative intent is safe. Dis Colon Rectum [Internet]. 2016;59(7):648–55. Available from: http://www.ncbi.nlm.nih.gov/pubmed/27270517.
136. Lambrichts DPV, Bolkenstein HE, van der Does DCHE, Dieleman D, Crolla RMPH, Dekker JWT, et al. Multicentre study of non-surgical management of diverticulitis with abscess formation. Br J Surg. 2019;106(4):458–66.
137. Elagili F, Stocchi L, Ozuner G, Dietz DW, Kiran RP. Outcomes of percutaneous drainage without surgery for patients with diverticular abscess. Dis Colon Rectum. 2014;57(3):331–6.
138. Devaraj B, Liu W, Tatum J, Cologne K, Kaiser AM. Medically treated diverticular abscess associated with high risk of recurrence and disease complications. Dis Colon Rectum. 2016;59(3):208–15.
139. Pittet O, Kotzampassakis N, Schmidt S, Denys A, Demartines N, Calmes J-M. Recurrent left colonic diverticulitis episodes: more severe than the initial diverticulitis? World J Surg [Internet]. 2009;33(3):547–52. Available from: http://www.ncbi.nlm.nih.gov/pubmed/19148697.
140. Ditzel M, Vennix S, Menon AG, Verbeek PCM, Bemelman WA, Lange JF. Severity of diverticulitis does not influence abdominal complaints during long-term follow-up. Dig Surg. 2019;36(2):129–36.
141. Gregersen R, Mortensen LQ, Burcharth J, Pommergaard H-C, Rosenberg J. Treatment of patients with acute colonic diverticulitis complicated by abscess formation: a systematic review. Int J Surg [Internet]. 2016;35:201–8. Available from: https://linkinghub.elsevier.com/retrieve/pii/S1743919116309542.
142. Moya P, Arroyo A, Pérez-Legaz J, Serrano P, Candela F, Soriano-Irigaray L, et al. Applicability, safety and efficiency of outpatient treatment in uncomplicated diverticulitis. Tech Coloproctol [Internet]. 2012;16(4):301–7. Available from: http://www.ncbi.nlm.nih.gov/pubmed/22706731.
143. Peláez N, Pera M, Courtier R, Sánchez J, Gil MJ, Parés D, et al. Applicability, safety and efficacy of an ambulatory treatment protocol in patients with uncomplicated acute diverticulitis. Cir Esp [Internet]. 2006;80(6):369–72. Available from: http://www.ncbi.nlm.nih.gov/pubmed/17192220.
144. Rose J, Parina RP, Faiz O, Chang DC, Talamini MA. Long-term outcomes after initial presentation of diverticulitis. Ann Surg [Internet]. 2015;262(6):1046–53. Available from: http://www.ncbi.nlm.nih.gov/pubmed/25654646.
145. Ho VP, Nash GM, Milsom JW, Lee SW. Identification of diverticulitis patients at high risk for recurrence and poor outcomes. J Trauma Acute Care Surg [Internet]. 2015;78(1):112–9. Available from: http://www.ncbi.nlm.nih.gov/pubmed/25539211.
146. Moreno AM, Wille-Jørgensen P. Long-term outcome in 445 patients after diagnosis of diverticular disease. Colorectal Dis [Internet]. 2007;9(5):464–8. Available from: http://www.ncbi.nlm.nih.gov/pubmed/17504345.
147. Anaya DA, Flum DR. Risk of emergency colectomy and colostomy in patients with diverticular disease. Arch Surg [Internet]. 2005;140(7):681–5. Available from: http://www.ncbi.nlm.nih.gov/pubmed/16027334.
148. Mäkelä JT, Kiviniemi HO, Laitinen ST. Spectrum of disease and outcome among patients with acute diverticulitis. Dig Surg [Internet]. 2010;27(3):190–6. Available from: http://www.ncbi.nlm.nih.gov/pubmed/20571265.

149. Li D, Baxter NN, McLeod RS, Moineddin R, Wilton AS, Nathens AB. Evolving practice patterns in the management of acute colonic diverticulitis: a population-based analysis. Dis Colon Rectum [Internet]. 2014;57(12):1397–405. Available from: http://www.ncbi.nlm.nih.gov/pubmed/25380006.
150. Masoomi H, Buchberg BS, Magno C, Mills SD, Stamos MJ. Trends in diverticulitis management in the United States from 2002 to 2007. Arch Surg [Internet]. 2011;146(4):400–6. Available from: http://www.ncbi.nlm.nih.gov/pubmed/21173283.
151. Regenbogen SE, Hardiman KM, Hendren S, Morris AM. Surgery for diverticulitis in the 21st century: a systematic review. JAMA Surg [Internet]. 2014;149(3):292–303. Available from: http://www.ncbi.nlm.nih.gov/pubmed/24430164.
152. Lanas A, Abad-Baroja D, Lanas-Gimeno A. Progress and challenges in the management of diverticular disease: which treatment? Ther Adv Gastroenterol. 2018;11:1–21.
153. Lembcke B. The gastroenterologist's view. Dig Dis [Internet]. 2012;30(1):122–8. Available from: http://www.ncbi.nlm.nih.gov/pubmed/22572699.
154. Altadill A, Eiró N, González LO, Junquera S, González-Quintana JM, Sánchez MR, et al. Comparative analysis of the expression of metalloproteases and their inhibitors in resected Crohn's disease and complicated diverticular disease. Inflamm Bowel Dis [Internet]. 2012;18(1):120–30. Available from: http://www.ncbi.nlm.nih.gov/pubmed/21438097.
155. Tursi A, Elisei W, Brandimarte G, Giorgetti GM, Inchingolo CD, Nenna R, et al. Mucosal expression of basic fibroblastic growth factor, Syndecan 1 and tumor necrosis factor-alpha in diverticular disease of the colon: a case-control study. Neurogastroenterol Motil [Internet]. 2012;24(9):836–e396. Available from: http://www.ncbi.nlm.nih.gov/pubmed/22680042.
156. Haboubi NY, Alqudah M. Pathology and pathogenesis of diverticular disease and patterns of colonic mucosal changes overlying the diverticula. Dig Dis [Internet]. 2012;30(1):29–34. Available from: http://www.ncbi.nlm.nih.gov/pubmed/22572682.
157. Boostrom SY, Wolff BG, Cima RR, Merchea A, Dozois EJ, Larson DW. Uncomplicated diverticulitis, more complicated than we thought. J Gastrointest Surg [Internet]. 2012;16(9):1744–9. Available from: http://www.ncbi.nlm.nih.gov/pubmed/22696233.

Nonoperative Treatment of Diverticular Abscess

8

Jason Hall

Introduction and Epidemiology

Diverticulitis is a common gastrointestinal disorder. The incidence of diverticular disease has increased significantly over the previous decades. In the early twentieth century, diverticula were reported on autopsy studies at a rate of 2–10% [1]. It is estimated that 10% of people under 40 years old and up to 70% of those over the age of 80 have diverticulosis [2]. In 2014, there were over 350,000 visits for diverticulitis to the Emergency Department (ED), which represented an increase of 45% compared to 2006 [3]. The total annual healthcare costs to care for patients with diverticulitis are estimated to be over 5 billion dollars in the United States [3]. However, fewer patients with diverticular disease are managed as inpatients. The rate of admission to the hospital for diverticulitis management has decreased from 58.0% in 2006 to 47.1% in 2013. The use of emergency colonic resection for the management of acute diverticulitis has also decreased. The number of patients undergoing bowel surgery per 100,000 ED visits for diverticulitis has decreased from 7278 in 2006 to 4827 in 2013 [4]. Thus, there are increasing numbers of patients with complicated presentations of diverticulitis who are being managed without operative intervention. This chapter focuses on the nonoperative management of patients who present with a diverticular abscess.

J. Hall (✉)
Tufts Medical Center, Boston, MA, USA
e-mail: jason.f.hall@lahey.org

Complicated Diverticulitis: Abscess Formation

The four stages of diverticulitis originally proposed by Hinchey were based upon intraoperative and pathologic findings [5]. With the advent of imaging-based diagnosis of diverticulitis, particularly the use of computed tomography (CT) scans, new guidelines for the classification of diverticular disease have been developed based on imaging findings [6]. The benefits of CT imaging for diagnosis include the ability to evaluate the severity of diverticular disease, to rule out other possible etiologies of abdominal pain, and to identify complications of diverticulitis including abscess [7]. Multiple prospective studies have confirmed the superiority of CT imaging with intravenous (IV) contrast compared to water or barium enema, reporting a sensitivity and specificity near 100% [8–10].

In one large study including over 3000 patients, complicated diverticulitis, defined as the presence of fistula, abscess, obstruction, or frank perforation, was present in 12% of patients. Among patients with complicated disease, 69% had an abscess [11]. Clinical signs of patients who may have an abscess include failure to improve with standard therapy for uncomplicated diverticulitis (i.e., antibiotics alone), fever,

M. Boutros et al. (eds.), *Diverticulitis*, https://doi.org/10.1007/978-3-032-21720-2_8

leukocytosis, or even a tender palpable mass on exam [12].

Historically, the initial treatment of diverticular abscess was a three-stage procedure. The first intervention was an open abscess drainage with creation of a proximal diverting colostomy. This was followed by delayed resection of the diseased segment of the colon. The third and final procedure was for colostomy closure [13]. In one of the earliest series describing the use of a diverting loop colostomy for perforated diverticulitis, the authors suggested that the distal infected limb should be flushed regularly to remove all infection. The affected segment of the colon could then be safely resected at a subsequent operation [14–16]. The three-stage approach to diverticular abscess was later abandoned after further studies documented the clinical deterioration of patients who did not undergo initial resectional therapy [16, 17]. Greif et al. [18] examined 510 patients who underwent surgery for perforated diverticulitis, and compared mortality rates among patients who had upfront resection of the diseased colon (mainly Hartmann's procedure) to patients where the diseased colon was left in situ and removed at a later time (if at all). The authors reported a mortality rate of 2% in the resection group compared to 12% in the nonresected group ($p < 0.05$). The American Society of Colon and Rectal Surgeons (ASCRS) soon recommended against the three-stage "non resection" procedure due to associated high morbidity and mortality. In addition, improvements in other percutaneous radiological procedures for the management of postoperative complications decreased the morbidity and mortality associated with primary resection seen in previous decades [19].

Percutaneous Drainage: Early Implementation

Percutaneous drainage (PCD) represents one of the more significant advances in the modern treatment of diverticulitis. The technique was first described in multiple other disease processes, including hemorrhagic pancreatitis, endometriosis and postappendectomy abscess, prior to its application in the management of complicated diverticulitis [20]. Case reports dating back to the 1970s described catheter-based drainage of appendiceal and hepatic abscesses as well as pancreatic pseudocysts [21]. Johnson et al. [22] published data comparing the outcomes of operative drainage and percutaneous drainage using ultrasound or CT imaging over the course of a10-year time period for intra-abdominal abscesses of various etiologies. The authors defined treatment as successful if the abscess completely resolved and did not recur shortly after and if the patient survived the episode. In all, 89% of cases managed by percutaneous drainage were deemed successful by these criteria compared to 70% in the traditional operative group. At the time of this published study, percutaneous drainage seldom used and was described as "a significant departure from the universally accepted but heretofore unchallenged surgical methods of operative incision and drainage for therapy of abdominal abscesses" [22].

The use of PCD in patients who were clinically unstable or in those with multiloculated, fistulizing, or poorly defined abscesses was described by van Sonnenberg et al. [20] in a series of 15 patients. Abscess location in this study population included kidney, pelvis, liver, and pancreas. The authors reported that within this group of critically ill patients with complicated abscesses who could not undergo a surgical intervention, PCD resulted in a significant decrease in patients' systemic signs of infection. Drainage allowed for surgery to be deferred to a more opportune time and was ultimately performed when indicated in 13 of these patients. The authors promoted that the combined radiological-surgical approach greatly benefited this group of patients with complicated abscesses, who were previously managed with a very high mortality risk due to ineffective surgical drainage alone [20, 23].

With the safety, feasibility, and benefits of PCD well established for the management of intra-abdominal collections, studies reporting the applicability of this technique to diverticulitis began to surface. Neff et al. [13] published a series of 16 patients with diverticular abscess initially treated with CT-guided PCD as opposed to operative intervention. The abscesses were 5–15 cm in diameter and located in the pelvis, paracolic area, and psoas muscle. The authors reported that all patients had resolution of fever within 72 h and no patients required an emergent operative intervention after PCD. Sixty-nine percent of patients underwent a single-stage sigmoid resection with anastomosis within 6 weeks after drainage [13].

Stabile et al. [24] reported similar results in a series of 19 patients who underwent PCD. In this series, mean size of abscess was 8.9 cm and only 2 of 19 patients had persistent leukocytosis or fever following catheter placement. Seventy-four percent of patients ultimately underwent a single-stage colectomy with primary anastomosis. The remaining patients either refused surgery or had fecal fistulas with inadequate infection control mandating operative intervention.

Mueller et al. [25] examined the role of PCD in a population of 111 patients with perforated diverticulitis, 24 of whom underwent PCD and 87 of whom underwent surgery. Of the 24 patients who underwent drainage first, 58% underwent a single-stage operation thereafter; the remainder of this subgroup either underwent a two-stage procedure or refused surgery. The authors also reviewed the imaging and outcomes of patients who did not undergo PCD and who had a two-stage procedure. They proposed that 50% of patients who underwent a two-stage procedure could be converted to a single-stage surgery if the use of a PCD was used preoperatively.

After percutaneous drainage of a diverticular abscess, drains are removed when the fluid drainage decreases in a significant manner with signs of resolution of the abscess, which usually takes several days. The decision of drain removal is made based on clinical assessment and a reduction in the drainage volume. Reimaging with CT scanning after percutaneous drainage is not routinely required unless the clinical condition of the patients does not show improvement or if there are concerns about complete drainage or complications. Reimaging can help guide management decisions, such as surgical intervention or the need for another drainage procedure [26].

Risk Factors for Treatment Failure After Percutaneous Drainage

A multicenter observational study [27] assessed the effect of percutaneous drainage on the outcome of diverticular abscess according to the abscess size. There were no significant differences in treatment failure rates between patients treated with or without percutaneous drainage when the abscess size was 3–5 cm (35.7% vs. 28.4%; $p = 0.200$), or ≥5 cm (35% vs. 28%, $p = 0.409$). Another study [28] reported that the presence of more than one abscess was not significantly associated with the risk of failure. The location of the abscess, whether local or distant, was also not significantly associated with failure. A recent study [29] confirmed that percutaneous drainage was not significantly associated with the risk of failure or success of the nonoperative treatment in abscesses >5 cm.

Which Patients Should Undergo PCD Versus Antibiotics Alone?

While the use of PCD in diverticulitis can provide source control and bridge patients to an operation if indicated, there remains a possibility that some patients may be treated with the use of antibiotics alone. The selection of patients to undergo PCD in conjunction with antibiotic therapy has been the target of many research studies.

Kumar et al. [30] reported a series of 114 patients with intra-abdominal abscesses (26% were diverticular) who were all initially treated with conservative therapy including bowel rest, antibiotics, and fluid resuscitation. Fifty-four percent of the total patient population responded to conservative management alone, 95% of whom had no documented recurrence. Conversely, 44% of the study population underwent PCD due to failure to respond to conservative management, which included continued fevers, leukocytosis, and abdominal pain. The average abscess size was larger in patients who failed medical therapy alone (6.5 cm vs. 4 cm, $p < 0.001$). After multivariate regression, only fever ($p = 0.0067$) and abscess size greater than 6.5 cm ($p < 0.0001$)

were associated with failure of conservative management.

Siewert et al. [31] published a series of 31 patients with diverticular abscess out of 181 patients diagnosed with diverticulitis by CT imaging. Of these, 73% had an abscess smaller than 3 cm, and all were successfully treated with antibiotics alone, either as an inpatient or outpatient.

In a prospective study of 73 cases of diverticular abscess, Ambrosetti et al. [32] examined isolated mesocolic or pelvic abscess documented by CT imaging. All patients were hospitalized and offered an intervention, either surgery or PCD, if no improvement on IV antibiotics was appreciated within 48 h. Within this study population, 25% underwent an operation at the first hospitalization, 34% of patients required an operation 2 months to 9 years later, and 41% of patients never required any intervention beyond antibiotic therapy. PCD was required more often with an abscess size >5 cm ($p = 0.03$) [32].

More recently, Lambrichts et al. [27] examined the outcomes of patients who underwent nonoperative management (antibiotics with or without PCD) of diverticular abscess in a multicenter retrospective study of 447 patients with CT-proven diverticulitis. They also aimed to identify risk factors associated with adverse outcomes, to help guide patient selection during nonoperative therapy. Median abscess diameter was larger in patients who underwent PCD. Abscess size >3 cm was predictive of treatment failure with antibiotic only, defined as complications, readmissions, persistent symptoms, or need for PCD. No other factors including age, body mass index (BMI), comorbidities, leukocytosis, or C-reactive protein level were predictive of treatment failure. Nonetheless, the majority of patients were treated without PCD, with only 4.8% requiring drainage due to treatment failure.

From this data, it is clear that antibiotics alone can be used for the management of patients with diverticular abscess [33]. The principal factor associated with treatment failure identified in most of these studies was abscess size. In their 2020 practice parameters for the treatment of sigmoid diverticulitis, the ASCRS stated that image-guided PCD is usually recommended for stable patients with abscesses >3 cm in size. Antibiotic treatment alone for abscesses <3 cm is typically successful and, in stable patients, treatment can usually be administered in the outpatient setting [34]. However, another study found that surgical treatment was associated with a lower risk of recurrence in patients with abscess >4 cm, compared to antibiotics [35].

Laparoscopic Lavage and Abscess Drainage

Some patients are not candidates for PCD due to anatomic constraints and/or abscess location. However, in patients who fail antibiotic therapy alone, source control is needed for the patient to improve. In such instances, laparoscopic lavage and abscess drainage have emerged as a potential management strategy [36]. The literature on laparoscopic lavage mostly consists of patients with Hinchey III diverticulitis, which differs from diverticular abscess (Hinchey I/II) in that the abscess has ruptured and caused purulent peritonitis. However, the presentation and management of patients with Hinchey II disease can at times overlap with that Hinchey III diverticulitis. Therefore, a review of recent randomized controlled trials (RCTs) examining the use of laparoscopic lavage in the management of acute diverticulitis is useful.

Multiple randomized trials have examined the use of laparoscopic lavage. In the SCANDIV trial [37], 172 patients were randomized to either undergo laparoscopic lavage or primary resection and followed for multiple outcomes including need for further intervention, stoma formation, and surgical site infections. Severe complications and overall mortality were not significantly different between the two groups. Deep surgical site infections were more common in patients who underwent laparoscopic lavage ($p = 0.006$). Patients who underwent primary resection were more likely to have a stoma at 1 year ($p < 0.001$). While not significant, complications in the laparoscopic lavage group were more commonly related to the retained diseased colon segment including continued abdominal infection sequelae and patients who underwent lavage were more likely to require reoperation.

The LADIES [38] RCT has two major components, one of which was the LOLA arm that compared laparoscopic peritoneal lavage to sigmoidectomy in perforated diverticulitis. The major endpoint was major morbidity and mortality at 12 months, defined as surgical reintervention, abdominal wall dehiscence, abscesses needing percutaneous drainage, urosepsis, myocardial infarction, renal failure, and respiratory failure. The study was terminated early due to early-superiority determination with a significant amount of morbidity reported in the lavage group. In-hospital surgical reinterventions were more common in the lavage group compared to the sigmoidectomy group ($p = 0.011$). Combined major morbidity and mortality was 33% in the laparoscopic lavage group compared to 19% of patients who underwent sigmoidectomy ($p = 0.0427$) within 30 days of operation. However, there was no difference in combined morbidity and mortality at 12 months ($p = 0.58$). This study could not adequately show noninferiority of laparoscopic lavage due to the early ending of accrual.

The DILALA [39] trial was another trial of 87 patients randomized to either laparoscopic lavage or resection. Data analysis showed that more patients in the resection group required secondary operations compared to the laparoscopic lavage group ($p = 0.012$) and a risk reduction of 45 percent. There was no significant difference in the number of hospital readmissions or mortality between the two groups.

In a recent meta-analysis by Penna et al. [40], a total of 589 patients were analyzed from multiple RCTs including the ones described above. In this meta-analysis, the odds of developing an intra-abdominal abscess were three times as high in patients who underwent laparoscopic lavage. The authors reported that the major complication of laparoscopic lavage is continued intra-abdominal sepsis and peritonitis requiring emergency surgery. The complications of laparoscopic lavage have been compared to those seen in earlier surgeries for diverticular disease where the diseased segment of colon was not resected [41]. The meta-analysis by Penna et al. [40, 42] presents the question of whether laparoscopic lavage should be considered a definitive treatment or damage control procedure. A more recent study by Horesh et al. [43] concluded that long-term follow-up of patients who underwent emergency surgery for perforated diverticulitis showed that laparoscopic lavage had lower odds of long-term ostomy and reoperation, but more risk for disease recurrence when compared with resection in purulent peritonitis. Data suggest that although laparoscopic peritoneal lavage is an option for acute management of Hinchey III diverticulitis, it is associated with high rates of reintervention and therefore should be employed with caution.

Nondrainable Diverticular Abscess

Abscesses that are not amenable to percutaneous drainage due to location or multilocularity may require surgical drainage. Surgical drainage is also indicated when percutaneous drainage fails to drain the abscess adequately or if complications occur. Open surgical drainage of a diverticular abscess often involves an incision and drainage procedure and can be used as a bridge before definitive surgery or as a treatment option for large or complex abscesses [44].

Role of Elective Surgery Following Management of Initial Diverticular Abscess

There is a strong base of evidence for the use of image-guided PCD for the treatment of patients with diverticular abscesses, particularly those >5 cm. However, the surgical management of patients after successful nonoperative treatment with antibiotics alone or PCD is less clear. The current practice parameters recommend elective colectomy after recovery from an episode of complicated diverticulitis. This recommendation is based predominantly on retrospective studies showing high recurrence rates following

PCD. There is some more recent data that supports the possibility of managing diverticular abscesses without elective colectomy.

Garfinkle et al. [42] reported on 73 patients with complicated diverticulitis managed by PCD with or without antibiotics. Subsequent to resolution of initial episode, 30.1% (22/73) of patients went to the ED for symptoms and were found to have a recurrent episode of diverticulitis based on CT imaging. Two of these patients presented with generalized peritonitis and required emergency intervention while 7 other patients underwent an elective resection. Sixty-four patients (87.7%) never required an operation. These authors concluded that long-term nonoperative management for diverticulitis with abscess is associated with a low risk of emergency interventions or future resection. However, further studies are indicated particularly to evaluate the quality of life in patients who do not undergo surgery and the subset of patients who may benefit from elective resection [41].

Aquina et al. [45] reported on an overall study population of 10, 342 patients who were admitted to the hospital with a diagnosis of diverticulitis with abscess; 5412 of this larger population did not undergo elective colectomy. Data shows that, of the patient population that did not undergo elective colectomy, 24.8% had a recurrence of diverticulitis within 5 years, 7.4% had multiple episodes of recurrence, 13.6% had recurrence that was complicated, 18.5% underwent either emergent or elective colectomy. These authors suggested that close observation without elective colectomy is a reasonable course of action following PCD for diverticular abscess [40, 42].

Other studies reported that elective colectomy should be routine following complicated diverticulitis. Lamb et al. [46] reported on a meta-analysis of 22 studies which examined the management of diverticular abscesses. Seventy percent of these patients were initially managed nonoperatively and discharged from the hospital. In ten studies, recurrence of diverticular symptoms was tracked in patients who were awaiting elective surgery. Thirty-nine percent of patients had persistent or recurrent symptoms. Authors conclude that not offering an elective colectomy in the case of complicated diverticulitis is associated with an increased risk of recurrent diverticulitis episodes along with an increase in morbidity and mortality.

Gregersen et al. [47] published a large meta-analysis of 1723 screened studies, 42 of which were included in a final analysis examining multiple outcomes including PCD, antibiotic therapy, and the role of elective colectomy in the management of diverticular abscesses. The authors concluded that nonoperative treatment of a diverticular abscess does not require elective colectomy. However, since there are no "definitive indications for elective surgery…patients should be considered on case-by-case basis." The recurrence rate of abscess is 19% even after elective colectomy and the percentage of patients who developed incisional hernias and minimal improvement of long-term quality of life was not insignificant. The studies identified for this meta-analysis were predominantly observational and a randomized trial comparing antibiotics, abscess size as related to management, and elimination of elective colectomy altogether after successful treatment of diverticular abscesses requires further standardized investigation. More recent evidence shows that surgery can be avoided in 60% of diverticular abscesses and that abscess size was significantly associated with avoidance of surgery [28].

Conclusion

The management of complicated diverticulitis continues to be an evolving field of research. The nonoperative options for diverticular abscess have grown considerably with the advances in diagnostic radiological imaging and noninvasive treatments. For larger abscesses, PCD is recommended as opposed to antibiotic therapy alone. PCD has the ability to temporize the severity of a patient's disease so that a multistep operation can be converted into a one-stage surgery, thereby often obviating the need for stoma formation. Predicting when PCD will fail as sole management in complicated diverticulitis abscess management is less clear.

There are conflicting data regarding the use of elective colectomy following nonoperative resolution of a diverticular abscess. At the time of this publication, this remains an open question and the decision mandates thorough discussion of the risks and benefits associated with both options.

References

1. Weizman AV, Nguyen GC. Diverticular disease: epidemiology and management. Can J Gastroenterol. 2011;25(7):385–9.
2. Nally DM, Kavanagh DO. Current controversies in the management of diverticulitis: a review. Dig Surg. 2019;36:195–205.
3. Peery AF, Crockett SD, Murphy CC, Lund JL, Dellon ES, Williams JL, et al. Burden and cost of gastrointestinal, liver, and pancreatic diseases in the United States: update 2018. Gastroenterology. 2019;156:254–72.
4. Bollom A, Austrie J, Hirsch W, Nee J, Friedlander D, Ellingson K. Emergency department burden of diverticulitis in the United States: 2006 to 2013. Dig Dis Sci. 2017;62(10):2694–703.
5. Hinchey EJ, Schaal PG, Richards. Treatment of perforated diverticulitis of the colon. GK Adv Surg. 1978;12:85–109.
6. Klarenbeek B, Korte N, van der Peet D, Cuesta M. Review of current classifications for diverticular disease and a translation into clinical practice. Int J Color Dis. 2012;27:207–14.
7. DeStigter KK, Keating DP. Imaging update: acute colonic diverticulitis. Clin Colon Rectal Surg. 2009;22(3):147–55.
8. Liljegren G, Chabok A, Wickbom M, et al. Acute colonic diverticulitis: a systematic review of diagnostic accuracy. Color Dis. 2007;9:480–8. https://doi.org/10.1111/j.1463-1318.2007.01238.x.
9. Ambrosetti P, Jenny A, Becker C, et al. Acute left colonic diverticulitis—compared performance of computed tomography and water-soluble contrast enema: prospective evaluation of 420 patients. Dis Colon Rectum. 2000;43:1363–7. https://doi.org/10.1007/BF02236631.
10. Cho KC, Morehouse HT, Alterman DD, et al. Sigmoid diverticulitis: diagnostic role of CT—comparison with barium enema studies. Radiology. 1990;176:111–5.
11. Bharucha AE, et al. Temporal trends in the incidence and natural history of diverticulitis: a population based study. Am J Gastroenterol. 2015;110(11):1589–96. https://doi.org/10.1038/ajg.2015.302.
12. Stollman NH, Raskin JB. Diagnosis and management of diverticular disease of the colon in adults: Ad Hoc Practice Parameters Committee of the American College of Gastroenterology. Am J Gastroenterol. 1999;94:3110–21.
13. Neff C, vanSonnenberg E, Casola G, Wittich G, Hoyt D, Halasz N, Martini D. Diverticular abscesses: percutaneous drainage. Radiology. 1987;163:15–8.
14. Judd ES, Pollock LW. Diverticulitis. Ann Surg. 1924;80(3):425–38.
15. Smithwick R. Experiences with the surgical management of diverticulitis of the sigmoid. Ann Surg. 1942;115(6):969–85.
16. Vermeulen J, Lange JF. Treatment of perforated diverticulitis with generalized peritonitis: past, present, and future. World J Surg. 2010;34(3):587–93. https://doi.org/10.1007/s00268-009-0372-0.
17. Large JM. Treatment of perforated diverticulitis. Lancet. 1964;1:413–4.
18. Greif JM, Fried G, McSherry CK. Surgical treatment of perforated diverticulitis of the sigmoid colon. Dis Colon Rectum. 1980;23:483–7. https://doi.org/10.1007/BF02987083.
19. Wong WD, Wexner SD, Lowry A, et al. Practice parameters for the treatment of sigmoid diverticulitis–supporting documentation. The Standards Task Force. The American Society of Colon and Rectal Surgeons. Dis Colon Rectum. 2000;43:290–7.
20. Van Sonnenberg E, Wing VW, Casola G, et al. Temporizing effect of percutaneous drainage of complicated abscesses in critically ill patients. AJR Am J Roentgenol. 1984;142:821–6.
21. Gerzof SG, Robbins AH, Birkett DH, Johnson WC, Pugatch RD, Vincent ME. Percutaneous catheter drainage of abdominal abscesses guided by ultrasound and computed tomography. AJR Am J Roentgenol. 1979;133:1–8.
22. Johnson WC, Gerzof S, Robbins A, Nasbeth D. Comparative evaluation of operative drainage versus percutaneous catheter drainage guided by computed tomography or ultrasound. Ann Surg. 1981;194:4.
23. Fry DE, Garrison RN, Heitsch RC, Calhoun K, Polk HC. Determinants of death in patients with intraabdominal abscess. Surgery. 1980;88:517–23.
24. Stabile BE, Puccio E, Van Sonnenberg E, Neff CC. Pre-operative percutaneous drainage of diverticular abscesses. Am J Surg. 1990;159:99–104.
25. Mueller PR, Saini S, Wittenburg J, et al. Sigmoid diverticular abscesses: percutaneous drainage as an adjunct to surgical resection in 24 cases. Radiology. 1987;164:321–5.
26. National Guideline Centre (UK). Evidence review for percutaneous drainage versus resectional surgery for the management of abscesses: diverticular disease: diagnosis and management: evidence review N. London: National Institute for Health and Care Excellence (NICE); 2019. NICE Guideline, No. 147. Available from: https://www.ncbi.nlm.nih.gov/books/NBK558093/.
27. Lambrichts DPV, Bolkenstein HE, van der Does D, et al. Multicentre study of non-surgical management of diverticulitis with abscess formation. Br J Surg. 2019;106(4):458–66. https://doi.org/10.1002/bjs.11129.

28. Bachelani AM, Holton LA, Soliman Y. Short- and long-term outcomes in the nonoperative treatment of diverticular abscesses. Surg Pract Sci. 2023;13:100180. https://doi.org/10.1016/j.sipas.2023.100180. PMID: 39845384; PMCID: PMC11749905.
29. Podda M, Ceresoli M, Di Martino M, et al. Towards a tailored approach for patients with acute diverticulitis and abscess formation. The DivAbsc2023 multicentre case-control study. Surg Endosc. 2024;38(6):3180–94. https://doi.org/10.1007/s00464-024-10793-z. Epub 2024 Apr 17. PMID: 38632117; PMCID: PMC11133057.
30. Kumar RR, Kim JT, Haukoos JS, et al. Factors affecting the successful management of intra-abdominal abscesses with antibiotics and the need for percutaneous drainage. Dis Colon Rectum. 2006;49:183–9.
31. Siewert B, Tye G, Kruskal J, et al. Impact of CT-guided drainage in the treatment of diverticular abscesses: size matters. AJR Am J Roentgenol. 2006;186:680–6.
32. Ambrosetti P, Chautems R, Soravia C, Peiris-Waser N, Terrier F. Long term outcome of mesocolic and pelvic diverticular abscesses of the left colon: a prospective study of 73 cases. Dis Colon Rectum. 2005;48:787–91.
33. Mali J, Mentula P, Leppäniemi A, Sallinen V. Determinants of treatment and outcomes of diverticular abscesses. World J Emerg Surg. 2019;14:31. https://doi.org/10.1186/s13017-019-0250-5. PMID: 31320921; PMCID: PMC6615185.
34. Hall J, Hardiman K, Lee S, Prepared on behalf of the Clinical Practice Guidelines Committee of the American Society of Colon and Rectal Surgeons, et al. The American Society of Colon and Rectal Surgeons clinical practice guidelines for the treatment of left-sided colonic diverticulitis. Dis Colon Rectum. 2020;63(6):728–47. https://doi.org/10.1097/DCR.0000000000001679. PMID: 32384404.
35. Arezzo A, Nicotera A, Bonomo LD, Olandese F, Veglia S, Ferguglia A, Pentassuglia G, Mingrone G, Morino M. Outcomes of surgical treatment of diverticular abscesses after failure of antibiotic therapy. Updat Surg. 2023;75(4):855–62. https://doi.org/10.1007/s13304-023-01509-4. Epub 2023 Apr 24. PMID: 37093495; PMCID: PMC10284947.
36. Kaushik M, Bhullar JS, Bindroo S, Singh H, Mittal VK. Minimally invasive management of complicated diverticular disease: current status and review of literature. Dig Dis Sci. 2016;61:663–72.
37. Schultz JK, Wallon C, Blecic L, Forsmo HM, Folkesson J, Buchwald P, Kørner H, Dahl FA, Øresland T, Yaqub S. One-year results of the SCANDIV randomized clinical trial of laparoscopic lavage versus primary resection for acute perforated diverticulitis. Br J Surg. 2017;104:1382–92.
38. Vennix S, Musters GD, Mulder IM, Swank HA, Consten EC, Belgers EH, et al. Laparoscopic peritoneal lavage or sigmoidectomy for perforated diverticulitis with purulent peritonitis: a multicentre, parallel-group, randomised, open-label trial. Lancet. 2015;386:1269–77.
39. Kohl A, Rosenberg J, Bock D, Bisgaard T, Skullman S, Thornell A, Gehrman J, Angenete E, Haglind E. Two-year results of the randomized clinical trial DILALA comparing laparoscopic lavage with resection as treatment for perforated diverticulitis. Br J Surg. 2018;105:1128–34.
40. Penna M, Markar SR, Mackenzie H, Hompes R, Cunningham C. Laparoscopic lavage versus primary resection for acute perforated diverticulitis: review and meta-analysis. Ann Surg. 2018;267:252–8.
41. Zeitoun G, Laurent A, Rouffet F, et al. Multicentre, randomized clinical trial of primary versus secondary sigmoid resection in generalized peritonitis complicating sigmoid diverticulitis. Br J Surg. 2000;87:1366–74.
42. Garfinkle R, Kugler A, Pelsser V, Vasilevsky CA, Morin N, Gordon P, Feldman L, Boutros M. Diverticular abscess managed with long-term definitive nonoperative intent is safe. Dis Colon Rectum. 2016;59(7):648–55.
43. Horesh N, Emile SH, Khan SM, Freund MR, Garoufalia Z, Silva-Alvarenga E, Gefen R, Wexner SD. Meta-analysis of randomized clinical trials on long-term outcomes of surgical treatment of perforated diverticulitis. Ann Surg. 2023;278(5):e966–72. https://doi.org/10.1097/SLA.0000000000005909. Epub 2023 May 30. PMID: 37249187.
44. Brolin RE, Nosher JL, Leiman S, Lee WS, Greco RS. Percutaneous catheter versus open surgical drainage in the treatment of abdominal abscesses. Am Surg. 1984;50(2):102–8. PMID: 6703514.
45. Aquina CT, Becerra AZ, Xu Z, Justiniano CF, Noyes K, Monson JRT, Fleming FJ. Population-based study of outcomes following and initial acute diverticular abscess. Br J Surg. 2019;106:467–76.
46. Lamb MN, Kaiser AM. Elective resection versus observation after nonoperative management of complicated diverticulitis with abscess: a systematic review and meta-analysis. Dis Colon Rectum. 2014;57:1430–40.
47. Gregersen, et al. Treatment of patients with acute colonic diverticulitis complicated by abscess formation: a systematic review. Int J Surg. 2016;35:201–8.

Management of Smouldering (Chronic) Diverticulitis

9

Allison J. Pang and Carol-Ann Vasilevsky

Introduction

The diagnosis and management of chronic diverticulitis, also commonly referred to as smouldering diverticulitis, remains a challenging topic for surgeons and gastroenterologists alike. Traditionally, diverticulitis has been classified as either uncomplicated or complicated. This rather simplistic view, however, has been called into question with the increasing recognition of several variations in clinical presentation, such as smouldering diverticulitis, which do not fit the traditional mold. The natural history of acute diverticulitis following an initial episode is difficult to predict and may range from complete resolution to persistence of abdominal symptoms in up to 30% of patients [1–3]. Despite this, none of the current clinical practice guidelines issued by major societies [American Society of Colon and Rectal Surgeons (ASCRS), Society of American Gastrointestinal and Endoscopic Surgeons (SAGES)] address these atypical presentations. In addition, there is a paucity of literature pertaining to these entities and the terminology used is rather confusing which renders the management more challenging.

Defining the terminology of diverticular disease remains one of the biggest challenges. Differentiating between failed medical management, recurrence, chronicity of diverticular disease, and other inflammatory processes of the bowel is what makes the management and decision making of uncomplicated diverticulitis nuanced and challenging. Furthermore, when faced with a chronically inflamed colon, such as with smouldering diverticulitis, one must always be cautious about the possibility of an underlying cancer. This chapter will focus on the definition, pathophysiology, and management of smouldering diverticulitis, and although the literature is sparse, we will use three different clinical scenarios to highlight the nuances involved in its differentiation from other atypical presentations.

Clinical Scenario #1

Alexander, a healthy 44-year-old male, presents to the emergency department with left lower quadrant abdominal pain and fever. His past medical history includes occasional smoking, hypertension, and he has an elevated body mass index (BMI). He had been treated as an outpatient 20 days ago for acute uncomplicated diverticulitis with oral antibiotics. During this second visit to the hospital, he was found to have leukocytosis and a repeat computed tomography (CT)-scan demonstrated sigmoid diverticulosis with adjacent inflammation, but no abscess, in keeping with acute uncomplicated diverticulitis. No radiologic improvement was seen compared to

A. J. Pang · C.-A. Vasilevsky (✉)
Division of Colon and Rectal Surgery, Jewish General Hospital, Montreal, QC, Canada
e-mail: allison.pang@mcgill.ca; carol-ann.vasilevsky@mcgill.ca

M. Boutros et al. (eds.), *Diverticulitis*, https://doi.org/10.1007/978-3-032-21720-2_9

his index hospital visit. A colorectal surgeon was consulted to assist in the next steps of his management.

After further questioning, the patient admits that he never really improved to his baseline status after completing the full course of antibiotics that he had been previously prescribed. Since it has only been a short time since his index episode of diverticulitis, he was admitted to hospital for a course of intravenous antibiotics on the presumption that he was experiencing persistent disease due to failure of initial outpatient conservative treatment.

Terminology

When faced with a patient with ongoing symptoms following an index episode of uncomplicated diverticulitis, it is important to define the details of the clinical presentation. Having noted that acute uncomplicated diverticulitis could be associated with a spectrum of clinical presentations, Boostrom et al. [4] proposed three separate categories to describe uncomplicated diverticulitis: acute resolving, chronic/smouldering, and atypical (Table 9.1). They defined acute resolving diverticulitis as discrete episodes of left lower quadrant pain associated with fever, leukocytosis, and radiologic evidence of inflammation that resolve with conservative treatment. Chronic/smoldering uncomplicated diverticulitis was defined as left lower quadrant pain with evidence of inflammation as manifested by a leukocytosis, fever, and CT evidence of inflammation that fails to improve with traditional antibiotic treatment or rebounds after cessation of antibiotics and lasts for at least a 3-month duration. Atypical uncomplicated diverticulitis was defined as left lower quadrant pain with possible change in bowel habits of at least 3 months without the clinical and radiographic evidence of diverticulitis. Based on this categorization, they performed a retrospective study of patients who had undergone sigmoid resection for diverticulitis. They identified 82% as acute resolving diverticulitis, 10% as chronic or smouldering diverticulitis and 8% as atypical diverticular disease. Others have described smouldering diverticulitis as chronic left-lower quadrant pain, only partially improved on antibiotics and medical therapy without fever or elevated white blood cell count [5].

Chronic smoldering diverticulitis must also be differentiated from treatment failure and recurrent disease, which can be done using an arbitrary 60-day cut off from the index attack [6, 7]. Patients who are symptomatic after 60 days of the index episode are thought to have disease recurrence, assuming that there has been a period of symptom resolution. Those who continue to be symptomatic within the 60 days are more likely to be considered as treatment failures while patients with smouldering diverticulitis never have a significant period of time without abdominal symptoms. Interestingly, since a time-based interval definition of smoldering diverticulitis has not been suggested, some authors have defined smouldering diverticulitis as a more rapid recurrence of diverticulitis than in typical patients [8]. Regardless of the definition, the patient who is thought to have smouldering diverticulitis must have radiologic or endoscopic confirmation of diverticula with no evidence of complications such as stricture, abscess, perforation, or obstruction.

As is evident, the terminology for persistent uncomplicated diverticulitis is diverse and confusing. The lack of consensus makes the clinical differentiation between recurrent, treatment

Table 9.1 Classification of uncomplicated diverticulitis [4]

Classification	Patient symptoms	Clinical findings	Radiographic findings
Acute resolving	Pain, ABH	Fever, leukocytosis	Evidence of diverticulitis
Chronic or smouldering	Pain, ABH	Fever, leukocytosis	Evidence of diverticulitis
Atypical	Pain, ABH	None	None

ABH altered bowel habits

failure, and chronic smouldering diverticulitis a challenging feat for the treating physician.

Pathophysiology

Evolving research has elucidated that diverticular disease is not necessarily a progressive, episodic disease, but rather a chronic illness with a spectrum of manifestations [1]. The commonly held traditional theory espouses that diverticulitis originates from obstruction of a diverticulum by a fecalith causing subsequent ischemia, microperforation, and infection [9, 10]. However, this theory has been repeatedly challenged by data from several uncontrolled and randomized controlled trials (RCTs) that have failed to demonstrate that antibiotics may hasten recovery or improve outcomes in patients with uncomplicated diverticulitis [11, 12]. This has led to the proposition that the pathogenesis of diverticulitis is multifactorial and includes a complex interaction of diet, lifestyle factors, medications, genetics, and dysbiosis of the gut microbiome [1, 10]. Alterations to the gut microbiome may lead to defects in the mucosal barrier leading to a chronic inflammatory process and chronic hypersensitivity symptoms. It is therefore thought that chronic diverticulitis may morphologically and clinically overlap with other entities such as irritable bowel syndrome (IBS), inflammatory bowel disease (IBD), and symptomatic uncomplicated diverticular disease (SUDD). Interestingly, SUDD is a separate manifestation of diverticular disease that has been found to have microscopic inflammation with mucosal macrophage infiltration (*see* Chap. 7) [13]. Putting all of this together, it is not surprising that patients with uncomplicated diverticulitis may not only develop smouldering disease, but they may also be at a higher risk of IBS and functional bowel disease [14].

Considerable efforts have been made to better understand why some patients with uncomplicated diverticulitis develop smouldering diverticulitis despite the lack of complicated disease, such as abscess, obstruction, or fistula. The answer may lie in the discovery of unsuspected intramural and pericolic abscesses that are not apparent on CT scans but have been found at surgery and in pathologic examination following elective sigmoid resection in patients who have had symptomatic uncomplicated diverticulitis. One of the first studies to support this finding dates back to 1990 when Moreaux and Vons [15] studied their patients diagnosed with uncomplicated diverticulitis who had undergone sigmoid colectomy for chronic abdominal symptoms. Unsuspected abscesses were discovered in one--third of these patients, while long-term results were found to be excellent in 82% of the patients who had surgery for chronic symptoms. These findings were substantiated by other studies that looked at surgical outcomes in a population of smouldering diverticular disease, which not only showed that sigmoid resection was beneficial, but that the majority also had evidence of acute on chronic mucosal inflammation. On pathologic examination, 15% of patients also had an unsuspected pericolic abscess [5]. Furthermore, Boostrom et al. [16] found unsuspected abscesses in 4% of their patients either at operation or at pathologic analysis in both the smouldering and atypical groups of patients. Moreover, a recent, large multicenter prospective study investigating the incidence of pericolic or intramural abscesses in patients undergoing elective sigmoidectomy for all types of symptomatic uncomplicated diverticular disease found that an unexpected abscess was seen in 47.5% of these patients. The proportion of patients with these abscesses was greater for those in the smouldering group. These unsuspected pericolic abscesses could therefore be the cause of persistent symptoms in smouldering diverticulitis, suggesting that it is in fact a more complicated disease process than previously thought.

Clinical Scenario #2

Three months later, Alexander comes to see his colorectal surgeon for follow-up. He has been experiencing ongoing abdominal pain and discomfort that has never fully resolved. As a result, he has not been able to return to his usual daily activities. His bowel habits have not changed since his index case of diverticulitis, but he did admit to having two episodes of rectal bleeding. Although he has CT-documented diverticulitis, he has never had a colonoscopy. He wants to know what further management can be offered other than another trial of antibiotics.

Management

Work-Up

The goal of the work-up should focus on correctly identifying a case of smouldering diverticulitis and differentiating it from other similar clinical scenarios. Initially, a detailed history must be obtained to ascertain the timing, location, and description of the abdominal pain, and antibiotic history. The evidence of diverticulitis on CT or endoscopy must also be confirmed. Evidence of inflammation on blood work can also be helpful, such as leukocytosis or an elevated C-reactive protein (CRP). Although non-diagnostic on its own, an elevated CRP (a value usually >200) has been shown to be a predictor of worse outcome in uncomplicated cases of acute diverticulitis [17–19]. An elevation also indicates the possible presence of a complication (e.g., perforation) and is associated with an increased need for intervention. Stool analysis for *C. difficile* should also be entertained since these patients have been on multiple courses of antibiotics. To ensure that one is dealing with smoldering diverticulitis, other causes of abdominal pain such as IBD, bacterial infections, ischemic colitis, and IBS must be ruled out.

It is also important to differentiate symptoms from recurrence and failure of medical management. Furthermore, one must be aware of the overlap in symptoms of chronic diverticulitis and IBS, since it may be difficult to differentiate between these two entities [20]. Performing a surgical intervention on a patient with IBS often results in poor outcomes, including persistent pain, bowel hypersensitivity, and potentially, worse overall abdominal pain compared to their pre-operative state. Adding more of a challenge, there is now a growing body of research describing a postdiverticulitis syndrome that mimics IBD. This syndrome includes a picture of low-grade inflammation, sensory-motor nerve damage, and changes in the gut microbiome (dysbiosis) [21, 22]. Two other new entities associated with diverticular disease and persistent abdominal pain have also emerged—SUDD and 'IBS-like diverticular disease'—further complicating the definition and diagnosis of smouldering diverticulitis (*See* Chap. 16). It is for this reason that there must be a careful and detailed discussion with the patient about their symptomology.

The character of the pain is a key point of discussion (Table 9.2). The pain associated with smouldering diverticulitis is often described as a low level of constant pain lasting for long periods of time versus a cramping pain that is seen in IBS. Although both diagnoses may be associated with alterations in bowel habits, constipation alternating with diarrhea is typically seen in IBS and not with smouldering diverticulitis. SUDD, on the other hand, is defined by gastrointestinal symptoms with diverticulosis, but without diagnostic evidence of inflammation. Therefore, when conventional management of diverticulitis has failed, referral to a gastroenterologist for dietary evaluation, antispasmodics, and other pharmacologic agents may be useful. Lastly, an endoscopic evaluation is important, especially in smouldering diverticulitis, as will be discussed in the next section of this chapter.

Table 9.2 Important chronic pain characteristics differentiating SUDD from IBS from smouldering diverticulitis

Pain characteristics	SUDD	IBS	Chronic/smouldering diverticulitis
Diffuse/generalized	No	Yes	No
Localized	Yes	No	Yes
Relieved by passing stool or flatulence	No	Yes	No
Wakes the patient at night	No	No	Yes
Elevation of inflammatory markers	No	No	Yes

SUDD symptomatic uncomplicated diverticular disease, *IBS* irritable bowel syndrome

Treatment

For many years, antibiotics, dietary modification, and pain control have been the mainstays of treatment for patients with acute uncomplicated diverticulitis. A formal treatment algorithm for smouldering diverticulitis, however, has not been well described, and as a result, treatment is usually dependent on the expertise and anecdotal experience of the treating physician. Surgical intervention is not usually the first choice of treatment for any type of uncomplicated diverticulitis, but it is nonetheless offered when patients develop life-altering symptoms or when they do not improve with aggressive medical management.

For the initial treatment of smouldering diverticulitis, a trial of broad-spectrum antibiotics should be exhausted prior to considering surgery. At the beginning of treatment, oral antibiotics can be started; however, if there remains no clinical improvement, treatment can be upscaled to an antibiotic with greater bioavailability, which usually requires intravenous delivery. Eventually, if there is still no resolution of symptoms, a trial of long course out-patient intravenous antibiotics could be attempted, although evidence for this is lacking. Numerous studies have demonstrated the diagnostic and prognostic value of CRP for patients with acute diverticulitis; therefore, it should be recommended that CRP be included in the evaluation of patients who are being treated for smouldering diverticulitis [23].

If antibiotic treatment is successful, the next step is the management of the chronic disease. This is done by addressing modifiable risk factors, which include poor diet (high red meat, fat, and refined grains), decreased physical activity, central obesity, smoking, and an overall lack of fiber intake [22, 24]. Several medications have also been associated with increased risk of diverticulitis, most notably nonaspirin nonsteroidal anti-inflammatory drugs (NSAIDs) and opiate analgesics, and therefore should be avoided [24]. The use of mesalamine (5-ASA) has been recommended to control inflammation that may serve as the cause for persistent symptoms. However, the most recent SAGES and European Association of Endoscopic Surgery (EAES) expert opinions came to the consensus that the use of mesalamine is not supported in the prevention of recurrent diverticulitis nor in the improvement of chronic gastrointestinal symptoms [23]. In addition, the use of rifaximin, a poorly absorbed antibiotic that achieves high luminal concentrations, is not supported by current guidelines, either when used alone or in combination with mesalamine or fiber supplements.

If conservative management fails, and the patient continues to have chronic abdominal pain, elective surgery (sigmoidectomy) should be considered and offered in the context of the patient's medical comorbidities. Several retrospective reviews have looked at the results of surgery for patients with smouldering diverticulitis and have found that complete resolution of symptoms occurred in 76.5%–89% of patients. Surgery was also found to be safe with no mortality and a low morbidity rate of 4.2% [25]. However, the authors make the point that it is important to exclude other diagnoses such as functional bowel disorders in these patients since persistent symptoms following resection were most likely related to comorbid IBS. More recently, the DIRECT trial, a large multicenter randomized controlled trial, looked at conservative management versus elective sigmoidectomy specifically in patients with recurrent or chronic diverticulitis (chronicity defined as symptoms lasting ≥3 months, or having persistent abdominal complaints, pain, or change in bowel activity) [26]. Although the trial was terminated early due to difficulties in recruitment, the gastrointestinal quality of life score at 6 months was significantly higher for the patients who had surgery, despite an anastomotic leak rate of 15%. Of the patients who were initially assigned to the conservative group, 23% ultimately crossed over and underwent elective surgery. Furthermore, at 5-year follow-up, the group that underwent surgery continued to have a higher quality of life in comparison with the nonoperative group [27]. With the increasing evidence of unsuspected abscesses in patients with smouldering diverticulitis, earlier surgical intervention may play an important role in the management of this subgroup of patients. The current data suggest that surgery is effective in alleviating persistent symptoms following uncomplicated diverticulitis; however, this decision should be individualized through shared decision making with the patient (ASCRS guideline 2020) [28].

There is also a growing understanding that the gut microbiome plays an important role in the homeostasis of colonic health [22]. Studies have shown that colonic dysbiosis can lead to a chronic inflammatory state in the colon, thereby increasing the susceptibility of the colon to infection, and potentially, to diverticular disease recurrence or persistence [22]. During a state of dysbiosis, the use of fecal microbiota transplantation (FMT) may be able to clear pathogens from the intestine and re-establish colonization with commensal gut flora. For this reason, FMT has gained wide interest in the treatment of recurrent *C. difficile* infections, and it is now deemed an established safe and effective therapy [29]. With this in mind, the application of FMT to the management of other gastrointestinal disorders, such as recurrent or persistent diverticulitis, is an interesting concept. Although the data are still lacking, a recent case study reported the successful use of FMT for the treatment of a patient with chronic diverticulitis. The authors concluded that this could become a novel approach to the treatment of refractory diverticulitis [30].

To summarize, we describe a potential treatment algorithm for smouldering diverticulitis

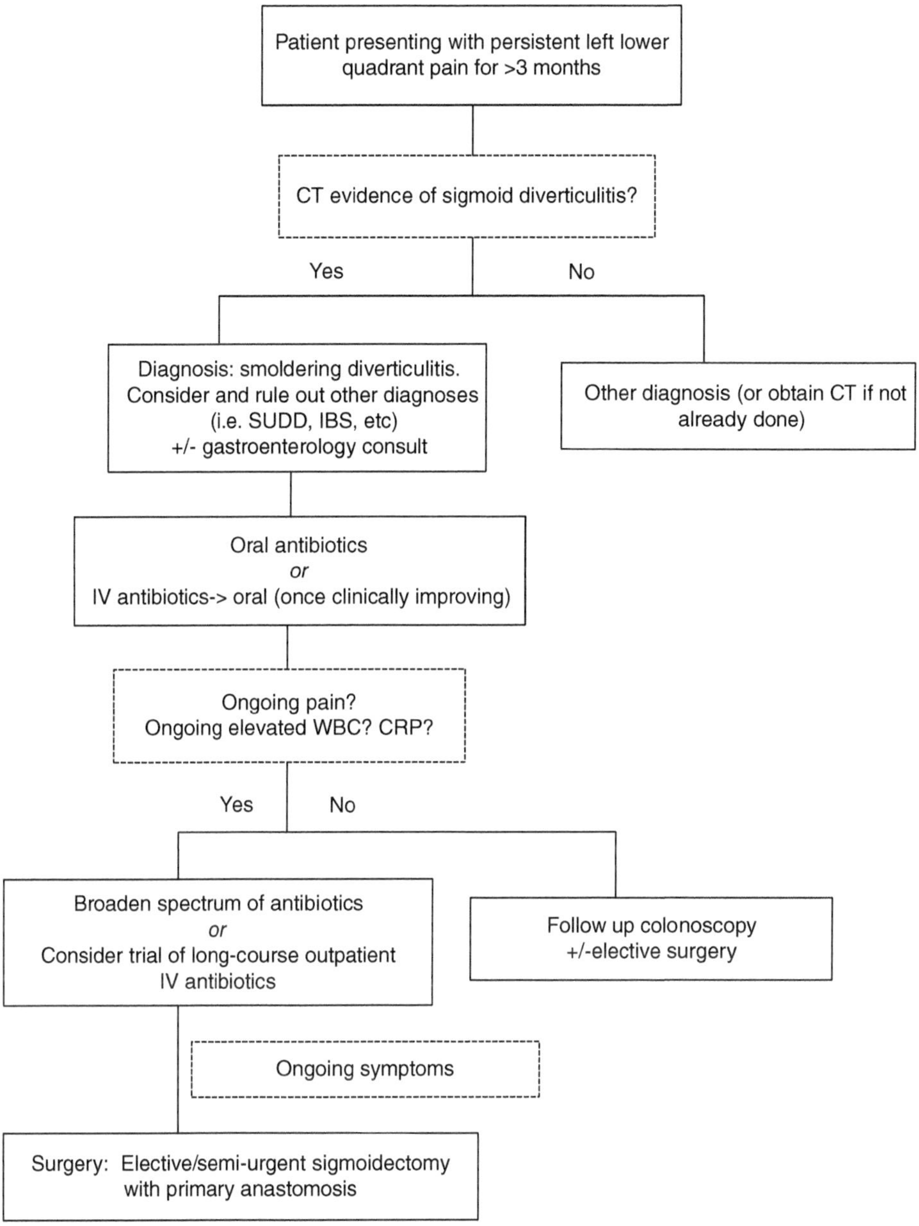

Fig. 9.1 Proposed treatment algorithm for smouldering diverticulitis

(Fig. 9.1). The first step in the management is carefully selecting the right subgroup of patients who have symptoms consistent with chronic, smouldering diverticulitis. After exhausting all other conservative treatment options (antibiotics, medications, and lifestyle changes), elective surgical resection is a safe option that yields effective results.

Scenario #3

Alexander has now experienced 6 months of ongoing left lower quadrant pain and now has altered bowel habits with the occasional blood in his stool. He has been meaning to schedule his colonoscopy, but due to scheduling issues it has been delayed. Despite modifying his diet, increasing his exercise, and stopping all use of NSAIDs, he continues to have pain that is altering his work and social life. Repeat CT scan continues to show inflammation and wall thickening of his sigmoid colon. His surgeon recommends that he have elective surgery to remove the affected piece of colon; however, before surgery, Alexander must first undergo a colonoscopy. At the time of colonoscopy, the endoscopist finds a circumferential mass in his distal sigmoid colon. Biopsies are taken and Alexander is brought back to clinic to discuss a likely new diagnosis of colon cancer.

Prevalence of Colorectal Cancer in Smouldering Diverticulitis

It remains controversial whether uncomplicated diverticulitis is a risk factor for colorectal cancer (CRC); however, the incidence of CRC is increased in the first year following diagnosis of an acute episode of diverticulitis. One study found a 4.3% incidence of CRC in a population with diverticulitis, including both uncomplicated and complicated cases, compared to 2.3% in a general population without diverticulitis [31]. Another smaller study that only looked at uncomplicated cases of diverticulitis found a 1.8% prevalence of CRC, but also found a 1.5% prevalence of advanced adenomas [32]. More recently, a large systematic review and meta-analysis of observational studies described a 1.9% pooled prevalence of CRC amongst diverticulitis cases. Although CT has a 98% accuracy of detecting diverticulitis with high sensitivity and specificity [33], this increased risk of CRC likely arises from the fact that imaging features between CRC and diverticulitis can overlap (Fig. 9.2). For this rea-

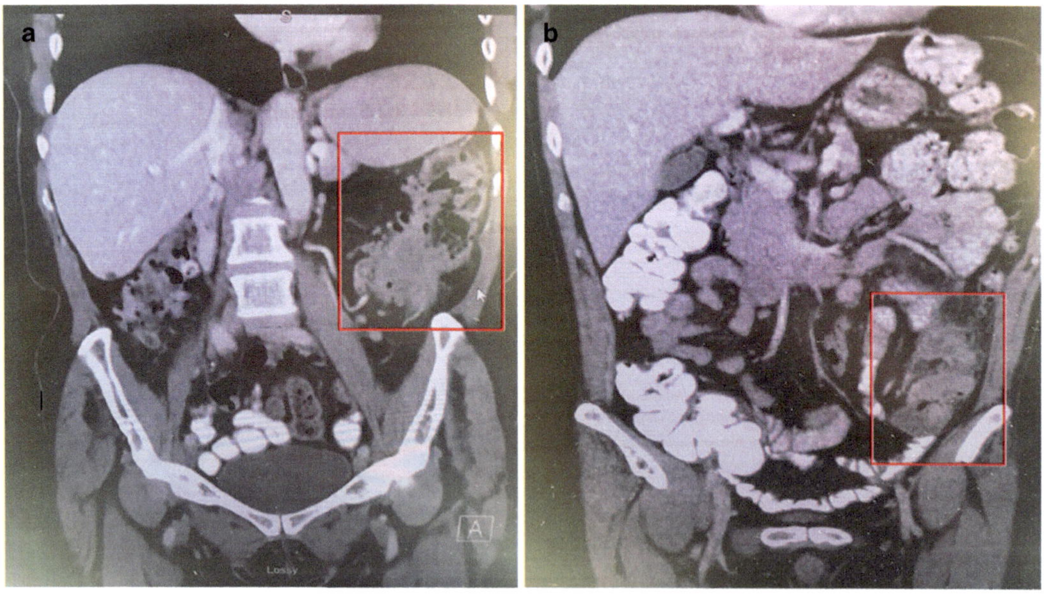

Fig. 9.2 CT images of two different patients who were diagnosed with smouldering diverticulitis and who eventually underwent elective colon resection. Pathology showed (**a**) diverticulitis (**b**) malignant tumor

son, practice guidelines from both surgical and gastrointestinal societies have recommended routine follow-up colonoscopy after an index episode of diverticulitis, specifically to exclude an occult malignancy [34, 35]. These recommendations are slowly changing and the most recent 2019 consensus (SAGES and EAES guideline) now recommend against routine colonic evaluation after successfully treated uncomplicated acute diverticulitis, unless high-risk features are present; however, the strength of this recommendation is still considered weak [23]. The most recent ASCRS Clinical Practice Guidelines recommend that patients with uncomplicated diverticulitis should undergo further assessment with colonoscopy if their clinical recovery is atypical [28].

Since smouldering diverticulitis represents only a small proportion of uncomplicated diverticulitis cases, there is limited literature available on the exact prevalence of CRC in this specific subgroup of patients. However, since we now know that smouldering diverticulitis consists of a persistent inflammatory state, which can be in itself a risk factor for cancer and is often associated with unsuspected abscesses, this subgroup of patients has the potential of being reclassified as 'complicated'. Since complicated diverticulitis has a significantly higher prevalence of misdiagnosed CRC (7.9% versus 1.9%) [36, 37], the role of colonoscopy is clearly important and the prevalence of CRC in smouldering diverticulitis may in fact be higher compared to other uncomplicated cases. Additionally, with the rise in both diverticulitis and CRC among younger patients [38–40], clinicians should be vigilant of the possibility of an occult CRC in a young patient presenting with chronic diverticulitis. Furthermore, any history of rectal bleeding should be taken seriously and prompt endoscopic evaluation.

Conclusion

Smouldering diverticulitis is a poorly defined and understood complex variation of uncomplicated diverticulitis. The persistent symptoms and inflammatory state not only affect a patient clinically but can also greatly impact a patient's quality of life. There is insufficient literature on the best practices and management of smouldering diverticulitis. We propose a stepwise approach. First, a correct diagnosis must be made based on a thorough medical history leukocytosis and elevated CRP with radiographic or endoscopic evidence of diverticulitis. Along with this, smouldering diverticulitis must be differentiated from recurrence, treatment failure, and other similar abdominal pain syndromes. Second, antibiotics should be used as initial treatment, and if there is no clinical improvement, the spectrum, route of administration, and duration of the antibiotics should be broadened. Third, if antibiotics fail, surgery should be recommended as it has been shown that elective surgery is safe and effective. Lastly, a baseline colonoscopy for every patient who is diagnosed with smouldering diverticulitis should be performed prior to surgery in order to rule out an occult malignancy.

References

1. Strate LL, Morris AM. Epidemiology, pathophysiology, and treatment of diverticulitis. Gastroenterology. 2019;156:1282–98.e1.
2. Daniels L, Unlu C, de Korte N, et al. Randomized clinical trial of observational versus antibiotic treatment for a first episode of CT-proven uncomplicated acute diverticulitis. Br J Surg. 2017;104:52–61.
3. van Dijk ST, Daniels L, de Korte N, et al. Quality of life and persistent symptoms after uncomplicated acute diverticulitis. Dis Colon Rectum. 2019;62:608–14.
4. Boostrom SY, Wolff BG, Cima RR, et al. Uncomplicated diverticulitis, more complicated than we thought. J Gastrointest Surg. 2012;16:1744–9.
5. Horgan AF, McConnell EJ, Wolff BG, et al. Atypical diverticular disease: surgical results. Dis Colon Rectum. 2001;44:1315–8.
6. Garfinkle R, Kugler A, Pelsser V, et al. Diverticular abscess managed with long-term definitive nonoperative intent is safe. Dis Colon Rectum. 2016;59:648–55.
7. Etzioni DA, Chiu VY, Cannom RR, et al. Outpatient treatment of acute diverticulitis: rates and predictors of failure. Dis Colon Rectum. 2010;53:861–5.
8. Simianu VV, Fichera A, Bastawrous AL, et al. Number of diverticulitis episodes before resection and factors associated with earlier interventions. JAMA Surg. 2016;151:604–10.

9. Simpson J, Scholefield JH, Spiller RC. Origin of symptoms in diverticular disease. Br J Surg. 2003;90:899–908.
10. Humes DJ, Spiller RC. Review article: the pathogenesis and management of acute colonic diverticulitis. Aliment Pharmacol Ther. 2014;39:359–70.
11. Chabok A, Pahlman L, Hjern F, et al. Randomized clinical trial of antibiotics in acute uncomplicated diverticulitis. Br J Surg. 2012;99:532–9.
12. Isacson D, Smedh K, Nikberg M, Chabok A. Long-term follow-up of the AVOD randomized trial of antibiotic avoidance in uncomplicated diverticulitis. Br J Surg. 2019;106(11):1542–8.
13. Barbara G, Scaioli E, Barbaro MR, et al. Gut microbiota, metabolome and immune signatures in patients with uncomplicated diverticular disease. Gut. 2017;66:1252–61.
14. Cohen E, Fuller G, Bolus R, et al. Increased risk for irritable bowel syndrome after acute diverticulitis. Clin Gastroenterol Hepatol. 2013;11:1614–9.
15. Moreaux J, Vons C. Elective resection for diverticular disease of the sigmoid colon. Br J Surg. 1990;77:1036–8.
16. Mari GM, Crippa J, Borroni G, et al. Symptomatic uncomplicated diverticular disease and incidence of unexpected abscess during sigmoidectomy: a multicenter prospective observational study. Dig Surg. 2020;37(3):199–204.
17. Jaung R, Kularatna M, Robertson JP, et al. Uncomplicated acute diverticulitis: identifying risk factors for severe outcomes. World J Surg. 2017;41:2258–65.
18. Tan JP, Barazanchi AW, Singh PP, et al. Predictors of acute diverticulitis severity: a systematic review. Int J Surg. 2016;26:43–52.
19. Kechagias A, Sofianidis A, Zografos G, et al. Index C-reactive protein predicts increased severity in acute sigmoid diverticulitis. Ther Clin Risk Manag. 2018;14:1847–53.
20. Alamo RZ, Quigley EMM. Irritable bowel syndrome and colonic diverticular disease: overlapping symptoms and overlapping therapeutic approaches. Curr Opin Gastroenterol. 2019;35:27–33.
21. Ambrosetti P. Acute left-sided colonic diverticulitis: clinical expressions, therapeutic insights, and role of computed tomography. Clin Exp Gastroenterol. 2016;9:249–57.
22. Strate LL, Modi R, Cohen E, Spiegel BM. Diverticular disease as a chronic illness: evolving epidemiologic and clinical insights. Am J Gastroenterol. 2012;107:1486–93.
23. Francis NK, Sylla P, Abou-Khalil M, et al. EAES and SAGES 2018 consensus conference on acute diverticulitis management: evidence-based recommendations for clinical practice. Surg Endosc. 2019;33:2726–41.
24. Strate LL, Liu YL, Huang ES, et al. Use of aspirin or nonsteroidal anti-inflammatory drugs increases risk for diverticulitis and diverticular bleeding. Gastroenterology. 2011;140:1427–33.
25. Wolff BG, Boostrom SY. Prophylactic resection, uncomplicated diverticulitis, and recurrent diverticulitis. Dig Dis. 2012;30:108–13.
26. van de Wall BJM, Stam MAW, Draaisma WA, et al. Surgery versus conservative management for recurrent and ongoing left-sided diverticulitis (DIRECT trial): an open-label, multicentre, randomised controlled trial. Lancet Gastroenterol Hepatol. 2017;2:13–22.
27. Bolkenstein HE, Consten ECJ, van der Palen J, et al. Long-term outcome of surgery versus conservative management for recurrent and ongoing complaints after an episode of diverticulitis: 5-year follow-up results of a multicenter randomized controlled trial (DIRECT-Trial). Ann Surg. 2019;269:612–20.
28. Hall J, Hardiman K, Lee S, et al. The American Society of Colon and Rectal Surgeons clinical practice guidelines for the treatment of left-sided colonic diverticulitis. Dis Colon Rectum. 2020;63:728–47.
29. Kelly CR, Khoruts A, Staley C, et al. Effect of fecal microbiota transplantation on recurrence in multiply recurrent Clostridium difficile infection: a randomized trial. Ann Intern Med. 2016;165:609–16.
30. Meyer DC, Hill SS, Bebinger DM, et al. Resolution of multiply recurrent and multifocal diverticulitis after fecal microbiota transplantation. Tech Coloproctol. 2020;24:971.
31. Mortensen LQ, Burcharth J, Andresen K, et al. An 18-year nationwide cohort study on the association between diverticulitis and colon cancer. Ann Surg. 2017;265:954–9.
32. Soh NYT, Chia DKA, Teo NZ, et al. Prevalence of colorectal cancer in acute uncomplicated diverticulitis and the role of the interval colonoscopy. Int J Color Dis. 2018;33:991–4.
33. Werner A, Diehl SJ, Farag-Soliman M, Duber C. Multi-slice spiral CT in routine diagnosis of suspected acute left-sided colonic diverticulitis: a prospective study of 120 patients. Eur Radiol. 2003;13:2596–603.
34. Feingold D, Steele SR, Lee S, et al. Practice parameters for the treatment of sigmoid diverticulitis. Dis Colon Rectum. 2014;57:284–94.
35. Stollman N, Smalley W, Hirano I, Committee AGAICG. American Gastroenterological Association Institute guideline on the management of acute diverticulitis. Gastroenterology. 2015;149:1944–9.
36. Lau KC, Spilsbury K, Farooque Y, et al. Is colonoscopy still mandatory after a CT diagnosis of left-sided diverticulitis: can colorectal cancer be confidently excluded? Dis Colon Rectum. 2011;54:1265–70.
37. Meyer J, Orci LA, Combescure C, et al. Risk of colorectal cancer in patients with acute diverticulitis: a systematic review and meta-analysis of observational studies. Clin Gastroenterol Hepatol. 2019;17:1448–56.e17.

38. Brenner DR, Heer E, Sutherland RL, et al. National trends in colorectal cancer incidence among older and younger adults in Canada. JAMA Netw Open. 2019;2:e198090.
39. Mauri G, Sartore-Bianchi A, Russo AG, et al. Early-onset colorectal cancer in young individuals. Mol Oncol. 2019;13:109–31.
40. Weizman AV, Nguyen GC. Diverticular disease: epidemiology and management. Can J Gastroenterol. 2011;25:385–9.

10 Emergency Surgery for Diverticulitis: From Primary Anastomosis to Damage Control Surgery

Simone Arolfo and Alberto Arezzo

Introduction

Left-sided colonic acute diverticulitis represents one of the most common diseases of surgical interest in the emergency department. Admission rates are increasing, especially in people under 40 years of age [1, 2]. An accurate diagnosis and proper risk stratification are required to identify patients who need emergency surgery for sepsis control. The Hinchey classification remains a practical tool to guide therapeutic decisions, with Hinchey 3 and 4 diverticulitis (purulent or feculent diffuse peritonitis) representing critical conditions with a mortality rate reaching 30% (see Fig. 6.1).

The clinical presentation of perforated diverticulitis can be extremely variable, ranging from pneumoperitoneum and peritonitis to frank hemodynamic instability and septic shock. In the emergency setting, it is extremely difficult to plan and execute randomized clinical trials, so clear guidelines from the literature with a high level of evidence are often lacking. Although many authors have attempted to accurately predict the indications and timing of surgery for acute complicated diverticulitis, there is minimal consensus beyond a patient with hemodynamic compromise or diffuse peritonitis, which are the two most important indicators for urgent surgery. Extracolonic air on abdominal computed tomography (CT) scan (Fig. 10.1), which has a sensitivity of 76–100% and specificity of 83–91% in detecting colonic perforation particularly when found at a distance from the site of the perforation, is a radiological sign predictive of diffuse peritonitis and was commonly considered an indication for urgent operation [4]. However, Costi et al. [3] published a series of patients with the presence of extradigestive air on CT scan who were managed safely by antibiotic therapy alone in 36 out of 39 patients. Currently, the American Society of Colon and Rectal Surgeons (ASCRS) Practice Parameters do not consider the presence of extracolonic air alone ("microperforation") as an indication for urgent surgery, as most of these patients improve with medical management [5].

This chapter is an overview on the current literature evaluating different management options for patients requiring emergency surgical treatment of complicated acute diverticulitis. Some of the topics discussed include the decision to perform a primary anastomosis after resective surgery, the use of colonic stents for obstructing disease, and the safety of laparoscopic surgery in the emergency setting. Laparoscopic lavage, which is a controversial and often debated procedure in emergency diverticulitis surgery, will be discussed separately in Chap. 12.

S. Arolfo (✉) A. Arezzo
Department of Surgical Sciences, Molinette Hospital and University of Torino School of Medicine, Turin, Italy
e-mail: simone.arolfo@unito.it; alberto.arezzo@unito.it

M. Boutros et al. (eds.), *Diverticulitis*, https://doi.org/10.1007/978-3-032-21720-2_10

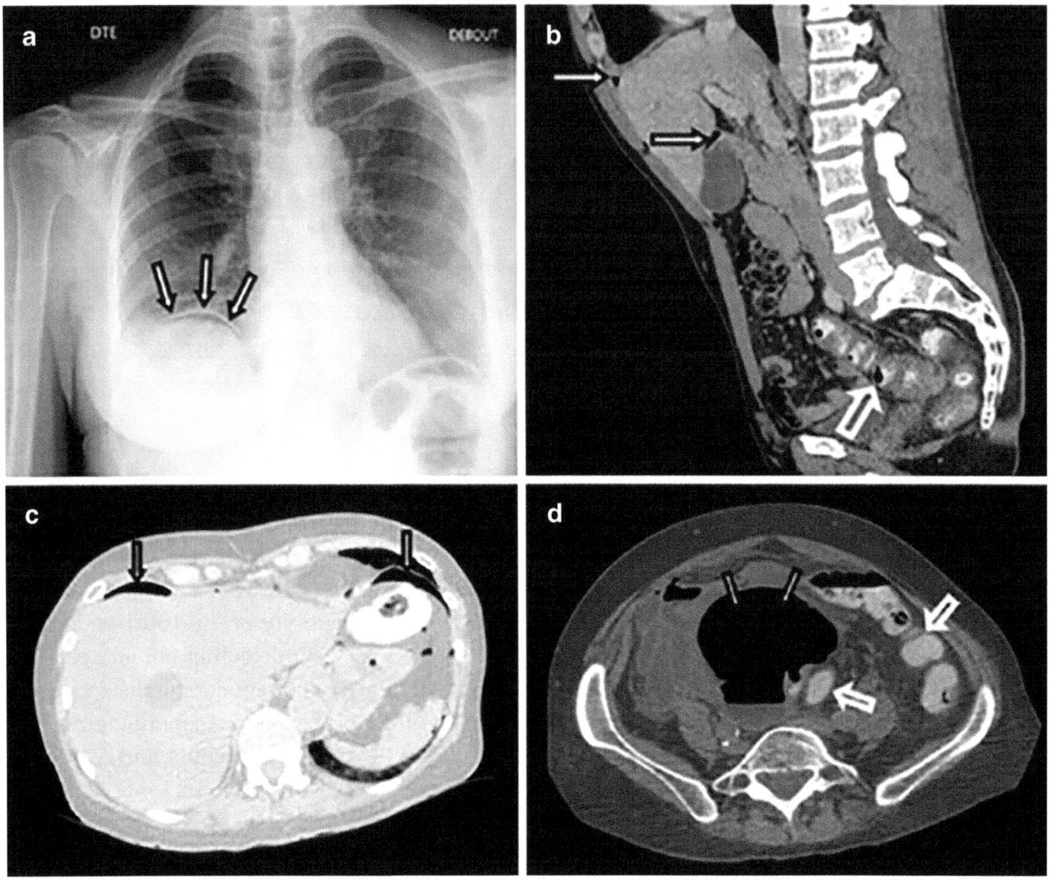

Fig. 10.1 Extracolonic air showed by X-ray (**a**) and CT scan (**b–d**). (Modified and used with permission from Costi et al. [3]. © 2012 Springer Nature)

Emergency Surgery: Options and Strategy

In a critically ill patient with a large pelvic abscess or diffuse peritonitis, it is often difficult to decide on the best operation for the patient. Typically, the most challenging question is whether or not to restore bowel continuity, balancing among other aspects the risks of anastomotic leak associated with a primary anastomosis (PA) with the low closure rate after a Hartmann's procedure (HP). The optimal surgery for perforated diverticulitis in the emergent setting is currently debated. The patient's clinical status is the most important factor to consider with regard to the type of operation performed [6].

Suture and Diversion Alone Versus Primary Resection

In the setting of purulent or feculent peritonitis with a free perforation, it is always preferable to resect the diseased segment of bowel. While once an accepted operation, ligation of the colonic perforation and diversion alone has fallen out of favor compared to primary resection, with or without fecal diversion. In a meta-analysis [7] of three studies [6, 8, 9], the pooled overall 30-day mortality rate with diversion and preservation of the perforated diseased segment of colon was 24.6% (18/73) compared to 13.6% (20/147) in the primary resection with anastomosis group. The duration of in-hospital postoperative length of stay was also lower among patients who underwent colonic resection (33 ± 3 days) compared to diversion alone (42 ± 7 days). Thus, when possible, the goal of emergency diverticulitis surgery in the setting of a free perforation should be resection of the offending segment of bowel.

Resection with Primary Anastomosis Versus Hartmann's Procedure

In 1921, Henri Hartmann proposed a new surgical procedure for rectal cancer in order to reduce the morbidity associated with an abdominoperineal resection [10]. The operation included resection of the rectosigmoid, while the distal rectum (rectal stump) and the sphincters were left in place, and a terminal colostomy was constructed in the left flank. The Hartmann's procedure (HP) was quickly adopted, not only for the treatment of rectal cancer but also for that of left-sided colonic perforations. Historically, the HP has been considered the treatment of choice in perforated left-sided colonic diverticulitis, mainly for the following reasons: (1) the splenic flexure mobilization is not required, avoiding any injury to the spleen and allowing for a shorter, simpler operation; (2) there is no anastomosis, and consequently no risk of postoperative leak and intra-abdominal fecal spillage, leading to ostensibly reduced postoperative morbidity and mortality. Indeed, a recent Japanese population-based propensity-score matched study reported higher 30-day mortality rates in the PA group without proximal diversion (9.6%) vs. HP group (7.7%) [11]. Despite these considerations, recent data support that in selected patients, sigmoid resection with PA and diverting ileostomy is associated with lower mortality compared to HP, as well as lower permanent stoma rates, lower re-intervention rates and shorter hospital stays [9, 12–14]. A recent meta-analysis [15] of 17 studies included 1060 patients: 392 who underwent a PA with diverting loop ileostomy and 624 had a HP. The level of evidence was assessed to be 2b [observational studies and low-quality randomized controlled trials (RCTs)]. Eleven studies included patients with Hinchey III–IV diverticulitis only. Overall mortality, defined as 30-day mortality after both emergency surgery and ostomy reversal rate, was 7.9% (29/366) after PA vs. 19.5% (103/529) after HP. The overall morbidity rate, defined as 30-day postoperative morbidity after both emergency surgery and ostomy reversal, was 41.1% (122/297) in PA vs. 48.8% (230/471) in HP. The morbidity rate after ostomy reversal alone was 13.5% (13/96) in PA vs. 28.6% (28/98) in HP. Reoperation rates were also significantly lower after PA (6.2%) compared with HP (16.3%), and importantly, ostomy nonreversal rates were significantly lower after PA (13.6%) than after HP (31.8%). This study was limited by the inclusion of observational studies, as there is an inherent selection bias with regard to the operation offered by a surgeon. A more recent meta-analysis of three RCTs confirmed similar findings. Acuna et al. [16] reported a similar rate of major complications (RR = 0.88, 95% CI 0.49–1.55) and post-operative mortality (RR = 0.58, 95% CI 0.20–1.70) with PA compared to HP, but were more likely to be ostomy-free at 12 months (RR = 1.40, 95% CI 1.18–1.67) and to experience fewer complications after ostomy closure (RR = 0.26, 95% CI 0.07–0.89) with a PA. These findings remained unchanged with the publication of the DIVA arm of the LADIES trial in 2019 [17], the fourth such RCT to compare these two operations. In the majority of the RCTs, the decision to perform a diverting loop ileostomy among patients who underwent PA was left to the discretion of the treating surgeon. While limited data exist, the omission of a diverting loop ileostomy appears safe [12], but the evidence is scant and highly subject to selection bias. Until stronger evidence emerges, diverting loop ileostomy should be strongly considered when PA is performed in the setting of perforated diverticulitis (Table 10.1). The European Association of Endoscopic Surgery (EAES) and SAGES recommendations are to consider sigmoid resection with PA and proximal diversion over HP in patients with Hinchey III/IV diverticulitis, in the appropriate clinical setting [18]. The ASCRS Clinical Practice Guidelines published in 2020 underline how the decision to restore bowel continuity should incorporate patient factors, intraoperative factors, and surgeon preference. Both recommendations are based on a moderate level of evidence (Fig. 10.2) [20].

Table 10.1 RCT comparing primary anastomosis (PA), primary anastomosis with diverting ileostomy (PA + DI) and Hartmann procedure (HP)

Author	Publication	Study design	Primary endpoint	Intervention strategy Hinchey III/IV diverticulitis (n)			Morbidity			Mortality			12-month stoma free survival rate		
				PA	PA + DI	HP	PRA (%)	HP (%)	*p*	PRA (%)	HP (%)	*p*	PRA (%)	HP (%)	*p*
Binda	Color Dis. 2012	RCT accrual of 15% of its sample size	Mortality/ morbidity	0	34	56	35.3	46.4	0.38	2.9	10.7	0.25	65	60	0.66
Oberkofler	Ann Surg. 2012	RCT accrual of 50% of its sample size	Morbidity	0	32	30	84	80	0.76	9	13	0.70	90	57	<0.01
Bridoux	J Am Coll Surg. 2017	RCT accrual of 42% of its sample size	Mortality	15	35	52	54	42.3	0.24	4	7.7	0.42	96	65	<0.01
Lambrichts	Lancet. 2019	RCT accrual of 55% of its sample size	12-month stoma-free survival	17	47	66	39	44	0.60	6	3	0.44	95	72	<0.01

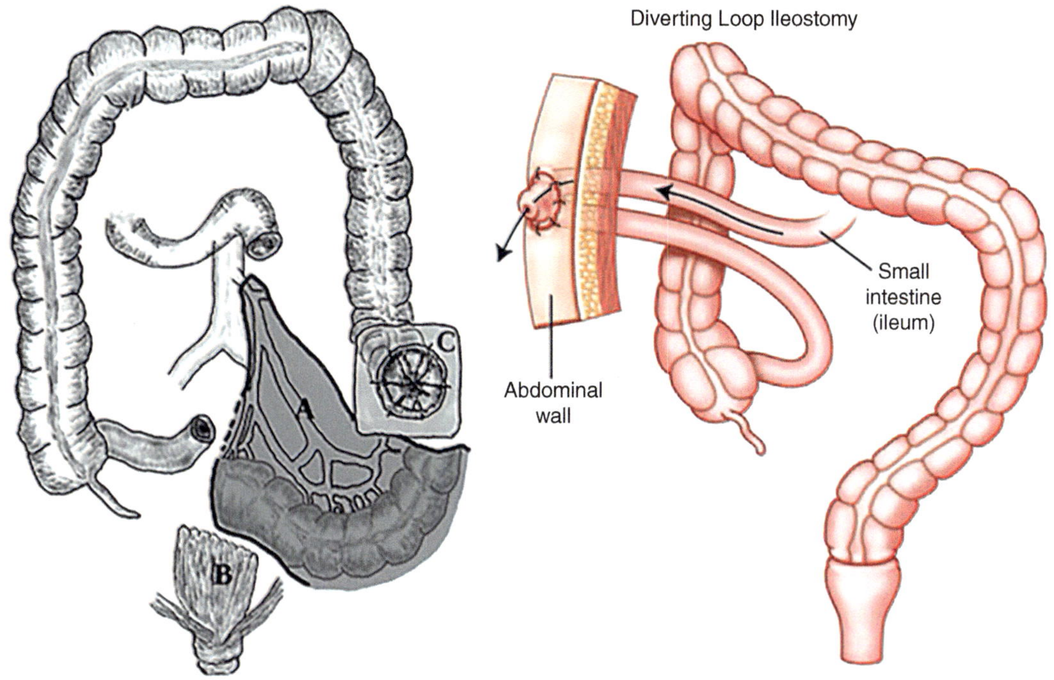

Fig. 10.2 Hartmann's procedure vs primary anastomosis and diverting ileostomy. (Used with permission from Hunt and Silviera [19])

While the pendulum has begun to swing in favor of PA, it may take some time to transition into clinical practice as the more commonly performed operation, and the HP has certainly not been abandoned. PA is a more difficult and longer operation compared to HP, and one that requires more colorectal surgical expertise. A population-based study showed that, in the United States, patients undergoing urgent surgery for left-sided diverticulitis who are admitted on a weekend have a higher risk for undergoing a HP and worse short-term outcomes compared with patients who are admitted on a weekday [21]. A statewide retrospective analysis conducted in the state of New York also showed that PA with proximal diversion for perforated diverticulitis was associated with increased postoperative morbidity and mortality when performed by general surgeons [22]. Most recently, an analysis of the American College of Surgeons (ACS) National Surgical Quality Improvement Program (NSQIP) data reported that the majority of emergency operations performed for perforated diverticulitis are HPs, with only 7.6% of cases including an anastomosis [23]. However, the study years were 2012–2016, preceding the publication of the two most recent RCTs. It will likely take several years to properly appreciate whether any shift in practice has transpired.

It is also important to use clinical judgment when operating for diverticulitis. In the setting of feculent peritonitis, septic shock, hemodynamic instability, chronic steroid therapy and poor baseline of the patient, HP may still be the most appropriate operation [24]. Despite the presence of RCT evidence to suggest short-term equivalence between patients undergoing HP and PA, there may be some unmeasured confounders biasing the conclusions from these studies. Furthermore, the two most recent studies only randomized (approximately) 50 and 65 patients to either group, respectively, and several of the RCTs were terminated early after interim analyses or due to poor recruitment. Thus, the quality

	1	2	3
Age years)	= 70	> 20	
ASA grade	I-II	III	IV
Preop. organ failure	None		One or more
Immunosuppression	No	Yes	
Ischaemic colitis	No	Yes	
Peritonitis stage	I-II	III_IV	

Fig. 10.3 Peritonitis severity score. ASA, American Society of Anesthesiologists. (Modified from Golda et al. [25])

of these trials must be scrutinized. The peritonitis severity score (PSS) (Fig. 10.3) is one assessment tool that can help in decision-making on whether to perform a PRA or an end colostomy [25]. According to PSS scoring, postoperative mortality risk was considered low for PSS 6–8, intermediate for PSS 9–11 and high for PSS scoring 12–14 [25]. Primary anastomosis may still be appropriate in some cases of limited fecal contamination, whereas an HP may be warranted with more widespread fecal contamination, especially in the presence of poor hemodynamic conditions.

As highlighted in the meta-analysis, the morbidity following Hartmann's reversal is not negligible. Hartmann's reversal is a challenging operation, with mortality rates up to 5% and morbidity rates up to 44% [26]. Furthermore, despite HP often being considered a two-stage operation, bowel continuity is not restored in a significant number of patients, ranging from 53% [27] to 59% [28]. These data come from selected centers with high experience in colorectal surgery, but the nationwide reversal rates are probably even lower in all European, US, and Canadian hospitals. In addition to the technical difficulties of Hartmann's reversal, the majority of these patients are old and frail, with several medical morbidities, increasing the risk of post-reversal anastomotic leakage and other morbidities. Therefore, perhaps the HP should be regarded as a one-stage operation, keeping in mind that less than 50% of patients undergo reversal. For all of the reasons listed above, we believe that HP should be reserved for select patients who are critically ill or when intraoperative findings do not allow for a safe primary anastomosis.

Damage Control Surgery

Patients with severe sepsis and hemodynamic impairment represent a surgical dilemma. Surgery is mandatory to remove the septic focus, but at the same time may worsen hemodynamic and physiologic balance. In critically ill patients, a complete and definitive operation may not be advisable. In the early 1980s, the concept of damage control surgery was introduced in trauma surgery. It centers on an abbreviated initial laparotomy, whereby the goal of surgery is to only control contamination and hemorrhage. Once this is achieved, the abdomen is temporarily closed with one of several possible methods, and the patient is resuscitated in the Intensive Care Unit. Once hemodynamic stability and normal physiology are restored, a planned second-look operation is performed, with definitive repair. This simple concept significantly improved outcomes in critically ill trauma patients [29] and was introduced in the management of critically ill patients with abdominal sepsis with encouraging results [30].

In patients affected by complicated acute diverticulitis who are hemodynamically unstable, damage control strategies (resection without anastomosis, temporary closure and second look) should be considered. This would include a limited resection of the diseased colon (leaving the remaining colon stapled-off in situ without reconstruction or ostomy maturation), temporary vacuum-assisted abdominal closure, followed by definite reconstruction at a second surgery 24–48 h later. Other authors have performed colonic resection with colostomy maturation in all cases (HP), avoiding leaving the remaining colon stapled off in situ. Nevertheless, they managed the abdomen with temporary closure and planned a second look within 48 h [31]. Temporary closure is usually achieved by means of a vacuum device (ABThera™) (Fig. 10.4). A protective layer is placed in the open abdomen

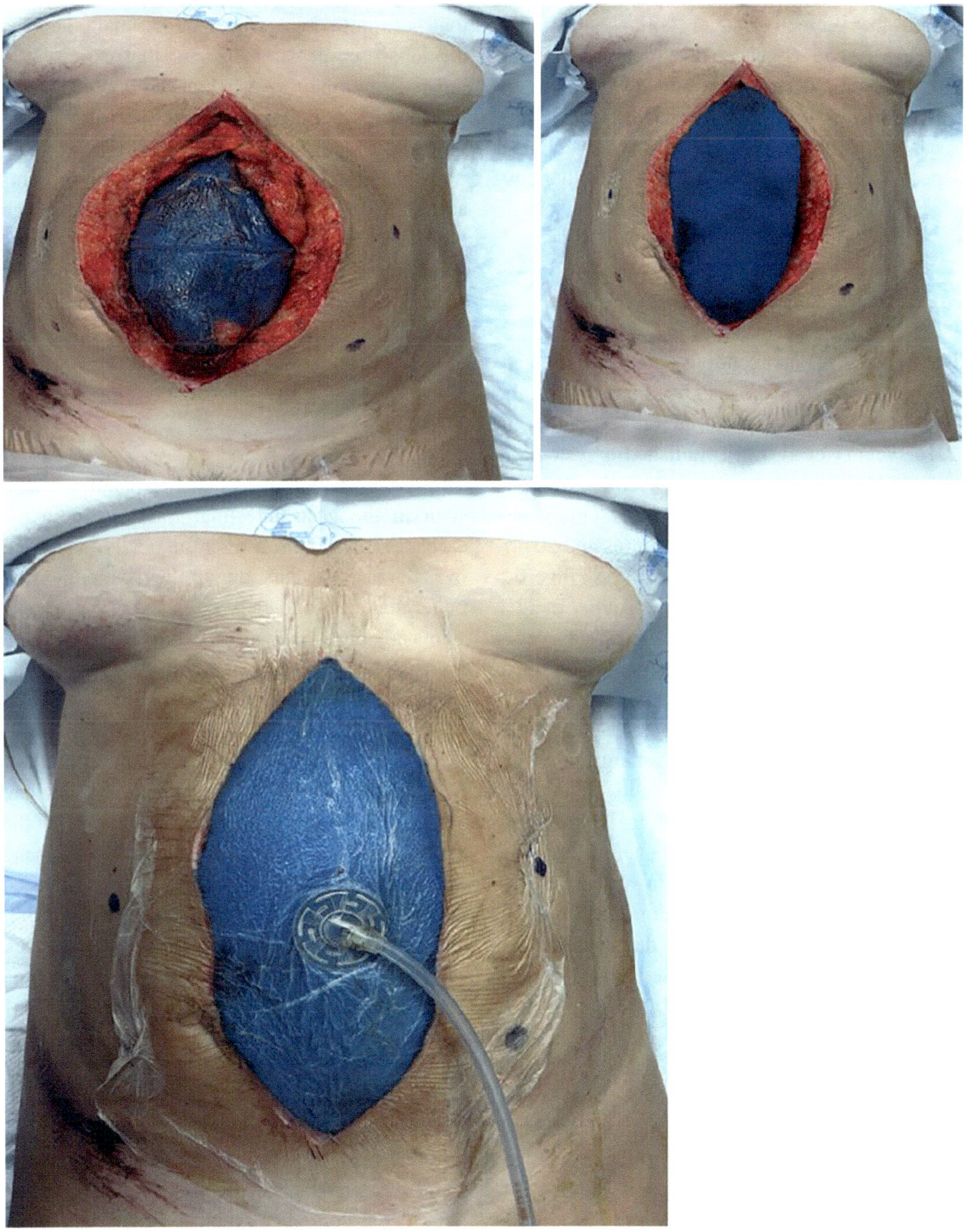

Fig. 10.4 Vacuum-assisted closure ABThera™. Open abdomen negative pressure therapy. (Used with permission from Khasawneh and Zielinskiu [32]. © 2016 Springer Nature)

close to the viscera and covered by a foam connected to the vacuum. When negative pressure is applied, the foam transfers negative pressure from the therapy unit to the visceral protective layer. Exudate and infectious material throughout the abdomen are removed. At the same time, the perforated foam and the encapsulated foam within the protective layer collapse medially, drawing fascial edges closer together, helping minimize fascial retraction and loss of domain. The use of negative-pressure devices for temporary abdominal closure, as well as other technical aspects of damage control surgery, is further covered in Chap. 11.

Minimally Invasive Surgery

The benefits of laparoscopic surgery in elective colorectal surgery have also been apparent in the emergency setting of perforated diverticulitis. In 2016, Vennix et al. [33] published a systematic review of retrospective studies collecting 104 patients who underwent laparoscopic emergency resections (84 Hartmann's procedures and 20 primary anastomoses) with Hinchey 3 or 4 diverticulitis. They reported an overall morbidity of 21% with no reports of anastomotic leaks, an overall mortality of 2.9%, and a conversion rate up to 20%. Several other individual retrospective studies have compared laparoscopic versus open resections in the emergency setting, reporting comparable morbidity and mortality [34, 35] or lower morbidity and mortality in laparoscopic group [36–38]. One consistent benefit of laparoscopy in these observational data was the reduction in length of hospital stay compared to open surgery (6–7 days versus 8.5–9 days). Care must be taken when interpreting these data as some of these series may be affected by selection bias, including patients with a lower grade of peritonitis in the laparoscopic group compared to the open group [37, 39]. In 2017, a Cochrane review was published including 392 patients from 3 trials [40]. There was little or no difference in length of hospital stay, postoperative pain, 30-day postoperative mortality, early overall morbidity, major and minor complications, surgical complications, postoperative times to liquid and solid diets, and reoperations due to anastomotic leak. The authors concluded that evidence to support or refute the safety and effectiveness of laparoscopic surgery versus open surgical resection for the treatment of patients with acute diverticular disease is insufficient. Furthermore, they stress that peritonitis brings on specific challenges for the laparoscopic surgeon, and that expertise in laparoscopy and diverticular colorectal resections is required to safely perform these procedures.

Laparoscopic Hartmann's reversal represents a feasible option even after an open HP. Although the level of evidence is low, a laparoscopic approach is feasible option in centers with high expertise, which is discussed in more detail in Chap. 21.

Stents

The experimental use of self-expanding metal stent in the gastrointestinal tract began in the early 1990s. Their use dramatically increased over the last 30 years, due to the development of better materials and endoscopic expertise. Plastic stents are almost only used in pancreatic and biliary duct decompression. In the gastrointestinal tract, self-expanding metallic stent (SEMS) are widely used, in order to obtain a more effective decompression (Fig. 10.5). The main property of SEMS is shape memory: unexpanded SEMS are small enough to enter the operative channel of the endoscope and once delivered, they expand through a deployment device and are placed against the luminal surface of interest. Several materials are available, including stainless steel, elgiloy, and nitinol, the latter being the most commonly used because of its flexibility [42].

SEMS represent a valuable therapeutic option in malignant large bowel obstruction, both for palliative and for bridge to surgery purposes. Conversely, the role of SEMS in colonic obstruction due to benign stricture, including diverticular disease, is unclear. In the presence of acute left-sided colonic benign obstruction, only small case series reporting the use of SEMS are avail-

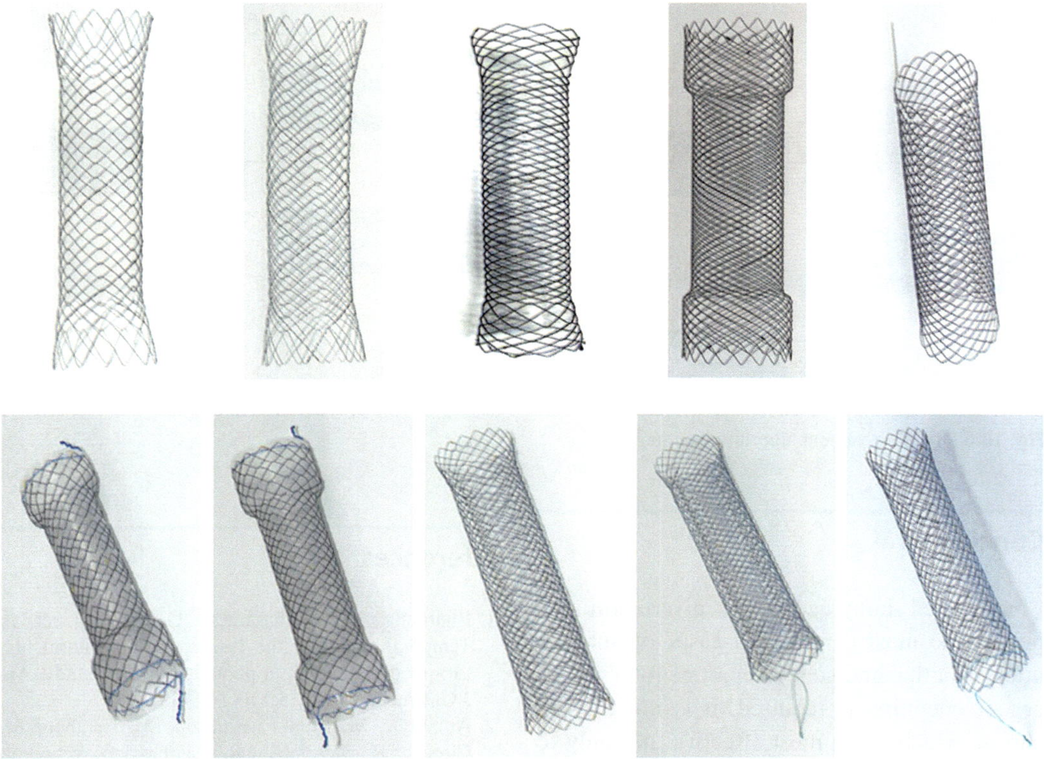

Fig. 10.5 Market available self-expanding metal stent. (Reused with permission from Baron [41])

able in the literature. Paul et al. [43] placed a colonic stent in two cases of acute diverticulitis complicated by a large abscess. The abscess resolved in both cases, but both developed a colonic fistula. Meisner et al. [44] published a series of 38 patients with acute colonic obstruction, of which eight patients had benign strictures. These eight patients accounted for several of the reinterventions, and only three patients truly gained benefit from stenting. Small et al. [45] published a series of 23 patients with benign obstructive disease treated with SEMS placement. The clinical success rate was 95%, but the major complication rate, including migration, reobstruction, and perforation, was 38%. A recent meta-analysis [46] reported 122 cases of benign colorectal strictures treated with SEMS placement, of which 64 cases were due to diverticular disease. For palliative procedures, clinical success was achieved in 54/68 (79%), whereas clinical success occurred in 44/54 (81%) patients in the bridge to surgery group. The most common reasons for clinical failure were perforation (10 patients), persisting obstruction in the presence of a technically successful stent (eight patients) and excessive pain after insertion (three patients). SEMS for benign lesions remains a matter of debate but has been included in some treatment algorithms in the US (Fig. 10.6). Based on the current data, SEMS can be an option for the management of benign colorectal obstructive lesions as a bridge to surgery in good surgical candidates, or as definitive treatment in patients at risk for surgery. Its role is limited for benign strictures, especially in the emergency setting, due to the reported high complications rate. Upfront surgery remains the standard of care in left-sided complicated colonic diverticulitis, but SEMS placement can be considered in extremely selected patients.

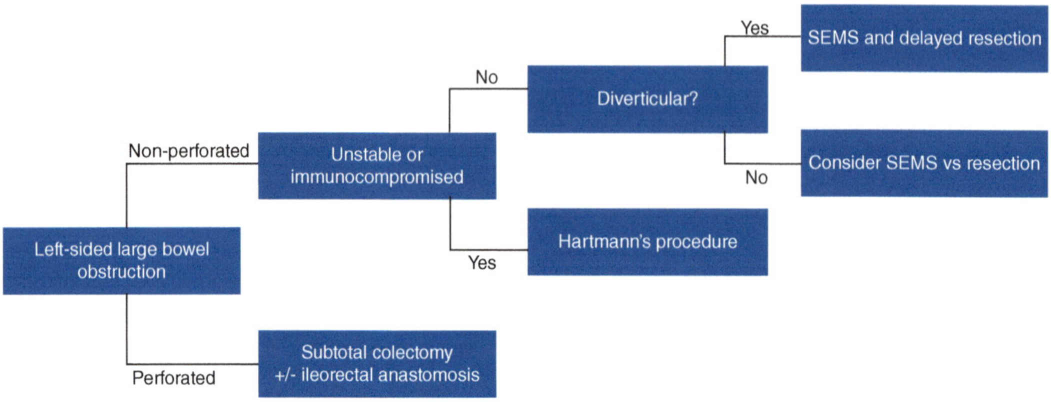

Fig. 10.6 SEMS treatment algorithms in the US

Conclusion

Complicated left-sided acute diverticulitis is one of the most common diseases of surgical interest in the emergency department. When an urgent operation is required, it is not easy to choose which is the most effective, not only to avoid mortality but also to warrant a good quality of life in the long term. Literature suggests that resection with primary anastomosis and diverting ileostomy represents the treatment of choice whenever patient's clinical condition and surgical expertise allow to do that. In patients with septic shock, abbreviated laparotomy and second look (damage control surgery) seem to be a valuable option. Hartmann's procedure remains a life-saving operation, but stoma reversal rate is extremely low and burdened by high morbidity, so that HP should be considered a one-stage operation. In case of large bowel obstruction due to diverticular stricture, a self-expanding metal stent as bridge to surgery could be an option, even if strong evidence is still lacking. A tailored treatment following these principles depicts the modern good clinical practice in emergency surgery for acute diverticulitis.

References

1. Bharucha AE, Parthasarathy G, Ditah I, et al. Temporal trends in the incidence and natural history of diverticulitis: a population-based study. Am J Gastroenterol. 2015;110(11):1589–96.
2. Amato A, Mataloni F, Bruzzone M, Carabotti M, Cirocchi R, Nascimbeni R, Gambassi G, Vettoretto NP, Pinnarelli L, Cuomo R, Annibale B, Fontana V, Binda GA. Hospital admission for complicated diverticulitis is increasing in Italy, especially in younger patients: a national database study. Tech Coloproctol. 2020;24(3):237–45.
3. Costi R, Cauchy F, Le Bian A, Honart JF, Creuze N, Smadja C. Challenging a classic myth: pneumoperitoneum associated with acute diverticulitis is not an indication for open or laparoscopic emergency surgery in hemodynamically stable patients. A 10-year experience with a nonoperative treatment. Surg Endosc. 2012;26:2061–71.
4. Gielens MPM, Mulder IM, van der Harst E, Gosselink MP, Kraal KJ, Teng HT, Lange F, Vermeulen J. Preoperative staging of perforated diverticulitis by computed tomography scanning. Tech Coloproctol. 2012;16:363–8.
5. Feingold D, Steele SR, Lee S, Kaiser A, Boushey R, Buie WD, Rafferty JF. Practice parameters for the treatment of sigmoid diverticulitis. Dis Colon Rectum. 2014;57(3):284–94.
6. Finlay IG, Carter DC. A comparison of emergency resection and staged management in perforated diverticular disease. Dis Colon Rectum. 1987;30:929–33.

7. Cirocchi R, Trastulli S, Desiderio J, Listorti C, Boselli C, Parisi A, Noya G, Liu L. Treatment of Hinchey stage III-IV diverticulitis: a systematic review and meta-analysis. Int J Color Dis. 2013;28(4):447–57.
8. Nagorney DM, Adson MA, Pemberton JH. Sigmoid diverticulitis with perforation and generalized peritonitis. Dis Colon Rectum. 1985;28:71–5.
9. Kronborg O. Treatment of perforated sigmoid diverticulitis: a prospective randomized trial. Br J Surg. 1993;80:505–7.
10. Ronel D, Hardy M. Henri Albert Hartmann: labor and discipline. Curr Surg. 2002;59:59–64.
11. Tsuchiya A, Yasunaga H, Tsutsumi Y, et al. Mortality and morbidity after Hartmann's procedure versus primary anastomosis without a diverting stoma for colorectal perforation: a nationwide observational study. World J Surg. 2018;42:866–75.
12. Bridoux V, Regimbeau JM, Ouaissi M, Mathonnet M, Mauvais F, Houivet E, Schwarz L, Mege D, Sielezneff I, Sabbagh C, Tuech JJ. Hartmann's procedure or primary anastomosis for generalized peritonitis due to perforated diverticulitis: a prospective multicenter randomized trial (DIVERTI). J Am Coll Surg. 2017;225(6):798–805.
13. Oberkofler CE, Rickenbacher A, Raptis DA, Lehmann K, Villiger P, Buchli C, Grieder F, Gelpke H, Decurtins M, Tempia-Caliera AA, Demartines N, Hahnloser D, Clavien PA, Breitenstein S. A multicenter randomized clinical trial of primary anastomosis or Hartmann's procedure for perforated left colonic diverticulitis with purulent or fecal peritonitis. Ann Surg. 2012;256(5):819–27.
14. Binda GA, Karas JR, Serventi A, Sokmen S, Amato A, Hydo L, Bergamaschi R, for the Study Group on Diverticulitis. Primary anastomosis vs nonrestorative resection for perforated diverticulitis with peritonitis: a prematurely terminated randomized controlled trial. Color Dis. 2012;14:1403–10.
15. Gachabayov M, Oberkofler CE, Tuech JJ, Hahnloser D, Bergamaschi R. Resection with primary anastomosis vs nonrestorative resection for perforated diverticulitis with peritonitis: a systematic review and meta-analysis. Color Dis. 2018;20:753–70.
16. Acuna SA, Wood T, Chesney TR, Dossa F, Wexner SD, Quereshy FA, Chadi SA, Baxter NN. Operative strategies for perforated diverticulitis: a systematic review and meta-analysis. Dis Colon Rectum. 2018;61(12):1442–53.
17. Lambrichts DPV, Vennix S, Musters GD, Mulder IM, Swank HA, Hoofwijk AGM, Belgers EHJ, Stockmann HBAC, Eijsbouts QAJ, Gerhards MF, van Wagensveld BA, van Geloven AAW, Crolla RMPH, Nienhuijs SW, Govaert MJPM, di Saverio S, D'Hoore AJL, Consten ECJ, van Grevenstein WMU, Pierik REGJM, Kruyt PM, van der Hoeven JAB, Steup WH, Catena F, Konsten JLM, Vermeulen J, van Dieren S, Bemelman WA, Lange JF, LADIES Trial Collaborators. Hartmann's procedure versus sigmoidectomy with primary anastomosis for perforated diverticulitis with purulent or faecal peritonitis (LADIES): a multicentre, parallel-group, randomised, open-label, superiority trial. Lancet Gastroenterol Hepatol. 2019;4(8):599–610.
18. Francis NK, Sylla P, Abou-Khalil M, Arolfo S, Berler D, Curtis NJ, Dolejs SC, Garfinkle R, Gorter-Stam M, Hashimoto DA, Hassinger TE, Molenaar CJL, Pucher PH, Schuermans V, Arezzo A, Agresta F, Antoniou SA, Arulampalam T, Boutros M, Bouvy N, Campbell K, Francone T, Haggerty SP, Hedrick TL, Stefanidis D, Truitt MS, Kelly J, Ket H, Dunkin BJ, Pietrabissa A. EAES and SAGES 2018 consensus conference on acute diverticulitis management: evidence-based recommendations for clinical practice. Surg Endosc. 2019;33(9):2726–41.
19. Hunt SR, Silviera ML. Anastomotic construction. In: Steele S, Hull T, Read T, Saclarides T, Senagore A, Whitlow C, editors. The ASCRS textbook of colon and rectal surgery. Springer; 2016.
20. Hall J, Hardiman K, Lee S, Lightner A, Stocchi L, Paquette IM, Steele SR, Feingold DL, Prepared on behalf of the Clinical Practice Guidelines Committee of the American Society of Colon and Rectal Surgeons. The American Society of Colon and Rectal Surgeons clinical practice guidelines for the treatment of left-sided colonic diverticulitis. Dis Colon Rectum. 2020;63(6):728–47.
21. Worni M, Schudel IM, Østbye T, et al. Worse outcomes in patients undergoing urgent surgery for left-sided diverticulitis admitted on weekends vs weekdays: a population-based study of 31 832 patients. Arch Surg. 2012;147(7):649–55.
22. Goldstone RN, Cauley CE, Chang DC, Kunitake H, Ricciardi R, Bordeianou L. The effect of surgical training and operative approach on outcomes in acute diverticulitis: should guidelines be revised? Dis Colon Rectum. 2019;62(1):71–8.
23. Lee JM, Bai P, Chang J, El Hechi M, Kongkaewpaisan N, Bonde A, Mendoza AE, Saillant NN, Fagenholz PJ, Velmahos G, Kaafarani HM. Hartmann's procedure vs primary anastomosis with diverting loop ileostomy for acute diverticulitis: nationwide analysis of 2,729 emergency surgery patients. J Am Coll Surg. 2019;229(1):48–55.
24. Biondo S, Lopez Borao J, Millan M, Kreisler E, Jaurrieta E. Current status of the treatment of acute colonic diverticulitis: a systematic review. Color Dis. 2012;14:e1–e11.
25. Golda T, Kreisler E, Rodriguez G, Miguel B, Biondo S. From colorectal to general surgeon in the management of left colonic perforation: a cohort study. Int J Surg. 2018;55:175–81.
26. Vermeulen J, Coene PP, Van Hout NM, Van Der Harst E, Gosselink MP, Mannaerts GH, Weidema WF, Lange JF. Restoration of bowel continuity after surgery for acute perforated diverticulitis: should Hartmann's procedure be considered a one-stage procedure? Color Dis. 2009;11:619–24.
27. Hallam S, Mothe BS, Tirumulaju R. Hartmann's procedure, reversal and rate of stoma-free survival. Ann R Coll Surg Engl. 2018;100(4):301–7.

28. Horesh N, Lessing Y, Rudnicki Y, Kent I, Kammar H, Ben-Yaacov A, Dreznik Y, Tulchinsky H, Avital S, Mavor E, Wasserberg N, Kashtan H, Klausner JM, Gutman M, Zmora O. Considerations for Hartmann's reversal and Hartmann's reversal outcomes—a multicenter study. Int J Color Dis. 2017;32:1577.
29. Chovanes J, Cannon JW. Nunez TC the evolution of damage control surgery. Surg Clin N Am. 2012;92(4):859–75.
30. Waibel BH, Rotondo MF. Damage control for intra-abdominal sepsis. Surg Clin N Am. 2012;92(2):243–57.
31. Cirocchi R, Arezzo A, Vettoretto N, et al. Role of damage control surgery in the treatment of Hinchey III and IV sigmoid diverticulitis: a tailored strategy. Medicine (Baltimore). 2014;93(25):e184.
32. Khasawneh MA, Zielinskiu MD. Optimum methods for keeping the abdomen open. Curr Trauma Rep. 2016;2:189–95.
33. Vennix S, Boersema GS, Buskens CJ, Menon AG, Tanis PJ, Lange JF, Bemelman WA. Emergency laparoscopic sigmoidectomy for perforated diverticulitis with generalised peritonitis: a systematic review. Dig Surg. 2016;33(1):1–7.
34. Rea JD, Herzig DO, Diggs BS, Cone MM, Lu KC. Use and outcomes of emergent laparoscopic resection for acute diverticulitis. Am J Surg. 2012;203(5):639–43.
35. Zdichavsky M, Kratt T, Stüker D, Meile T, Feilitzsch MV, Wichmann D, Königsrainer A. Acute and elective laparoscopic resection for complicated sigmoid diverticulitis: clinical and histological outcome. J Gastrointest Surg. 2013;17:1966.
36. Vennix S, Lips DJ, Di Saverio S, van Wagensveld BA, Brokelman WJ, Gerhards MF, van Geloven AA, van Dieren S, Lange JF, Bemelman WA. Acute laparoscopic and open sigmoidectomy for perforated diverticulitis: a propensity score-matched cohort. Surg Endosc. 2016;30(9):3889–96.
37. Letarte F, Hallet J, Drolet S, Boulanger-Gobeil C, Bouchard A, Grégoire RC, Gagné JP, Thibault C, Bouchard P. Laparoscopic versus open colonic resection for complicated diverticular disease in the emergency setting: a safe choice? A retrospective comparative cohort study. Am J Surg. 2015;209(6):992–8.
38. Turley RS, Barbas AS, Lidsky ME, Mantyh CR, Migaly J, Scarborough JE. Laparoscopic versus open Hartmann procedure for the emergency treatment of diverticulitis: a propensity-matched analysis. Dis Colon Rectum. 2013;56(1):72–82.
39. Titu LV, Zafar N, Phillips SM, Greenslade GL, Dixon AR. Emergency laparoscopic surgery for complicated diverticular disease. Color Dis. 2009;11:401–4.
40. Abraha I, Binda GA, Montedori A, Arezzo A, Cirocchi R. Laparoscopic versus open resection for sigmoid diverticulitis. Cochrane Database Syst Rev. 2017;11(11):CD009277.
41. Baron TH. Technique of colonic stenting. Tech Gastrointest Endosc. 2014;16:108–11.
42. Kim EJ, Kim YJ. Stents for colorectal obstruction: past, present, and future. World J Gastroenterol. 2016;22(2):842–52.
43. Paúl L, Pinto I, Gómez H, Fernández-Lobato R, Moyano E. Metallic stents in the treatment of benign diseases of the colon: preliminary experience in 10 cases. Radiology. 2002;223:715–22.
44. Meisner S, Hensler M, Knop FK, West F, Wille-Jørgensen P. Self-expanding metal stents for colonic obstruction: experiences from 104 procedures in a single center. Dis Colon Rectum. 2004;47(4):444–50.
45. Small AJ, Young-Fadok TM, Baron TH. Expandable metal stent placement for benign colorectal obstruction: outcomes for 23 cases. Surg Endosc. 2008;22:454–62.
46. Currie A, Christmas C, Aldean H, Mobasheri M, Bloom IT. Systematic review of self-expanding stents in the management of benign colorectal obstruction. Color Dis. 2014;16:239–45.

11 The Sick Patient: Feculent Peritonitis

Michael S. Truitt, Muhammad Ghanem, and Karalyn R. Bentley

Introduction

The cause of diverticulitis is thought to be inflammatory or infectious in nature. It is one of the most common causes of abdominal pain, contributing to over 312,000 hospital admissions in the United States alone [1]. Diverticulitis is no longer solely a disease of the Western world. Right--sided diverticulitis is typically more common in Asian countries; however, left-sided diverticulitis is increasing in incidence, due, in part, to the pervasiveness of the Western diet [2]. Diverticulosis, and subsequently diverticulitis, has an age-dependent distribution. Approximately two-thirds of the general population will have diverticulosis by the age of 85 [3], and the incidence of diverticulitis in younger patients is increasing [4]. Management of patients with feculent peritonitis differs from that of patients with uncomplicated diverticulitis. Patients with feculent peritonitis frequently have multiple comorbidities, often present in critical condition, and universally need operative intervention. The most commonly performed procedure for the treatment of feculent peritonitis is a Hartmann's procedure [5]. However, more recently, studies have shown a decreasing role of Hartmann's procedure [6, 7]. In addition to surgery, high-quality perioperative care, including fluid resuscitation, hemodynamic support, and antibiotic treatment, is an important aspect of management and has contributed to positive patient outcomes.

Clinical Presentation

Diverticula are outpouchings of the mucosa through the muscularis propria. The colon is predisposed to develop diverticulosis at the weakest points in the bowel wall, namely, where the vasa recta penetrate the circular muscle layer [8]. Diverticula of the colon are false diverticula as they do not contain all layers of the bowel wall. Pulsion diverticula typically form as a result of increased intraluminal pressure, which leads to herniation of the mucosa.

Not all patients with diverticulosis develop diverticulitis. The vast majority of diverticulosis patients remain asymptomatic throughout their lifetime; estimates indicate <5% of patients develop symptoms [9]. Those who develop diverticulitis classically present with abdominal pain usually located in the left lower quadrant of the abdomen, with fever and leukocytosis often accompanying these symptoms. A contained, or walled-off, perforation presents as a paracolic

M. S. Truitt (✉)
Department of Surgery, TCU School of Medicine, Medical City Plano, Plano, TX, USA

M. Ghanem
Orlando Health Weight Loss and Bariatric Surgery Institute, Orlando, FL, USA

K. R. Bentley
Baton Rouge General Hospital, Advanced Robotics Institute of Louisiana, Baton Rouge, LA, USA

M. Boutros et al. (eds.), *Diverticulitis*, https://doi.org/10.1007/978-3-032-21720-2_11

abscess. Clinically, these patients have abdominal pain, fever, and localized peritonitis along with leukocytosis. Imaging of the abdomen shows a paracolic abscess with no or minimal free air. The abscess can progress to purulent peritonitis if it ruptures and subsequently progresses to feculent peritonitis if fecal spillage occurs [10]. Progression to complicated diverticulitis occurs in fewer than 25% of patients, and a small portion of these develop feculent diverticulitis [11]. Such patients present with abdominal pain and an acute abdomen with diffuse peritonitis. Hemodynamic instability and septic shock can follow.

Diagnosis

The diagnosis of feculent diverticulitis is challenging and can sometimes only be made in the operating theater. Morbidly obese patients can be particularly challenging, as peritonitis may not be present on exam. Immunosuppressed patients, including those with organ transplantation, may not develop signs of sepsis until late in their presentation. Patients with end-stage renal disease may also require special consideration. Diagnosis of a patient with suspected diverticulitis starts with an initial evaluation, including a thorough history and physical exam, a complete blood count, urinalysis, and plain abdominal films. Patients with feculent peritonitis benefit from plain abdominal films as they are easily obtained, noninvasive, low cost, and may demonstrate free intraperitoneal air.

Commonly, diverticulitis patients undergo computerized tomography (CT), which is highly sensitive and specific [12]; oral or rectal contrast can further enhance sensitivity and can aid in distinguishing a free perforation from a sealed perforation. While a CT scan can be a helpful modality, hemodynamically unstable patients should not be assessed in this manner. Additionally, the acquisition of a CT scan should not delay operative intervention. A history typical of diverticulitis, along with pneumoperitoneum on abdominal films in a critically ill patient, should prompt timely operative intervention. A diagnosis of feculent peritonitis is confirmed in the operating room by the presence of fecal matter in the peritoneal cavity along with a thickened and edematous colon and associated diverticula. The culprit diverticulum can often be difficult to identify in purulent diverticulitis; however, a frank bowel perforation is often observed with feculent diverticulitis.

Treatment

General Intervention Guidelines

Patients with peritonitis and associated diverticulitis should be treated expeditiously. Any delay in treatment can have a significant impact on morbidity and mortality. Unnecessary diagnostic testing should be eschewed. Treatment should be initiated with intravenous (IV) antibiotics (Gram--negative/anaerobic bacteria) and fluid resuscitation as soon as the diagnosis is made. Patients with feculent diverticulitis/peritonitis should undergo immediate operative intervention. Traditionally, the surgical procedure of choice is a Hartmann's procedure, which involves resection of the diseased and perforated segment of the colon with a proximal end colostomy. Hartmann's procedure remains the gold standard and is considered the safest and most prudent approach in the unstable patient [11]. Other surgical options to consider when treating a patient with feculent diverticulitis are resection and primary anastomosis with proximal diversion [13] or damage control surgery [14]. Resection and primary anastomosis without diversion is not typically indicated in feculent diverticulitis and has been associated with worse outcomes [15]. A laparoscopic approach in the hemodynamically stable patient has been demonstrated to decrease overall complications [15]. The World Society of Emergency Surgery (WSES) suggest performing an emergency laparoscopic sigmoidoscopy only if technical skills and equipment are available (weak recommendation base on low-quality evidence, 2C) [16]. A surgeon skilled in laparoscopy with a patient sufficiently stable to tolerate pneumoperitoneum may benefit from a laparoscopic

Hartmann's resection or sigmoid resection with primary anastomosis and proximal diversion [17]. Laparoscopy should be eschewed in the hypotensive patient requiring intraoperative resuscitation or vasopressors. In the setting of Hinchey IV diverticulitis, the diseased colon is unlikely to be treated with drain placement or diversion alone due to the presumed size of the perforation in the bowel wall. Appropriate intervention must be tailored to the individual patient; failure to do so is likely to negatively impact outcomes.

A Hartmann's procedure resects the perforated segment of the colon to provide source control. An end colostomy avoids the morbidity associated with a primary anastomosis in the context of peritoneal spillage and hemodynamic instability. An end colostomy is usually performed through a midline laparotomy, mobilizing the sigmoid colon from the retroperitoneum along the white line of toldt in a typical lateral-to--medial approach. The proximal margin does not need to include every diverticulum, but should be composed of soft, healthy colon devoid of induration. The distal margin should be at the rectosigmoid junction distal to where the taenia coalesce at the sacral promontory; however, in the emergency setting in an unstable patient, limiting the resection to the acutely affected segment of bowel is acceptable [15]. Mobilization of the left colon and splenic flexure should only be performed as necessary to mature an end colostomy. If the proximal end of the colon reaches the abdominal wall easily and without tension, then this step is unnecessary and may disrupt tissue planes for subsequent colostomy reversal. The left ureter should be identified and preserved. Preoperative placement of ureteral stents does not decrease the incidence of ureteral injury, but it may help identify the injury when it occurs [18]. Ureteral stent placement may not be feasible in the acute setting and should not delay operative intervention in the unstable patient. The use of indocyanine green and subsequent visualization with near infrared light is a recent development that may aid in the identification of the ureter. Thorough irrigation is performed for all cases, and a drain may be left in the peritoneal cavity at the surgeon's discretion. There is no significant evidence to support the use or disuse of drains in the setting of perforated diverticulitis [17, 19]. Although a HP is the gold standard in a patient with feculent peritonitis, recent literature has focused on the morbidity of the subsequent colostomy care or takedown. Wound infection, anastomotic leak, and abdominal wall hernias are not uncommon and must be considered in the holistic evaluation of which operation to employ. Reversal procedures can be challenging, and some patients may best be served with a permanent colostomy.

Primary Anastomosis and Diverting Loop Ileostomy in Hinchey IV Diverticulitis?

Given the morbidity of a traditional Hartmann's procedure, recent attention has focused on identifying a procedure with similar upfront results and decreased late morbidity. As a result, some have advocated for primary anastomosis with proximal diversion (ileostomy) in select patients. Studies have indicated similar rates of short-term morbidity [13, 20]; however, the ostomy reversal rate is demonstrably higher with a loop ileostomy than with an end colostomy [20], and the morbidity is slightly lower. However, care must be taken when interpreting the results of recent RCTs comparing primary anastomosis and diverting loop ileostomy to Hartmann's procedure, as the majority of the patients included in these trials had Hinchey III disease at the time of operative exploration [21]. A patient with normal to mildly altered hemodynamics, a small degree of fecal contamination, and a younger age may be considered for this operation. In contrast, a patient with significantly altered physiology and hemodynamic instability is not an ideal candidate for an anastomosis, and an HP or damage control surgery should be strongly considered. Emergent resection of the colon is associated with significant risks. The procedural complication rate can be as high as 65% and includes respiratory and cardiac morbidities [22]. Risk factors significantly associated with increased morbidity and mortality include age, shock, delay in operative treatment, and increased operative duration [22]. Together, these factors highlight the importance of timely intervention in patients with Hinchey IV diverticulitis. According to the WSES guidelines, Hartmann's procedure should be performed for managing diffuse peritonitis in critically ill patients and in select patients with multiple comorbidities (strong recommendation based on low-quality evidence (2B)). In critically ill patients, the WSES suggests primary resection with anastomosis with or without a diverting stoma (weak recommendation based on low--quality evidence (2B)) [17]. According to the ASCRS guidelines, following resection, the decision to restore bowel continuity should incorporate patient factors and surgeon preference (strong recommendation based on moderate quality evidence (1B)) [23].

Damage Control Surgery

Damage control surgery (DCS) is another approach for patients with Hinchey IV diverticulitis presenting in extremis. DCS was initially described following severe abdominal injury in trauma. However, the concepts of staged laparotomy can be applied to any patient who is too physiologically deranged to tolerate typical operative strategies.

The five principles of DCS are as follows [24]:

Phase 0: Triage
Phase 1: Damage control surgery (source control only without anastomosis)
Phase 2: Intensive care unit (ICU) resuscitation
Phase 3: Definitive surgery (restoration of continuity)
Phase 4: Closure of abdominal wall/fascia

Indications for DCS include hypothermia, coagulopathy, tissue ischemia (pH $<$ 7.2; base deficit $>$15; lactate $>$5 mmol/L), large volume resuscitation, inability to close the abdomen due to tissue edema, and arrhythmias [25]. Operative intervention should be expeditious. Contamination is controlled by resecting the perforated colon and leaving the bowel in discontinuity. An anastomosis is not performed at the index operation, and an ostomy may not be mature. The peritoneal cavity is then lavaged, and the abdomen is left open or temporarily closed with a vacuum closure device (KCI AbThera™) (Figs. 11.1, 11.2, 11.3, and 11.4). WSES guidelines suggest DCS with staged laparotomies in select unstable patients with diffuse peritonitis due to diverticular perforation (weak recommendation based on low-quality evidence (2C)) [16].

Definitive intervention includes restoring continuity of the bowel or maturing ostomies with abdominal closure and is typically performed 24–48 h after the initial DCS. The specific timing of the follow-up procedure is dependent on the patient's physiologic status. While leaving the

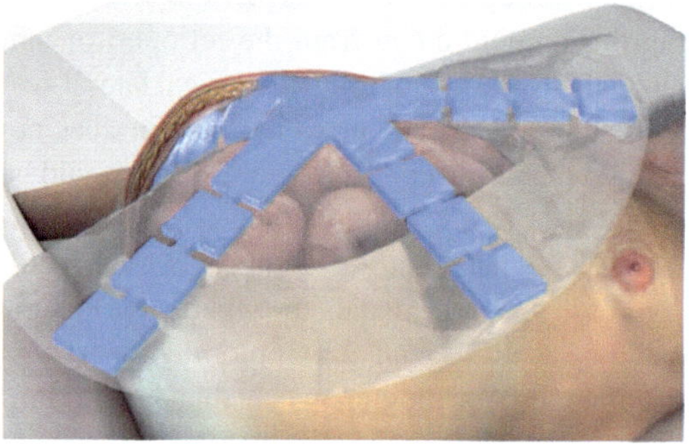

Fig. 11.1 Application of the ABThera™ Open Abdomen NPT System. Place the ABThera drape. (Reused with permission from Shah and Chiu [26]. © 2021 Springer Nature)

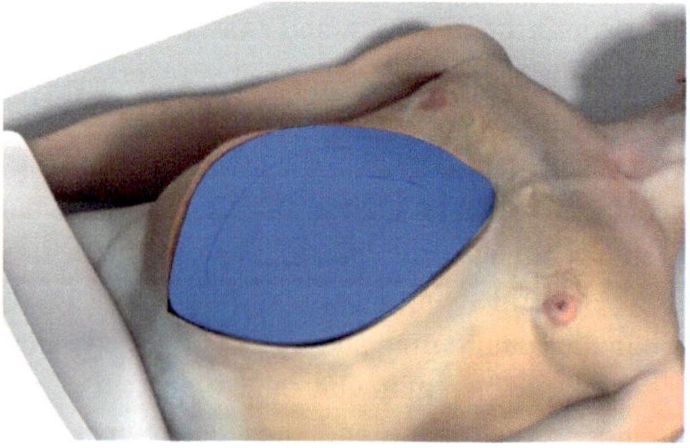

Fig. 11.2 Application of the ABThera™ Open Abdomen NPT System. Size and position the perforated foam. (Reused with permission from Shah and Chiu [26]. © 2021 Springer Nature)

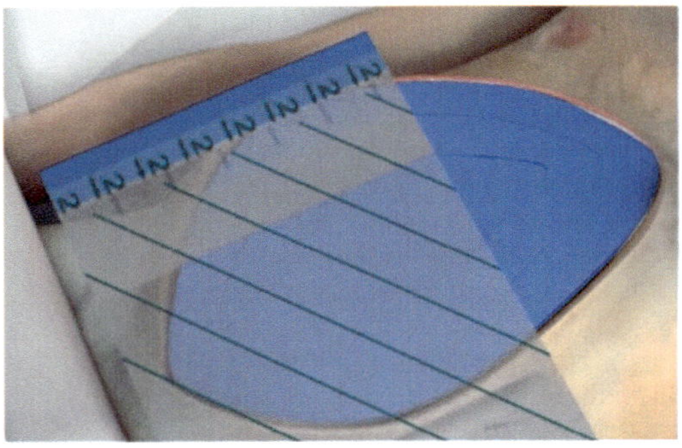

Fig. 11.3 Application of the ABThera™ Open Abdomen NPT System. Drape and seal the dressing. (Reused with permission from Shah and Chiu [26]. © 2021 Springer Nature)

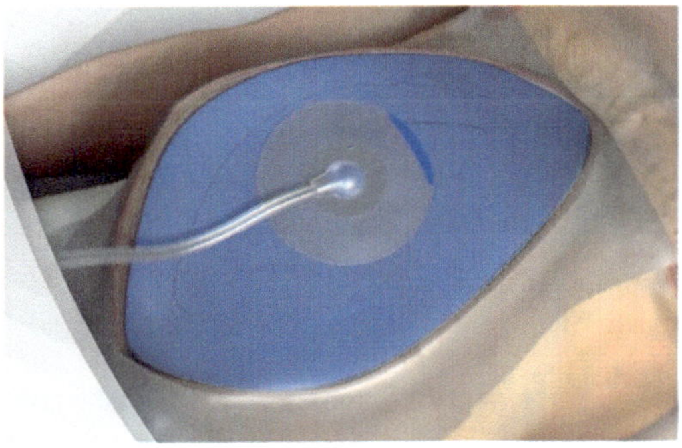

Fig. 11.4 Application of the ABThera™ Open Abdomen NPT System. Connect and start negative pressure suction. (Reused with permission from Shah and Chiu [26]. © 2021 Springer Nature)

abdomen open can be beneficial in allowing for repeated irrigation of the abdomen with reassessment of the bowel, it can lead to additional morbidity if not carefully managed. Complications include fluid loss, fistula formation, and loss of domain [27]. If 1–2 washouts are required, the associated risks are small and clinically insignificant; however, when a patient requires multiple washouts or the abdomen is too tense to close safely, several options may be considered. The temporary patch closure and utilization of a negative pressure wound device with sequential primary fascial closure with interrupted sutures are two valid options in patients requiring multiple washouts. The patch involves suturing a Velcro® sheet to each edge of the fascia and abdominal wall (Fig. 11.5). The medial portion of the patch

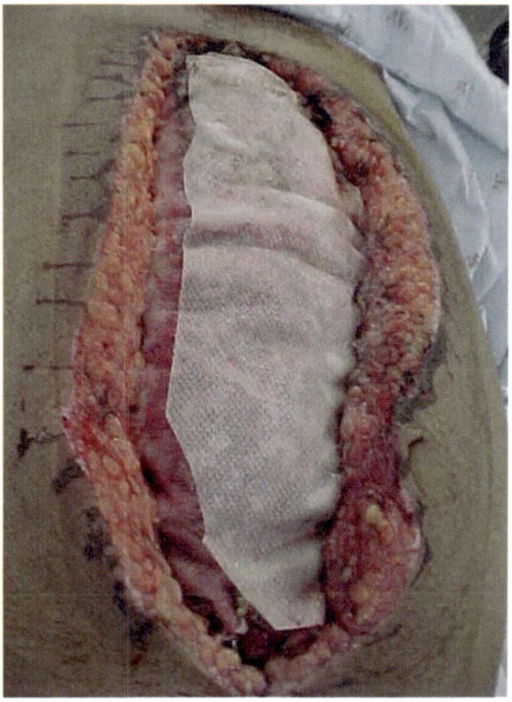

Fig. 11.5 Temporary patch closure. Velcro sheet is sutured to each edge of the fascia and abdominal wall

consists of a Velcro®-like material, facilitating gradual approximation of the edges through readjustment while maintaining fascial tension. Similarly, a wound vacuum applies negative pressure to the edges of the fascia in order to maintain tension and facilitate closure. Without a concentrated effort to maintain tension on the fascia, rapid loss of abdominal domain with retraction of the fascial edges will ensue. This makes fascial closure increasingly difficult and increases the risk of fistula. Patients with an open abdomen are typically managed in the intensive care unit (ICU). The presence of an open abdomen in and of itself is not an indication for mechanical ventilation or a contraindication to enteral nutrition. Patients are typically taken back to the operating room every 24–48 h, wherein the patch is tightened, the negative pressure dressing is exchanged, and sequential interrupted suture closure is performed. Some studies have reported a high primary fascial closure rate with the use of a wound vacuum device, along with lower 30-day mortality [28]. One study has pointed to better outcomes for the Wittmann patch (temporary foreign body) in the absence of sepsis, the wound vac technique was preferred in the presence of abdominal sepsis [29].

The abdomen is definitively closed at the earliest opportunity, but is dictated by patient physiology and time. It may require more than one trip to the operating room, and the surgeon must avoid the temptation to close the fascia under excessive tension and precipitate abdominal compartment syndrome [30]. Multiple methods can be used to close the abdomen. Primary closure of the fascia when feasible is often the best course as it is the simplest method with the lowest complication rate [31]. If the fascial edges cannot be safely approximated, two important principles must be considered: time and tension. With time and tension on the fascia, most patients can obtain primary fascial closure, and the remainder will be left with a significantly smaller wound (Figs. 11.6, 11.7, and 11.8). Tension can be facilitated by the Whitman patch and vacuum assist device as described above. Another option is the abdominal re-approximation anchor system, or ABRA® (Surgical Innovation) (Fig. 11.9). This is a device that uses the same concept of time and pressure to slowly approximate the fascial edges. It consists of elastomers that are anchored through the full thickness of the abdominal wall, hence keeping constant tension on both edges and preventing the fascia from retracting. This can be tightened gradually, allowing for gradual re-approximation of the fascial edges, and eventual closure. One retrospective study showed that combining the ABRA® with a vacuum closure device achieved closure in 92% of patients [33]. Another demonstrated 100% fascial closure rates using a technique that involved placing sutures to keep the fascia under tension and an occlusive dressing [34]. In the rare case when the physician cannot obtain reapproximation of the fascia using the techniques above, the skin should be closed over the viscera whenever possible. This method guarantees a hernia but decreases the risk of enteroatmospheric fistula. If the overlying skin cannot be closed, a split thickness skin graft applied directly to the bowel is a

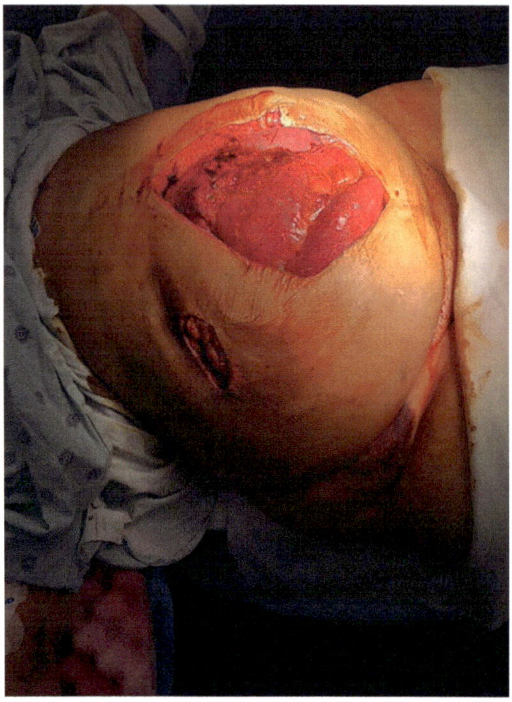

Fig. 11.6 Open abdomen closure

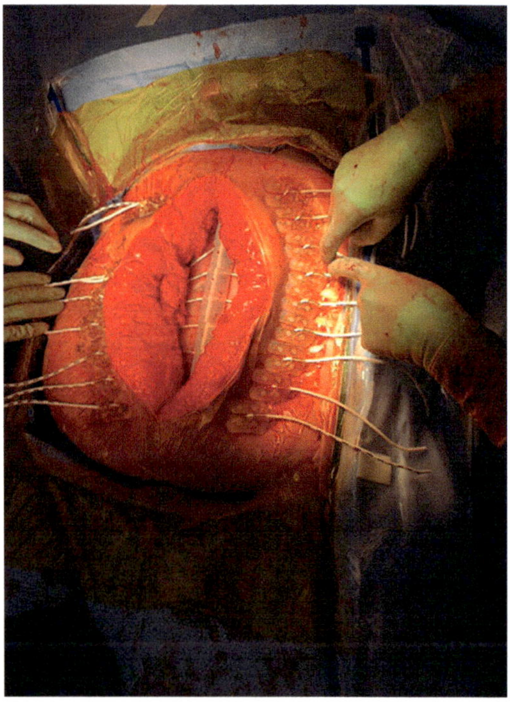

Fig. 11.7 Progressive fascial closure

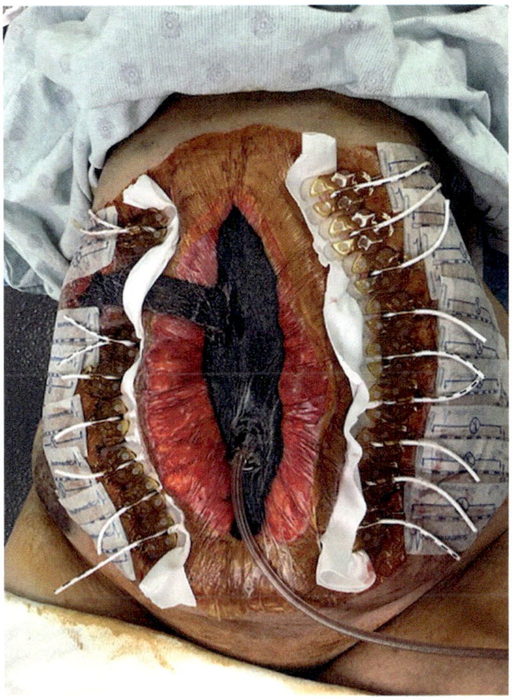

Fig. 11.8 Progressive fascial closure with negative pressure therapy

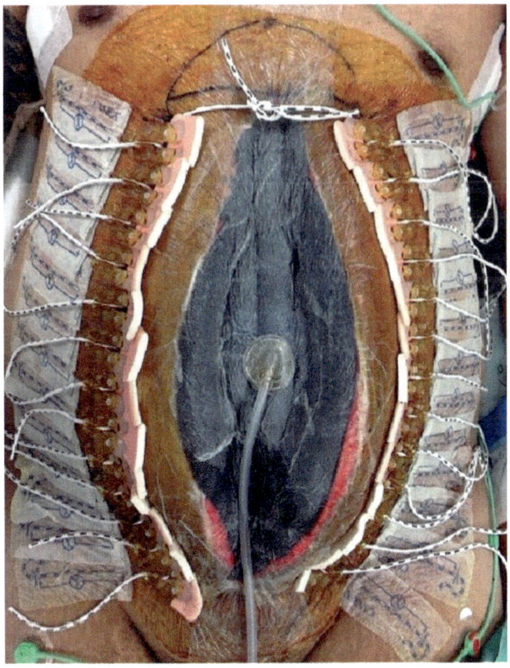

Fig. 11.9 Abdominal re-approximation anchor device with overlying vacuum-assisted closure dressings in situ. (Used with permission from Okullo et al. [32]. Copyright © 2017, Sage Publications)

final consideration. It can be tempting to employ the silver bullet of abdominal wall reconstruction, a component separation (CS), in the acute setting. However, CS should almost never be used during the index hospitalization as it has inferior results in the acute setting. In addition, it can only be performed once and should be preserved for definitive hernia repair once the primary disease process has resolved.

The first randomized controlled trial regarding DCS in 2020 concluded that damage control surgery in perforated diverticulitis Hinchey III and IV enhances the reconstruction of bowel continuity and can reduce the stoma rate at discharge [35].

Complications

DCS can be associated with a spectrum of complications, and hence it is extremely important to achieve closure of the abdomen when possible. This includes enteroatmospheric fistula, intra-abdominal abscesses, fascial retraction, and the formation of adhesions. This needs to be weighed against early overaggressive closure of the abdomen that can lead to intra-abdominal hypertension (IAH) and subsequently abdominal compartment syndrome (ACS). IAH is classified based on the intra-abdominal pressure (IAP):

1. Grade 1: 12–15 mmHg
2. Grade 2: 16–20 mmHg
3. Grade 3: 21–25 mmHg
4. Grade 4: ˃ 25 mmHg

ACS is defined as IAP of more than 20 mmHg associated with end-organ dysfunction [29]. Bladder pressures are used to mirror the IAPs. Early management of IAH includes fluid restriction, decompression of the abdomen with a nasogastric tube, removal of excess fluid if present (e.g., paracentesis), laying the patient flat, and neuromuscular blockade. ACS eventually develops as a result of decreased venous return, and urgent surgical decompression is required [36].

Reversal of a Hartmann's colostomy can be a challenging procedure, as there are often adhesions from the previous peritonitis. The earliest this procedure should be performed is 6–8 weeks after the HP, and often much later. A colonoscopy should be done through the colostomy to ensure the absence of synchronous malignancy. Also, a rectal stump barium enema or endoscopic evaluation is advised to ensure the rectal stump is intact and there are no strictures or other pathology. This can also provide valuable information on the length of the rectal stump; a very low anastomosis is associated with complications, including higher morbidity, decreased quality of life, higher leak rate, and increased bowel movements [37].

Conclusions

Patients with feculent peritonitis often present with significant baseline comorbidities and septic shock. Management of the patient should be expeditious, concentrating initially on resuscitation with IV fluid and antibiotics, followed by expeditious operative intervention. The gold standard for patients with feculent diverticulitis remains a Hartmann's procedure. Other operative interventions, such as primary anastomosis with diversion and laparoscopy, may be considered based on the surgeon's skill and the physiologic status of the patient. DCS is a lifesaving tool when indicated. Closure of the abdomen is performed as soon as physiology is restored, and bowel viability is confirmed. Surgeon skill and patient/disease factors are paramount in obtaining the best possible outcomes in the patient with feculent diverticulitis.

References

1. Kozak LJ, DeFrances CJ, Hall MJ. National hospital discharge survey: 2004 annual summary with detailed diagnosis and procedure data. Vital Health Stat. 2006;13:1–209.
2. Fischer MG, Farkas AM. Diverticulitis of the cecum and ascending colon. Dis Colon Rectum. 1984;27:454.
3. Parks TG. Natural history of diverticular disease of the colon. Clin Gastroenterol. 1975;4:53.
4. Etzioni DA, Mack TM, Beart RW, Kaiser AM. Diverticulitis in the United States: 1998–2005: changing patterns of disease and treatment. Ann Surg. 2009;249:210.
5. Cirocchi R, Trastulli S, Desiderio J, Listorti C, Boselli C, Parisi A, Noya G, Liu L. Treatment of Hinchey stage III-IV diverticulitis: a systematic review and meta-analysis. Int J Color Dis. 2013;28(4):447–57. https://doi.org/10.1007/s00384-012-1622-4. Epub 2012 Dec 15.
6. Horesh N, Emile SH, Khan SM, et al. Meta-analysis of randomized clinical trials on long-term outcomes of surgical treatment of perforated diverticulitis. Ann Surg. 2023;278(5):e966–72. https://doi.org/10.1097/SLA.0000000000005909. Epub 2023 May 30. PMID: 37249187.
7. Nascimbeni R, Amato A, Cirocchi R, et al. Management of perforated diverticulitis with generalized peritonitis. A multidisciplinary review and position paper. Tech Coloproctol. 2021;25(2):153–65. https://doi.org/10.1007/s10151-020-02346-y. Epub 2020 Nov 5. PMID: 33155148; PMCID: PMC7884367.
8. Meyers MA, Alonso DR, Gray GF, Baer JW. Pathogenesis of bleeding colonic diverticulosis. Gastroenterology. 1976;71(4):577–83.
9. Strate LL, Morris AM. Epidemiology, pathophysiology, and treatment of diverticulitis. Gastroenterology. 2019;156:1282–1298.e1. https://doi.org/10.1053/j.gastro.2018.12.033.
10. Moore FA, Moore EE, Burlew CC, et al. Western Trauma Association critical decisions in trauma: management of complicated diverticulitis. J Trauma Acute Care Surg. 2012;73(6):1365–137.
11. Morris AM, Regenbogen SE, Hardiman KM, Hendren S. Sigmoid diverticulitis: a systematic review. JAMA. 2014;311(3):287–97. https://doi.org/10.1001/jama.2013.282025.
12. Ambrosetti P, Jenny A, Becker C, Terrier TF, Morel P. Acute left-colonic diverticulitis: compared performance of computed tomography and water-soluble contrast: prospective evaluation of 420 patients. Dis Colon Rectum. 2000;43(10):1363–7.
13. Bridoux V, Regimbeau JM, Ouaissi M, et al. Hartmann's procedure or primary anastomosis for generalized peritonitis due to perforated diverticulitis: a prospective multicenter randomized trial (DIVERTI). J Am Coll Surg. 2017;225:798.
14. Cirocchi R, Arezzo A, Vettoretto N, et al. Role of damage control surgery in the treatment of Hinchey III and IV sigmoid diverticulitis: a tailored strategy. Medicine (Baltimore). 2014;93(25):e184. https://doi.org/10.1097/MD.0000000000000184.
15. Francis NK, Sylla P, Abou-Khalil M, et al. EAES and SAGES 2018 consensus conference on acute diverticulitis management: evidence-based recommendations for clinical practice. Surg Endosc. 2019;33(9):2726–41. https://doi.org/10.1007/s00464-019-06882-z. Epub 2019 Jun 27. PMID: 31250244; PMCID: PMC6684540.

16. Sartelli M, Weber DG, Kluger Y, et al. 2020 update of the WSES guidelines for the management of acute colonic diverticulitis in the emergency setting. World J Emerg Surg. 2020;15(1):32. https://doi.org/10.1186/s13017-020-00313-4. PMID: 32381121; PMCID: PMC7206757.
17. Ryan OK, Ryan ÉJ, Creavin B, Boland MR, Kelly ME, Winter DC. Systematic review and meta-analysis comparing primary resection and anastomosis versus Hartmann's procedure for the management of acute perforated diverticulitis with generalised peritonitis. Tech Coloproctol. 2020;24(6):527–43. https://doi.org/10.1007/s10151-020-02172-2. Epub 2020 Mar 2. PMID: 32124112.
18. Bothwell WN, Bleicher RJ, Dent TL. Prophylactic ureteral catheterization in colon surgery. A five-year review. Dis Colon Rectum. 1994;37(4):330–4.
19. Garoufalia Z, Wexner SD. Ureter identification utilizing indocyanine green (ICG) imaging in colorectal surgery: a systematic review of the literature. Mini Invasive Surg. 2022;6:51.
20. Oberkofler CE, Rickenbacher A, Raptis DA, et al. A multicenter randomized clinical trial of primary anastomosis or Hartmann's procedure for perforated left colonic diverticulitis with purulent or fecal peritonitis. Ann Surg. 2012;256:819.
21. Lambrichts DPV, Vennix S, Musters GD, et al. LADIES Trial Collaborators. Hartmann's procedure versus sigmoidectomy with primary anastomosis for perforated diverticulitis with purulent or faecal peritonitis (LADIES): a multicentre, parallel-group, randomised, open-label, superiority trial. Lancet Gastroenterol Hepatol. 2019;4:599–610. https://doi.org/10.1016/S2468-1253(19)30174-8.
22. McGillicuddy EA, Schuster KM, Davis KA, et al. Factors predicting morbidity and mortality in emergency colorectal procedures in elderly patients. Arch Surg. 2009;144(12):1157–62.
23. Hall J, Hardiman K, Lee S, Lightner A, Stocchi L, Paquette IM, Steele SR, Feingold DL, Prepared on behalf of the Clinical Practice Guidelines Committee of the American Society of Colon and Rectal Surgeons. The American Society of Colon and Rectal Surgeons clinical practice guidelines for the treatment of left-sided colonic diverticulitis. Dis Colon Rectum. 2020;63(6):728–47. https://doi.org/10.1097/DCR.0000000000001679. PMID: 32384404.
24. Johnson JW, Gracias VH, Schwab CW, et al. Evolution in damage control for exsanguinating penetrating abdominal injury. J Trauma. 2001;51:261.
25. Roberts DJ, Bobrovitz N, Zygun DA, et al. Indications for use of damage control surgery in civilian trauma patients: a content analysis and expert appropriateness rating study. Ann Surg. 2016;263:1018.
26. Shah PK, Chiu WC. Indications and techniques for trauma laparotomy. In: Scalea TM, editor. The shock trauma manual of operative techniques. Cham: Springer; 2021. https://doi.org/10.1007/978-3-030-27596-9_4.
27. Mayberry JC, Burgess EA, Goldman RK, et al. Enterocutaneous fistula and ventral hernia after absorbable mesh prosthesis closure for trauma: the plain truth. J Trauma. 2004;57:157.
28. Miller PR, Meredith JW, Johnson JC, Chang MC. Prospective evaluation of vacuum-assisted fascial closure after open abdomen: planned ventral hernia rate is substantially reduced. Ann Surg. 2004;239(5):608–16. https://doi.org/10.1097/01.sla.0000124291.09032.bf.
29. Quyn AJ, Johnston C, Hall D, et al. The open abdomen and temporary abdominal closure systems—historical evolution and systematic review. Color Dis. 2012;14(8):e429–38. https://doi.org/10.1111/j.1463-1318.2012.03045.x.
30. Huang Q, Li J, Lau WY. Techniques for abdominal wall closure after damage control laparotomy: from temporary abdominal closure to early/delayed fascial closure – a review. Gastroenterol Res Pract. 2016;2016:2073260. https://doi.org/10.1155/2016/2073260.
31. Patel NY, Cogbill TH, Kallies KJ, Mathiason MA. Temporary abdominal closure: long-term outcomes. J Trauma. 2011;70:769.
32. Okullo A, Siriwardhane M, Pang TC, Sinclair JL, Lam VW, Richardson AJ, Pleass H, Johnston E. The abdominal reapproximation anchor device. Surg Innov. 2017;24(1):49–54. https://doi.org/10.1177/1553350616671640. Epub 2016 Sept 27. PMID: 27678383.
33. Mukhi AN, Minor S. Management of the open abdomen using combination therapy with ABRA and ABThera systems. Can J Surg. 2014;57(5):314–9. https://doi.org/10.1503/cjs.026613.
34. Burlew CC, Moore EE, Biffl WL, Bensard DD, Johnson JL, Barnett CC. One hundred percent fascial approximation can be achieved in the postinjury open abdomen with a sequential closure protocol. J Trauma Acute Care Surg. 2012;72(1):235–41. https://doi.org/10.1097/TA.0b013e318236b319.
35. Kafka-Ritsch R, Zitt M, Perathoner A, Gasser E, Kaufman C, Czipin S, Aigner F, Öfner D. Prospectively randomized controlled trial on damage control surgery for perforated diverticulitis with generalized peritonitis. World J Surg. 2020;44(12):4098–105. https://doi.org/10.1007/s00268-020-05762-1. Epub 2020 Sept 8. PMID: 32901323; PMCID: PMC7599157.
36. Kirkpatrick AW, Roberts DJ, De Waele J, et al. Intra-abdominal hypertension and the abdominal compartment syndrome: updated consensus definitions and clinical practice guidelines from the World Society of the Abdominal Compartment Syndrome. Intensive Care Med. 2013;39:1190–206. https://doi.org/10.1007/s00134-013-2906-z.
37. Grumann MM, Noack EM, Hoffmann IA, Schlag PM. Comparison of quality of life in patients undergoing abdominoperineal extirpation or anterior resection for rectal cancer. Ann Surg. 2001;233(2):149–56.

12 Laparoscopic Lavage: When, How, and Should We?

Daniël P. V. Lambrichts, Johan F. Lange, and Willem A. Bemelman

Abbreviations

ASA American Society of Anesthesiologists
CI Confidence interval
MPI Mannheim Peritonitis Index
OR Odds ratio
pOR Pooled odds ratio

Introduction

Diverticulosis, defined as the presence of colonic diverticula, is common in developed countries. It is known to have an age-dependent prevalence with rates ranging from 5% at the age of 40 years up to 65% at the age of 85 or older [1, 2]. In contrast to Asian populations, diverticulosis is typically located in the left colon, and in up to 99% of individuals, diverticula are present in the sigmoid colon [3]. The majority of diverticula pass through weak points in the circular muscle layer, where blood vessels penetrate, and are "false" diverticula, as not all bowel layers are involved [4]. Formerly, it was estimated that individuals with diverticulosis had a lifetime risk of up to 25% of progression towards diverticulitis [5, 6]. However, more recent studies have found these rates to be lower, with an actuarial risk that approximates 4–7% [7, 8].

Diverticular disease can be complicated by a pericolic or distant abscess(es), perforation (Fig. 12.1) with peritonitis, as well as late complications such as fistulas or colonic obstruction [9]. Although the majority of patients with acute diverticulitis will have uncomplicated disease, a smaller proportion of these patients will suffer from complicated diverticular disease. The proportion of patients who present with complicated diverticulitis was estimated to be 12% in a population-based study [10], even though earlier data have also shown it to be present in up to 20% [11]. A recent Swedish population study found an overall standardised incidence rate of 8.7 per 100.000 person-years of first-time surgery for diverticular disease [12]. Interestingly, most patients presenting with complicated diverticular

Supplementary Information The online version contains supplementary material available at https://doi.org/10.1007/978-3-032-21720-2_12.

D. P. V. Lambrichts
Department of Surgery, Erasmus University Medical Center, Rotterdam, The Netherlands

Department of Surgery, Amsterdam University Medical Center, Amsterdam, The Netherlands
e-mail: d.lambrichts@erasmusmc.nl

J. F. Lange
Department of Surgery, Erasmus University Medical Center, Rotterdam, The Netherlands
e-mail: j.lange@erasmusmc.nl

W. A. Bemelman (✉)
Department of Surgery, Amsterdam University Medical Center, Amsterdam, The Netherlands
e-mail: w.a.bemelman@amsterdamumc.nl

M. Boutros et al. (eds.), *Diverticulitis*, https://doi.org/10.1007/978-3-032-21720-2_12

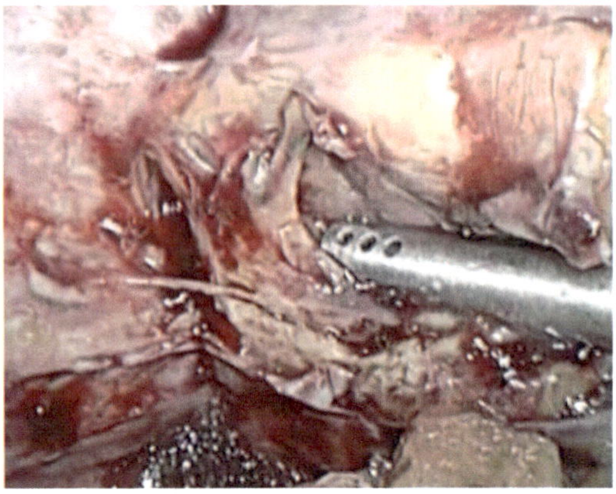

Fig. 12.1 Perforation

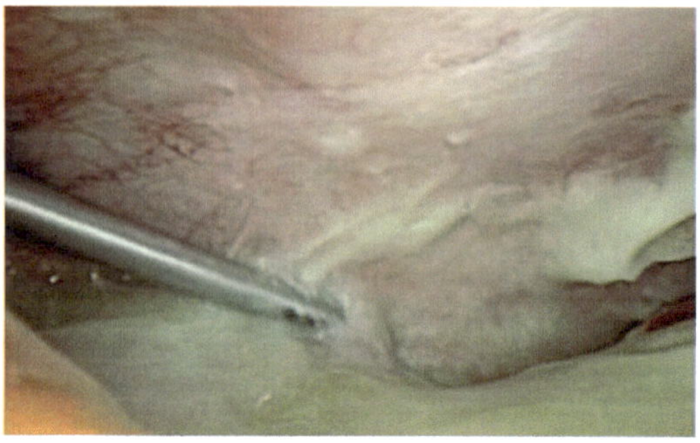

Fig. 12.2 Purulent peritonitis

disease have had no prior episodes of acute diverticulitis [13].

The overall incidence of diverticulitis has increased in the past decades, with a higher relative increase in patients under the age of 50 [10]. Moreover, the incidence of complicated diverticulitis has also increased [14, 15]. Specifically, the incidence of perforated diverticulitis has been known to have increased substantially in the last few decades [13]. These statistics highlight the impact of diverticulitis in terms of healthcare burden. In the United States, colonic diverticulitis is the third most common gastrointestinal discharge diagnosis [16], it is associated with estimated healthcare costs of 2.1 billion US dollars per year, and it results in more than 2.7 million outpatient visits and 200,000 inpatient admissions yearly [17].

In order to grade the severity of diverticular disease, several classifications have been proposed [18], such as those by Hansen et al. [19] and Köhler et al. [20]. However, the most widely used classifications are the Hinchey classification, as introduced in 1979 by Hinchey and colleagues [21], and its modified version, as proposed by Wasvary et al. [22] (see Fig. 6.1).

Historically, surgical strategies for perforated diverticulitis with generalised peritonitis have dramatically evolved over the course of the past century. Treatment recommendations have shifted from three-staged procedures to two-staged procedures with primary resection, resection with primary anastomosis, and, most recently, non-resectional approaches laparoscopic lavage [23]. Since its introduction in the 1990s, laparoscopic lavage has been increasingly investigated as a promising treatment strategy for perforated diverticulitis with purulent peritonitis (Fig. 12.2). Several case series and cohort studies evaluating its outcomes have since been published, followed by randomised clinical trials comparing laparoscopic lavage to sigmoid resection [24, 25].

The proposed advantages of laparoscopic lavage over resectional treatment, being either a Hartmann's procedure or sigmoid resection with primary anastomosis, are the avoidance of stoma construction, stoma-related complications, and the potential morbidity and mortality associated with the restoration of intestinal continuity [26]. Nevertheless, these advantages need to be weighed against the disadvantages related to leaving the perforated colon in situ as a potential septic focus and source of ongoing contamination [23]. In addition, after the acute attack, diverticulitis might persist with ongoing complaints, potentially mandating surgical resection. In recent years, several meta-analyses have been published on this topic, weighing potential advantages and disadvantages of laparoscopic lavage based on the published evidence, which, interestingly, have come to different conclusions [27, 28]. Hence, the question remains as to whether laparoscopic lavage should be considered in perforated diverticulitis, and if so, in which patients and under what circumstances does lavage result in optimal outcomes.

Currently, laparoscopic lavage is still a much-debated topic in the surgical scientific literature. Therefore, this chapter focuses on the different aspects of laparoscopic lavage as a treatment option for perforated diverticulitis and aims to provide answers to the questions: if, when, and how should laparoscopic lavage be performed?

History of Surgical Treatment for Perforated Diverticulitis

The first scientific report of surgical treatment for perforated diverticulitis dates back to the beginning of the twentieth century, when Mayo et al. [29] published a case series of five patients undergoing colonic resection for diverticulitis. As primary resection in the acute setting was considered too difficult, a three-stage procedure was standard practice and consisted of drainage of intra-abdominal sepsis and diverting colostomy, followed by colon resection 3–6 months later, and closure of the colostomy as the third stage [30–32].

During the second half of the twentieth century, surgical practice gradually shifted towards a two-staged approach, and primary resection of the involved colon became increasingly advocated [23]. The two-staged procedure has been known as Hartmann's procedure and involves resection of the diseased colonic segment, construction of a colostomy with closure of the distal rectal stump, followed by restoration of intestinal continuity during the second stage. Interestingly, Dr. Hartmann himself performed these procedures for rectal carcinoma and did not specifically recommend stoma reversal [33]. As Hartmann's procedure gradually became the "gold standard" of surgical treatment for perforated diverticulitis, interest in one-stage procedures with resection and primary anastomosis gradually increased in the 1990s [23]. Over the last two decades, several prospective trials comparing Hartmann's procedure to sigmoid resection with primary anastomosis, with or without diverting ileostomy, were conducted [34–37].

In the same period, the first reports on laparoscopic lavage were published. In 1996, O'Sullivan et al. [38] first reported on the outcomes of laparoscopic lavage in eight patients with perforated diverticulitis and purulent peritonitis. This initial report was followed by results from several other case series on laparoscopic lavage [39–41]. After these early studies, a large prospective multi-institutional study was published in 2008, which showed a postoperative morbidity and mortality rate of 4% and 3% in 92 patients with Hinchey II and III diverticulitis ($n = 25$ and $n = 67$, respectively) [26]. Evidence from these studies was systematically reviewed by Toorenvliet et al. [42], who concluded laparoscopic lavage showed promising results and seemed to be an important potential treatment for selected patients with perforated diverticulitis, excluding those with Hinchey IV diverticulitis. Nevertheless, the authors also stated that cautious interpretation of their findings was needed, as the included studies were heterogeneous and at high risk for selection bias, publication bias, and confounding. Hence, to avoid the risk of selection bias and to gather high-quality evidence, several randomised trials (e.g. SCANDIV, DILALA, LapLAND, and Ladies) comparing laparoscopic lavage with sigmoid resection for the treatment of perforated diverticulitis with purulent peritonitis were initiated [43–45]. The outcomes of these trials have since been published, which will be discussed further on in this chapter.

Technical Considerations

In the various published studies on the outcomes of laparoscopic lavage, several different techniques for performing the procedure have been described. In a systematic review, Gregori et al. [46] made an attempt to summarise the available evidence on the different technical aspects of laparoscopic lavage, but they were unable to define and propose a standardised procedure due to the heterogeneity across studies. The different procedural steps of laparoscopic lavage include significant variations in operative steps, including patient positioning, method of gaining laparoscopic access, trocar positioning, extent of adhesiolysis and colonic mobilisation, volume of peritoneal fluid injected and drained, and placement of drains, as well as variations in preoperative and postoperative imaging and other diagnostic tests (Video 12.1).

With respect to patient positioning, patients are commonly placed in the Lloyd-Davies position, at an angle of 30° Trendelenburg and with the hips flexed 15°. One alternative includes the French position, with the right arm placed alongside the body and the operating surgeon and assistant standing on the right side of the patient.

Access to the abdominal cavity can be achieved with an open Hasson technique or the closed Veress needle technique, the latter of which is advocated by Franklin et al. [47]. Although the existing evidence is insufficient to support the use of any one specific technique, the Hasson technique might lower the risk of visceral or vascular injury [48]. In the SCANDIV trial, the preferred access method was with the open transumbilical technique [43].

It is advised to use a three-trocar approach to gain further laparoscopic access to the abdominal cavity. Although some authors use four trocars, the three-trocar approach is commonly described in the literature [46]. With the 12 mm umbilical or supraumbilical port being used for the camera, the other two 5 mm trocars can be placed in the right upper and lower quadrants under direct vision.

Once access to the abdominal cavity has been achieved, variations have been described in the extent of laparoscopic adhesiolysis and mobilisation of the involved colonic segment needed. Some advocate aggressive adhesiolysis in order to optimise washout of intra-abdominal sepsis and optimise exposure and control of the diseased segment. Moreover, this step might facilitate the identification of a possible perforation that can be treated appropriately. However, a feared outcome of extensive adhesiolysis and mobilisation is the risk of progression from purulent peritonitis to faecal peritonitis by breaking open a sealed perforation. In the SCANDIV trial, adhesions to the sigmoid were not routinely dissected [43]. In the protocol of the LOLA arm of the Ladies trial, a careful inspection of the stomach, duodenum, and sigmoid colon was recommended to identify the site of perforation. Moreover, in the case of clearly adherent small bowel or omentum to the diseased segment, it was advised to leave this adherence in place [44]. In general, it is recommended to perform a thorough evaluation of the abdominal cavity, including exploration of the Douglas pouch, and full retraction of the omentum to rule out other causes of perforation. The authors of the recently published LLO multicentre cohort study also recommended that adhesiolysis should be avoided [49]. Furthermore, hydropneumatic ("bubble") testing might be advised as it might help to identify unsuspected sites of perforation. This can be done by insufflating the colon.

Throughout the literature, several techniques have been described for managing colonic perforation found during laparoscopic lavage, such as primary repair with absorbable sutures, with or without fibrin glue, or omentoplasty [38, 46, 50, 51]. However, nowadays, it is generally believed that in cases of an overt perforation, it might be preferable to convert to a resectional strategy, such as sigmoid resection with primary anastomosis, when possible [46, 52–54]. In the Ladies trial, patients with an intraoperative diagnosis of overt perforation were no longer eligible to undergo laparoscopic lavage [44].

Peritoneal lavage itself should be performed with saline, at body temperature, and all four quadrants need to be extensively washed out. In the SCANDIV and DILALA trials, at least 3 and 4 L of saline were used, respectively [43, 45], whereas the Ladies trial recommended 6 L of warm saline [44]. Although the number of litres used during the procedure might vary, the most important aspect is the fact that lavage should not be stopped before clear fluid returns from all four quadrants.

Major variations in the number, position, and duration of percutaneous drainage have been reported. In most cases, only one drain is left in place [38, 52, 55], whereas others described the use of two or even three drains [26, 40, 41, 50, 54, 56]. Drains were positioned in the pouch of Douglas, or near the diseased colon [46]. The study protocol of the DILALA trial required the use of a pelvic drain for a minimum of 24 h, whereas in the SCANDIV trial, two drains were placed on each side of the pelvis [45, 57]. In the Ladies trial, the protocol described insertion of a drain through the right lateral port and positioning in the pouch of Douglas [44].

In cases of failure of lavage, with persisting abdominal sepsis, reoperation or percutaneous drainage may be indicated. An important factor in the prevention of failure of laparoscopic lavage seems to be the optimisation of the detection of faecal peritonitis and overt perforations, or perforations caused by underlying colorectal carcinoma. Although not a part of routine practice, Vennix et al. [58] proposed the use of a CT scan with rectal contrast to discriminate between purulent and faecal peritonitis, as the latter might show contrast extravasation. Moreover, intraoperative sigmoidoscopy might also facilitate achieving an accurate diagnosis of an overt perforation.

With regard to follow-up of patients treated with laparoscopic lavage, it is recommended to obtain a colonoscopy in order to rule out an underlying malignancy. Even though all trials reported on evaluating for an underlying malignancy in the follow-up period, there were variations in recommendations. All patients in the DILALA had to undergo colonoscopy, or computed tomography colonography, or double contrast barium enema within 12 months [45]. In the Ladies trial, a sigmoidoscopy was planned 4–6 weeks postoperatively, and in the SCANDIV trial, a colonoscopy was required within 3 months of surgery [57, 58].

Outcomes of Laparoscopic Lavage

Several case series, as well as retrospective and prospective cohort studies assessing the outcomes of laparoscopic lavage, have been published. Moreover, three randomised controlled trials comparing laparoscopic lavage with sigmoid resection for perforated diverticulitis with purulent peritonitis have been published. While short-term outcomes have been reported, long-term outcomes are still relatively scarce. The following paragraphs summarise short- and long-term outcomes of laparoscopic lavage, as well as their interpretation in the abundance of recently published meta-analyses on the topic of laparoscopic lavage [28, 59, 67–70]. An overview of the available evidence on cost-effectiveness of this approach and patient-reported outcomes will also be provided.

RCTs of Laparoscopic Lavage: Study Designs

The first two trials to start enrolling patients in February 2010 were the SCANDIV and DILALA trials [43, 71]. Several months later, the LOLA arm of the Ladies trial also started accruing patients [58]. All three trials were multicentre superiority trials conducted in European populations (e.g. Sweden, Norway, Denmark, the Netherlands, Belgium, and Italy), and randomly allocated patients to laparoscopic lavage versus sigmoid resection. In the DILALA trial, only Hartmann's procedures were performed in the resection arm, whereas in the SCANDIV trial, the decision to proceed with open or laparoscopic Hartmann's procedure or primary anastomosis (with or without diverting ileostomy) was left to the discretion of the surgeon. To allow for additional comparison between resectional strategies, the Ladies trial was designed to allocate patients (2:1:1) between laparoscopic lavage, HP, and primary anastomosis (with or without diverting ileostomy). In the DILALA and LOLA studies, patients were randomised intraoperatively at the time of diagnostic laparoscopy, whereas patients in the SCANDIV were randomised preoperatively. Overall, only patients with purulent peritonitis caused by perforated diverticulitis were included and patients with faecal peritonitis or an overt perforation were excluded. Moreover, the Ladies trial specifically excluded patients on high-dose steroid use (≥20 mg daily), haemodynamic instability, and patients 85 or older. Primary outcome measures also differed between the studies: the SCANDIV main outcome measure was the number of severe diverticulitis-related complications at 1 year (Clavien-Dindo grade IIIa or more), whereas the primary outcome of the DILALA was the number of reoperations within 12 months follow-up. A composite endpoint of (predefined) major morbidity and mortality within 12 months was used in the LOLA arm of the Ladies trial. In addition, a wide range of secondary outcomes were collected in all studies.

RCTs: Short-Term and 12-Month Treatment Outcomes

In the DILALA study, 43 patients were allocated to laparoscopic lavage and 40 patients to HP [72]. The LOLA arm of the Ladies trial analysed 46 lavage patients and 42 sigmoidectomy patients [73]. However, the largest study population was enrolled in the SCANDIV trial, which overall randomised 101 patients to lavage and 98 to colonic resection [57]. Outcomes were assessed at 30 and 90 days postoperatively, as well as during the remaining 12-month follow-up.

During the 30-day follow-up period following index admission, the pooled risk ratio of reoperation derived from the three studies was 1.93 (95% confidence interval (CI) 0.71, 5.22) in favour of primary resection [61]. Additionally, in a meta-analysis, which also included non-randomised comparative studies, the pooled odds ratio (pOR) for 30-day emergency operations was found to be 2.474 (95% CI 0.900, 6.801, $p = 0.079$) [66]. It is of importance to note that the LOLA arm of the Ladies trial was terminated early by the data safety and monitoring board, because of an increased event rate in the lavage group. This was mainly driven by the higher number of in-hospital surgical reinterventions, with 18 such events in the lavage group versus 2 in the sigmoidectomy group ($p = 0.0011$) [58]. Only the SCANDIV trial reported the 90-day reoperation rates and found a weighted mean difference of 14.6% (95% CI 3.5, 25.6%, $p = 0.01$) in favour of resection ($n = 4/70$) over lavage ($n = 15/74$) [43, 61]. Overall, the rate of surgical reinterventions at 12 months, including stoma reversal procedures, was 32.5% ($n = 53/163$) for lavage versus. 47.4% ($n = 72/152$) for resection, with an associated risk ratio of 0.67 (95% CI 0.45, 1.02) [65].

The number of postoperative intra-abdominal abscesses at 90 days in the DILALA and SCANDIV trial was higher in the lavage group with a risk ratio of 2.54 (95% CI 1.34, 4.83) [61]. Moreover, the number of abscesses requiring percutaneous drainage during 30-day follow-up was higher in the lavage group of the Ladies trial, with nine patients in the lavage group requiring drainage versus three in the sigmoidectomy group (20% versus 7%, $p = 0.0027$) [58]. The meta-analysis of Penna et al. [66] demonstrated a pOR of 2.846 (95% CI 1.516, 5.344, $p = 0.001$) based on a 16.5% versus 6.6% rate of intra-abdominal abscesses in the lavage versus resectional group. Hence, the need for percutaneous drainage was also assessed, which showed an odds ratio (OR) of 5.414 (95% CI 1.618, 18.118, $p = 0.006$) for drainage associated with the lavage group [64]. In contrast, when results from both RCTs and non-randomised studies were combined, the number of wound infections was demonstrated to be lower in lavage patients, with a pOR of 0.151 (95% 0.052, 0.434, $p < 0.001$) in favour of lavage (1.2%) versus resection (10.7%) [66]. Based on randomised trial outcomes, lavage was associated with a significantly reduced incidence of wound infections, with an OR of 0.14 (95% CI 0.04, 0.45, $p = 0.0009$) [59].

Major complications, defined as Clavien-Dindo >IIIa [74], were reported at 90 days postoperatively and shown to lead to a relative risk of 1.47 (95% CI 0.99, 2.20) of laparoscopic lavage over resection [60], although Acuna and colleagues [65] found a relative risk of 1.68 (95% CI 1.10, 2.56) based on the same studies. This difference might potentially be explained by the discrepancy in the reported number of complications in the resection group of the DILALA trial between the two meta-analyses ($n = 10/35$ versus $n = 6/35$, respectively) [60, 65]. In addition, the meta-analysis of Penna and colleagues [66] found a POR for postoperative severe complications (Clavien-Dindo >IIIa) of 1.816 (95% CI). When major complications were assessed over the course of the 12-month follow-up period in the LOLA and SCANDIV studies, the risk ratio was 1.27 (95% CI 0.89, 1.80) and was no longer significantly different between lavage and resection [65]. In addition to postoperative complication rates, Shaikh et al. [64] also focused on the number of readmissions, but their analysis showed no difference between lavage and resection (OR 0.809, 95% CI 0.337, 1.945).

The composite primary endpoint of major morbidity and mortality used in the LOLA study was not significantly different between lavage and sigmoidectomy (67% versus 60%, OR 1.28, 95% CI 0.54, 3.03, $p = 0.58$) [58]. In addition, mortality was also assessed separately, as was also done in the other two trials. The postoperative mortality at index admission or within 30 days from the index intervention showed no statistically significant difference in favour of lavage or resection (4/148 (2.7%) versus 7/159 (4.4%), respectively) with a risk ratio of 1.33 (95% CI 0.37, 4.74) [61, 65]. In addition, at 90 days follow-up, no significant difference was found in mortality rates, with a relative risk of 0.86 (95% CI 0.40, 1.84) [60, 63]. Moreover, at the end of the 12-month follow-up period, no significant differences in mortality rates were found, with a relative risk of 0.89 (95% CI 0.49, 1.61) and OR of 0.86 (95% CI 0.416, 1.789, $p = 0.692$) [64, 65]. The 30-day, 90-day, and 12-month mortality rates were also assessed in the meta-analysis by Penna et al. [66], which also included non-randomised comparative studies. The PORs (lavage versus resection) for mortality at these time points were 0.863 (3.3% versus 3.9%, 95% CI 0.315, 2.363, $p = 0.774$), 0.464 (3.6% versus 5.7%, 95% CI 0.040, 5.325, $p = 0.538$), and 0.581 (6.5% versus 11.6%, 95% CI 0.249, 1.354, $p = 0.208$), respectively.

Since laparoscopic lavage was hypothesised to be associated with reduced stoma creation rates, decreased operative time, and shorter length of hospital stay, these outcomes were also analysed in the various published meta-analyses. The meta-analysis by Marshall et al. [63] reported a risk ratio of 0.50 (95% CI 0.14–1.76) for the presence of stoma at 12 months when lavage was compared to resection. However, the results of the SCANDIV trial were not included in their analysis, which demonstrated a significantly lower stoma rate in the lavage group at that time point (14% versus 42%, $p < 0.001$) [45]. Galbraith et al. [62] assessed the number of stomas formed within 90 days postoperatively in all three trials and found a pooled risk ratio of 0.18 (95% CI 0.12, 0.27, $p < 0.001$) when comparing laparoscopic lavage to colon resection. Penna et al. [66] stated that, overall, 90% of resection patients had a stoma constructed, of whom 74% underwent stoma reversal within 12 months. In comparison, 14% of patients treated with lavage required a stoma, of which 48% were reversed in this same period. As discussed by the authors, stoma construction in the lavage group was likely to be unplanned due to a complication or worsening of diverticulitis, thereby potentially diminishing the possibility of reversal.

The operative time and length of hospital stay were both demonstrated to be shorter for laparoscopic lavage. A pooled weighted mean difference of −78.5 min (95% CI −104.83, −52.18, $p < 0.001$) in operative time was found in favour of lavage [66], which was −72.105 min (95% CI −88.335, −55.876) when only randomised trials were assessed [64]. Similarly, laparoscopic lavage significantly shortened the length of hospital stay, with a pooled weighted mean difference of −8.3 days (95% CI −12.53, −4.08, $p < 0.001$) [66]. From a separate analysis of outcomes in the randomised trials, a weighted mean difference of −0.338 days (95% CI −0.565, −0.111, $p = 0.004$) was also found, favouring laparoscopic lavage [64].

Long-Term Treatment Outcomes

As described, most studies reported their outcomes at up to 12 months of follow-up. Nevertheless, some studies have also assessed outcomes of laparoscopic lavage over the course of a longer period of follow-up. One meta-analysis of long-term outcomes included five long-term follow-up studies of RCT comprising 499 patients. Three studies, excluding patients with faecal peritonitis, compared LL and colonic resection, and two compared PRA and Hartmann procedures. LL had lower odds of long-term ostomy [odds ratio (OR) = 0.133, 95% CI: 0.278–0.579; $p < 0.001$] and reoperation

(OR = 0.585, 95% CI: 0.365–0.937; p = 0.02) compared with colonic resection but higher odds of diverticular disease recurrence (OR = 5.8, 95% CI: 2.33–14.42; $p < 0.001$). Colonic resection with PRA had lower odds of long-term ostomy (OR = 0.02, 95% CI: 0.003–0.195; $p < 0.001$), long-term complications (OR = 0.195, 95% CI: 0.113–0.335; $p < 0.001$), reoperation (OR = 0.2, 95% CI: 0.108–0.384; $p < 0.001$), and incisional hernia (OR = 0.184, 95% CI: 0.102–0.333; $p < 0.001$). There was no significant difference in odds of mortality among the procedures [28].

The DILALA trial [75], one of the three RCTs including the LOLA [76] and the SCANDIV [24] to report results beyond the 12-month follow-up period, assessed the 2-year outcomes in 43 patients who underwent laparoscopic lavage versus 40 who underwent HP. Eighteen lavage patients (41.9%) had one or more reoperations versus 27 resection patients (67.5%), leading to an adjusted risk ratio of 0.49 (95% CI 0.30, 0.81). Additionally, the mean number of reoperations was 0.63 (±0.90) for laparoscopic lavage and 1.08 (±1.16) for HP, resulting in an adjusted risk ratio 0.47 (95% CI 0.27, 0.83). It should however be noted that not all reoperations were likely to be related to the index procedure. Although the differences in reoperations were significant, no difference was found in the mean number of admissions with 1.37 (±1.48) in lavage patients and 1.50 (±1.45) in resection patients (adjusted risk ratio 0.72, 95% CI 0.46, 1.11). Furthermore, at 24 months of follow-up, three lavage patients (7%) had a stoma as compared to nine resection patients (22.5%). Based on these outcomes, the authors concluded that laparoscopic lavage is a better option in the surgical management of perforated diverticulitis with purulent peritonitis relative to open HP.

In the retrospective multicentre international study conducted by Binda et al. [49], 231 patients who underwent laparoscopic lavage for purulent peritonitis across 24 centres in eight different countries were followed for a median of 22.4 months. During index admission and up to 60 days after discharge, 172 patients (74.5%) were treated successfully, as defined by being free of sepsis or not requiring reoperation. Among these successfully treated patients, a recurrent episode of acute diverticulitis was recorded in 46 patients (26.7%) during follow-up, with a mean time to recurrence of 11 (range 2–108) months, and 21 patients needed additional surgery. Interestingly, the majority of these recurrences presented as Hinchey stage I (35 patients). The authors concluded that, after excluding risk factors for failure of lavage (prior radiotherapy, steroids use, hemodynamic instability, feculent peritonitis), laparoscopic lavage appeared to be a reasonable option in selected patients presenting with Hinchey III diverticulitis.

In a smaller multicentre cohort study, Sneiders et al. [77] assessed long-term recurrence, reoperations, and readmissions in a previously established cohort of 38 patients treated with laparoscopic lavage [78]. At a median follow-up of 46 months (interquartile range 7–77), 17 episodes of recurrent diverticulitis were reported in 12 patients (32%), of which 7 were complicated and 10 were uncomplicated. Fifteen patients (39%) had a total of 50 readmissions and nine patients (24%) underwent sigmoidectomy during follow-up. Among the 31/38 patients successfully treated with laparoscopic lavage, 30 were alive at the beginning of the defined long-term follow-up period which started 90 days after the index procedure. Six patients (20%) required additional surgery, which included sigmoidectomy, as well as stoma reversal, parastomal hernia repair, and lysis of adhesions. Five of the seven patients who initially failed laparoscopic lavage were alive at the start of long-term follow-up with four patients requiring surgery during long-term follow-up (e.g. stoma reversal, incisional hernia repair, and ileosigmoid fistula treatment). Overall, a stoma could be avoided in 76% of patients who underwent laparoscopic lavage, and among those who underwent stoma construction, 78% eventually had their stomas reversed.

Costs

Several aspects of laparoscopic lavage, such as a shorter duration of surgery, reduced stoma rates, and stoma-related costs, might lead to a reduction in costs when compared to sigmoid resection. Two studies, the DILALA and LOLA trials, have performed an economic evaluation of their trial data [73, 79]. The health economic evaluation of the DILALA trial, as reported by Gehrman and colleagues [79], compared the costs associated with laparoscopic lavage (n = 43) with those associated with Hartmann's procedure (n = 40). During the 12-month study period, the mean total costs of laparoscopic lavage were €18,025 (±14,646) and €27,009 (±18,445) of Hartmann's procedure with a mean difference (lavage minus Hartmann's procedure) of €−8983 (95% CI −16,232, −1735, p = 0.016). Within these cost analyses, productivity loss from paid or unpaid work was not included. The cost analysis, as performed within the LOLA arm of the Ladies trial, reported by Vennix et al. [73], did include these indirect non-medical costs in addition to direct medical and non-medical expenses. The total costs in the lavage group (n = 46) were €27,125 and €33,425 in the sigmoid resection group (n = 42), with a cost difference of €−6300 (95% bias-corrected and accelerated CI −18,804, 6546). Interestingly, the authors stated that surgical reintervention increased the costs in the lavage group, while stoma reversal, stoma care, and productivity loss increased costs in the sigmoid resection group. The mean difference in total medical costs was €−3512 (95% bias-corrected and accelerated CI −16,020, 8149) and €−2789 (95% bias-corrected and accelerated CI −2798, 1810) in indirect non-medical costs. Consequently, the authors concluded that laparoscopic lavage was associated with lower costs.

Patient-Reported Outcomes

Evidence has shown that survivors of perforated diverticulitis have a worse quality of life than individuals in the general population, mainly after Hartmann's procedure. Moreover, the presence of a stoma seems to be an independent risk factor for worse quality of life, due to its effects on physical function and body image [80]. Subsequently, laparoscopic lavage, through a lower stoma rate, might lead to better quality of life as compared to sigmoid resection [28]. As part of their design, all three published trials have assessed patient-reported outcomes. In the SCANDIV trial, the 90-day postoperative quality of life was measured according to the Cleveland Global Quality of Life instrument, but no significant difference between lavage and resection was found [43]. By means of the EuroQol-5D and Short Form-36 questionnaires, the quality of life was measured in the DILALA trial at the time of discharge, and at 6- and 12-month follow-ups. No differences were found between groups in both questionnaires and at all time points [72]. Within the LOLA arm of the Ladies trial, quality of life was measured at 2, 4, 13, and 26 weeks postoperatively, through the use of the Short Form-36, Gastrointestinal Quality of Life Index, and EuroQol-5D questionnaires. However, also in this trial, no differences were found in any of the scores or subscales. Importantly, all three studies assessed patient-reported outcomes as secondary outcomes and might therefore have lacked statistical power to accurately detect differences between groups.

Interpretations of Meta-Analyses on Laparoscopic Lavage

Eight systematic reviews and meta-analyses have been published on outcomes of laparoscopic lavage [59–67]. However, the interpretation of the pooled data and, therefore, conclusions vary widely [27]. These differences are mostly accounted for by selection criteria for study inclusion, study endpoints, and the specific methodology to assess these endpoints. The long-term assessment in the follow-up SCANDIV trial also showed no significant differences in QoL [81].

Some authors have drawn relatively strong conclusions in favour of laparoscopic lavage, such as Angenete et al. [60], who considered laparoscopic lavage a valid alternative to sigmoid resection, based on their findings of a lower 12-month risk for reoperation, comparable overall morbidity and mortality, and reduced costs for lavage. Similarly, Shaikh et al. [64] stated lavage to be a safe and quick alternative in the management of perforated diverticulitis, mostly because of the fact that they did not find differences in perioperative mortality and serious morbidity.

In contrast, other authors have drawn less definite conclusions, mainly because of the lack of conclusive evidence in support or against the use of laparoscopic lavage, and the need for further research on the topic [59, 63]. Cirocchi et al. [61] stated that, "the fundamental flaw of this technique is the lack of a robust diagnosis". Hence, it is concluded by some that future research should focus on the identification of preoperative and intraoperative factors that may impact the success of lavage [63]. Accordingly, Galbraith et al. [62] stated that "as with all decisions in surgery, patient selection is key". Furthermore, some stated that data on long-term results should first be awaited before the widespread implementation of laparoscopic lavage [67].

Lastly, Acuna et al. [65] stated that lavage should not be considered as a treatment option for perforated diverticulitis with purulent peritonitis, as they have found evidence from their analyses that resection with primary anastomosis was the preferred treatment for these patients. This conclusion was based on the finding that laparoscopic lavage was associated with more major postoperative complications (Clavien-Dindo >IIIa) as compared to colon resection within data from RCTs. A risk ratio of 1.68 was derived (95% CI 1.10–2.56) from the comparison of such major complications in lavage patients (n = 47/158, 29.7%) compared to resection patients (n = 26/147, 17.7%).

Guideline Recommendations

Several international and national guidelines on the treatment of diverticular disease have been published. As laparoscopic lavage is a heavily debated topic, recommendations on the role of lavage differ throughout these guidelines. In several guidelines published prior to and up to 2013, laparoscopic lavage was considered a potentially appropriate treatment, such as guidelines from the Netherlands Surgical Society [81], the Danish Surgical Society [1], the European Association for Endoscopic Surgery (EAES) [82], the Association of Coloproctology of Great Britain and Ireland (ACPGBI) [83], and the 2013 guideline of the World Society for Emergency Surgery (WSES) [84]. This recommendation was based on recently published results from case series on laparoscopic lavage, and did not include data from RCTs. In more recent guideline updates, the 2020 WSES guidelines [85] suggest performing laparoscopic lavage and drainage only in very selected patients with generalised peritonitis. It is not considered the first-line treatment in patients with peritonitis from acute colonic diverticulitis (weak recommendation based on high-quality evidence, 2A). According to the ASCRS guidelines [86], laparoscopic lavage is not recommended in patients with feculent peritonitis; rather, colectomy should typically be performed in this situation (strong recommendation based on high-quality evidence, 1A). In patients with purulent peritonitis, colectomy is preferred over laparoscopic lavage. Laparoscopic lavage is associated with higher rates of secondary intervention in comparison with colectomy (strong recommendation based on high-quality evidence, 1A).

Since then, Galetin et al. [87] published a systematic review and comparison of ten guidelines and found that currently, laparoscopic lavage is not specifically recommended anymore within most guidelines.

The WSES guidelines for the management of acute left-sided colonic diverticulitis in the emergency setting, which were published in 2016, stated that laparoscopic lavage should not be considered the treatment of choice in patients with generalised peritonitis, mainly due to the discrepancy in results from RCTs [88]. More recently, in the summary of the 2018 emergency general surgery guidelines of the American Association for the Surgery of Trauma, laparoscopic lavage is stated to be no longer supported in the treatment of acute diverticulitis [89]. In contrast, an updated version of the Dutch guidelines on acute diverticulitis, revised in 2018, advised to consider laparoscopic lavage in patients with purulent peritonitis as an alternative to sigmoidectomy. However, the authors emphasised the importance of a thorough evaluation of the patient's clinical condition, characteristics, and preferences, as well as the importance of the surgeon's experience with the procedure. Moreover, higher short-term morbidity and rate of reinterventions need to be weighed against the long-term lower rate of reinterventions, stomas, and overall costs [90].

Laparoscopic lavage is also discussed in the evidence-based recommendations from the EAES and SAGES consensus conference on acute diverticulitis [91]. The authors state the recommendation that lavage may be considered in selected Hinchey III patients by surgeons with appropriate expertise. Also, they emphasise the importance of being able to closely watch for and manage complications. A comparable statement has been made within the guidelines for the management of diverticular disease as constructed by the European Society of Coloproctology, which states that lavage is feasible in selected patients with Hinchey III patients [92]. The recently published practice guidelines for the treatment of left-sided colonic diverticulitis, as constructed by the American Society of Colon and Rectal Surgeons, conclude otherwise, as a strong recommendation is provided that colectomy is preferred over laparoscopic lavage in patients with purulent peritonitis [93].

In summary, even in the most recent guidelines on diverticular disease, statements on the validity of laparoscopic lavage still vary.

Patient Selection

As laparoscopic lavage seems to be associated with an increased short-term reintervention rate as compared to sigmoid resection, an important potential way to improve outcomes is to identify preoperative and intraoperative factors associated with an increased risk of short-term treatment failure. Subsequently, these factors might facilitate the selection of patients who might benefit the most from laparoscopic lavage and who are at a lower risk of initial short-term treatment failure. Some studies have attempted to assess potential risk factors for failure to better define potential contraindications to laparoscopic lavage [49, 94–96].

The first reported study that aimed to appraise potential determinants of the outcomes of lavage was the prospective cohort study by Radé et al. [96] in which 71 patients underwent laparoscopic lavage, including 47 (66.2%) with Hinchey III and 24 (33.8%) with Hinchey I/II diverticulitis. Of note, any visible perforation was sutured during the procedure. The authors compared patients with ($n = 60$) and without ($n = 11$) treatment failure, which was defined as the need for reintervention for unresolved sepsis. Among potential risk factors for treatment failure that also included gender, BMI, history of abdominal surgery, history of diverticulitis, white blood cell count, C-reactive protein, Hinchey stage, and observed colonic perforation at presentation, the only factors that differed significantly between the groups by univariate analysis were age ≥ 80 years (3/60 versus 3/11, $p = 0.033$), immunosuppression (10/60 versus 5/11, $p = 0.028$), and ASA grade >II (4/60 versus 5/11, $p = 0.001$). The latter factor was the only one associated with treatment failure by multivariable analysis (OR 48.6, 95% CI 5.97, 395.19, $p < 0.010$).

In another study on risk factors for failure of laparoscopic lavage 71 consecutive patients who underwent laparoscopic lavage for Hinchey III diverticulitis were evaluated [94, 95]. Treatment failure, defined as reoperation or mortality within the first 30 postoperative days, occurred in 14 patients (19.7%), and several demographic, radiological, and intraoperative characteristics were compared between patients who failed treatment and those who were successfully treated. On univariate analysis, only immunosuppression (3% versus 29%, $p = 0.01$) and ASA grade >II (10% versus 36%, $p = 0.02$) were significantly associated with treatment failure. The use of immunosuppressive drugs was the only independent predictive factor for lavage failure on multivariable analysis (OR 17.1, 95% CI 1.416, 198.125, $p = 0.02$).

Lastly, the recent LLO study also assessed risk factors for failure of lavage and strict indications for resection [49]. From a total of 231

Hinchey III patients, 172 (74.5%) were successfully treated with laparoscopic lavage, as compared to 59 (25.5%) who failed lavage during short-term follow-up. Success was defined as the rate of patients alive and free from sepsis after the index episode, with no need for further surgery or death within 60 days after discharge. Several multivariable logistic regression models were used to assess a range of characteristics as risk factors for outcomes such as the identification of a free colonic perforation, conversion of lavage, in-hospital and 60-day reoperation, 30- and 60-day morbidity, and recurrence of acute diverticulitis.

Risk factors for the failure of lavage included the Mannheim Peritonitis Index (MPI) score ≥24 (OR 2.79, 95% CI 1.07, 7.28, $p = 0.036$), ASA grade (per unit increase, OR 1.84, 95% CI 1.08, 3.12, $p = 0.025$), extensive (versus limited) adhesiolysis (OR 2.94, 95% CI 1.14, 7.59, $p = 0.026$), and the identification of a free colonic perforation (OR 5.97, 95% CI 2.51, 13.74, $p < 0.001$). In this same logistic regression model, prior episode of diverticulitis was found to be an independent protective factor (OR 0.35, 95% CI 0.15, 0.82, $p = 0.016$). Interestingly, extensive adhesiolysis was also found to be an independent risk factor for the identification of a free colonic perforation (OR 3.17, 95% CI 1.30, 7.78, $p = 0.012$).

Risk factors for 30-day morbidity associated with laparoscopic lavage were also assessed. The time interval between admission and surgery (hours) was found to be an independent risk factor for postoperative complications (per unit increase, OR 1.04, 95% CI 1.02, 1.07, $p = 0.001$), as well as the identification of a free colonic perforation (OR 3.26, 95% CI 1.17, 9.14, $p = 0.024$), and the duration of surgery (per 15-min increase, OR 1.68, 95% CI 1.36, 2.08, $p < 0.001$). With respect to 60-day morbidity, an increased MPI score was identified as the only independent risk factor (per unit increase, OR 1.16, 95% CI 1.03, 1.29, $p = 0.012$) for complications. Lastly, an increased BMI (kg/m^2) (per unit increase, OR 1.39, 95% CI 1.04, 1.87, $p = 0.026$) or MPI score (per unit increase, OR 1.25, 95% CI 1.02, 1.54, $p = 0.035$) was independently associated with an increased risk of reoperation within the first 60 days. In contrast, previous abdominal surgery and previous diverticulitis were found to be protective factors with regard to this outcome (OR 0.07, 95% CI 0.01, 0.94, $p = 0.045$; OR 0.13, 95% CI 0.02, 1.00, $p = 0.049$, respectively). Overall, the authors conclude that high ASA grade, high MPI score, no prior history of diverticulitis, and finding of free perforation at the time of surgery are potential indications for resection, as they are strong predictors for failure of lavage.

Of note, although immunosuppression was found to be a risk factor for the failure of lavage in two of the three studies mentioned, the use of immunosuppressants was not assessed in the LLO study. Greilsamer et al. [94] defined immunosuppression as the use of steroids, chemotherapy, or anti-rejection drugs, whereas Radé et al. [96] classified patients with diabetes mellitus, and those taking steroids or "other immunosuppressive drugs" as immunosuppressed. Furthermore, in the LOLA arm of the Ladies trial, patients who used ≥20 mg of steroids daily were not eligible for inclusion [58]. In the SCANDIV and DILALA trials, immunosuppression was not considered a formal exclusion criterion [43, 71]. Only one patient (1%) in the lavage group of the SCANDIV trial was classified to have an "immunodeficiency or chronic hepatitis" and in the DILALA trial, 8.6% of lavage patients used immunosuppressants. Based on the above, the use of immunosuppressants should be considered a contraindication for laparoscopic lavage. In the Ladies trial, a history of pelvic irradiation was also used as an exclusion criterion and may represent a relative contraindication to lavage.

Lastly, it is of paramount importance to ensure that potential underlying colorectal malignancies are discovered in a timely fashion. A delayed diagnosis of colorectal cancer might lead to worse oncological outcomes, and because a perforated cancer might lead to failure of lavage. In the lavage group of the Ladies trial, one patient with persistent sepsis was diagnosed with an underlying carcinoma. In addition, one patient with a known perforated rectal carcinoma at the time of the index procedure was excluded [58]. Schultz et al. [57] cautioned that complications and reinterventions after lavage may be related to unsuspected perforated colorectal malignancy. In their cohort that underwent lavage, four of seven perforated sigmoid carcinomas were not detected at the index operation. Moreover, 12 patients with other concurrent diagnoses were excluded from their study, including three patients with tumours diagnosed intraoperatively and resected during the index operation. In the DILALA study, it is not entirely clear whether patients were diagnosed with cancer intraoperatively or during follow-up colonoscopy. Within the lavage groups in the Ladies, SCANDIV, and DILALA trials, 11% (n = 5/46), 5.4% (n = 4/74), and 6.9% (n = 3/43) of underlying malignancies were diagnosed intraoperatively [43, 58, 72].

Every effort should be made to diagnose potential colorectal malignancies in the preoperative setting, with a CT-scan with intravenous and rectal contrast and/or intraoperative sigmoidoscopy. Subsequently, all patients should undergo an interval colonoscopy. In addition to the intraoperative diagnosis of colorectal malignancy as a contraindication for laparoscopic lavage, other factors can be identified that contraindicate lavage as treatment. Such factors include haemodynamic instability, immunosuppression, and the presence of faecal peritonitis. Subsequently, the finding of multiple perforations or the presence of a fistula might require resection. Refer to Fig. 12.3 for a flowchart summarising potential treatment options for acute diverticulitis.

Next to patient selection, surgical expertise is of paramount importance in the context of laparoscopic lavage. Laparoscopic lavage should only be performed by those with experience in laparoscopic colorectal emergency procedures. Experience might also be an important factor in making an intraoperative distinction between Hinchey III and IV diverticulitis, as experience and technical skills are a requirement for meticulous lavage and ruling out free perforations that might be difficult to find [97]. Consequently, in case laparoscopic lavage is contraindicated

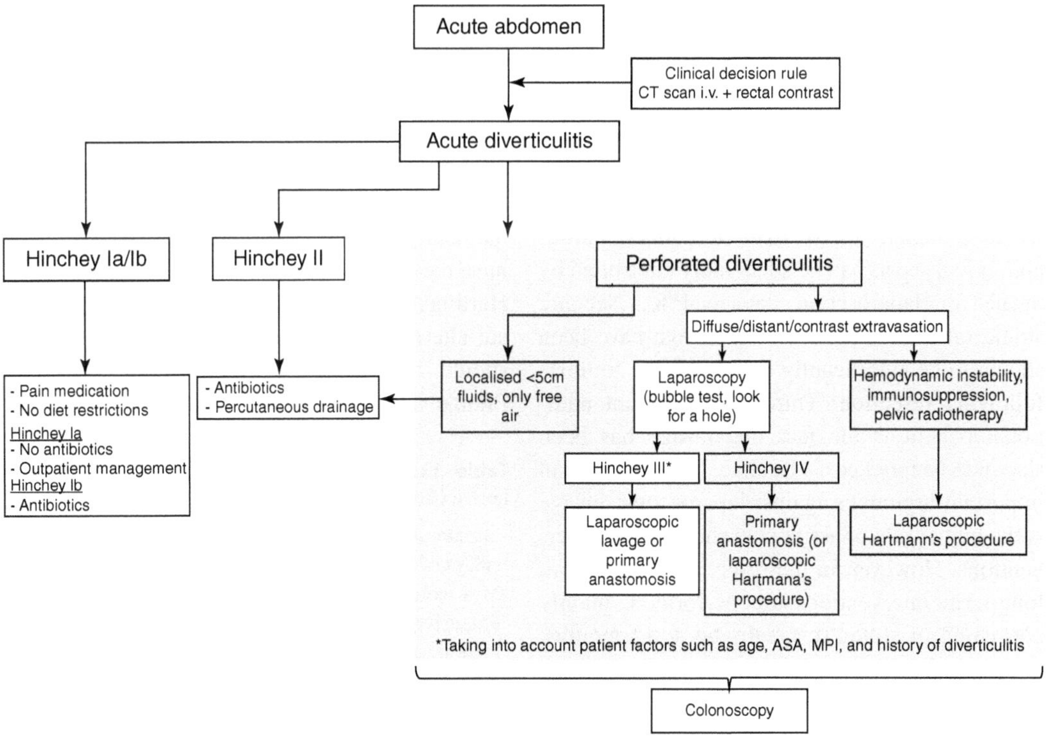

Fig. 12.3 Simplified flowchart summarising potential treatment options and indications

and conversion to a colon resection is required, experienced laparoscopic surgeons might more often choose a laparoscopic resectional strategy over an open procedure. Moreover, experience is of importance for the initial procedure, but also with regard to the timely recognition and correct management of complications of the procedure. Unfortunately, evidence on the learning curve of laparoscopic lavage for perforated diverticulitis is absent in the literature, and, therefore, eligibility criteria are difficult to define. However, it is evident that performing a significant number of laparoscopic and conventional emergency colorectal procedures is required. In a recent feasibility trial on the role of laparoscopic colorectal surgery in the acute setting, surgeon eligibility criteria included a minimum of 50 previously performed laparoscopic colorectal resections, with an annual rate of at least 20 elective laparoscopic resections, and with equivalent experience in the open setting [98].

Other Considerations

Although laparoscopic lavage has not conclusively proven to be superior to resectional treatment, several potential benefits support its use in carefully selected patients, and by surgeons with the appropriate expertise. First, in the vast majority of patients, up to 76% of patients, intra-abdominal sepsis can be adequately controlled by means of laparoscopic lavage [58]. Second, stoma rates after laparoscopic lavage have been shown to be significantly lower relative to those following resection. Third, an important additional benefit is the fact that lavage has been shown to be more cost-effective. Nevertheless, an important argument against laparoscopic lavage is the higher rate of associated short-term reinterventions. However, in the resection group, more long-term interventions are performed, mainly consisting of stoma reversal, and at 12 months, the morbidity and mortality rates seemed not be equivalent between non-resectional and resectional approaches. Hence, the dilemma remains as to whether the long-term adverse outcomes of resectional treatment outweigh the short-term adverse outcomes of laparoscopic lavage.

Since the misdiagnosis of Hinchey IV diverticulitis and underlying colorectal carcinoma seemed to have been the most frequent reasons for short-term failure, an important step towards reducing the rate of short-term failure of laparoscopic lavage in Hinchey III diverticulitis is to improve the accuracy of preoperative and intraoperative diagnostics. This may be best accomplished with a CT scan with intravenous and rectal contrast and/or intraoperative sigmoidoscopy. Another important strategy is to apply strict patient selection criteria for lavage. Several features have been found to be risk factors for the failure of laparoscopic lavage, such as a high ASA grade, older age, high MPI score, no prior history of diverticulitis, and finding of a free perforation at the time of surgery (Table 12.1). Moreover, it is important to stress that most of the evidence related to laparoscopic lavage has originated from randomised clinical trials, each with specific inclusion and exclusion criteria and selection biases.

For patients for whom laparoscopic lavage is not recommended, the optimal type of resection needs to be considered. Firstly, in complicated scenarios such as cases with an overt perforation or Hinchey IV diverticulitis, resection with primary anastomosis should be the procedure of choice. Secondly, in patients who are haemodynamically unstable, immunosuppressed, or who have received pelvic radiotherapy, a laparoscopic Hartmann's procedure would be a more appropriate alternative. In the latter cases, the specimen should be extracted via the stoma site or a Pfannenstiel incision when possible. An impor-

Table 12.1 Risk factors for failure of laparoscopic lavage (from multivariable analyses)

Immunosuppression [1, 94]
ASA grade >II [82, 96]
MPI score ≥24 [48, 49]
Extensive adhesiolysis [48, 49]
Identification of a free perforation [48, 49]
Smoking [49]
Steroid use [49]

ASA American Society of Anesthesiologists, *MPI* Mannheim Peritonitis Index

tant benefit of a laparoscopic versus open HP is its associated higher rate of stoma reversals as well as a higher chance of completing HP reversal laparoscopically [99].

Finally, to be able to address the questions "When, how, and should we?" with more certainty, more evidence on the long-term follow-up of laparoscopic lavage might be of relevance [28]. Such outcomes might benefit the discussion if long-term benefits outweigh the potential short-term disadvantages of laparoscopic lavage. Hence, long-term outcomes of the SCANDIV trial and the LOLA arm of the Ladies trial have been recently published. Moreover, the results of the randomised LapLAND trial, comparing laparoscopic lavage to bowel resection, have not yet been published and might add new insights to the existing evidence. In addition, individual patient-based meta-analyses might be able to identify predictive factors from the combined study populations. In addition, national registry studies or cross-sectional population-based studies might be able to provide novel insights into the outcomes of different strategies for the treatment of complicated diverticulitis, including laparoscopic lavage, particularly as they reflect true clinical practice.

Conclusion

Based on the evidence presented in this chapter, it can be stated that laparoscopic lavage is definitely a reasonable treatment option for patients with perforated diverticulitis with purulent peritonitis. However, it is important to rule out other diagnoses such as Hinchey IV and perforated colorectal cancer, which are a cause of treatment failure. Moreover, it should only be performed by surgical teams with significant experience in laparoscopic colorectal emergency surgery. In this respect, centralisation of colorectal care might be advantageous. Future evidence (e.g. more results from long-term studies) and future studies (e.g. national registries or cross-sectional population-based studies) will likely help to make more definitive statements on the role of laparoscopic lavage.

References

1. Andersen JC, Bundgaard L, Elbrond H, Laurberg S, Walker LR, Stovring J, et al. Danish national guidelines for treatment of diverticular disease. Dan Med J. 2012;59(5):C4453.
2. Andeweg CS, Mulder IM, Felt-Bersma RJ, Verbon A, van der Wilt GJ, van Goor H, et al. Guidelines of diagnostics and treatment of acute left-sided colonic diverticulitis. Dig Surg. 2013;30(4–6):278–92.
3. Heise CP. Epidemiology and pathogenesis of diverticular disease. J Gastrointest Surg. 2008;12(8):1309–11.
4. Vermeulen J, Van der Harst E, Lange JF. Pathophysiology and prevention of diverticulitis and perforation. Neth J Med. 2010;68(10):303–9.
5. Delvaux M. Diverticular disease of the colon in Europe: epidemiology, impact on citizen health and prevention. Aliment Pharmacol Ther. 2003;18(Suppl 3):71–4.
6. Hughes LE. Postmortem survey of diverticular disease of the colon. II. The muscular abnormality of the sigmoid colon. Gut. 1969;10(5):344–51.
7. Loffeld RJ. Long-term follow-up and development of diverticulitis in patients diagnosed with diverticulosis of the colon. Int J Color Dis. 2016;31(1):15–7.
8. Shahedi K, Fuller G, Bolus R, Cohen E, Vu M, Shah R, et al. Long-term risk of acute diverticulitis among patients with incidental diverticulosis found during colonoscopy. Clin Gastroenterol Hepatol. 2013;11(12):1609–13.
9. Vennix S, Morton DG, Hahnloser D, Lange JF, Bemelman WA. Research Committee of the European Society of Coloproctocology. Systematic review of evidence and consensus on diverticulitis: an analysis of national and international guidelines. Color Dis. 2014;16(11):866–78.
10. Bharucha AE, Parthasarathy G, Ditah I, Fletcher JG, Ewelukwa O, Pendlimari R, et al. Temporal trends in the incidence and natural history of diverticulitis: a population-based study. Am J Gastroenterol. 2015;110(11):1589–96.
11. Kaiser AM, Jiang JK, Lake JP, Ault G, Artinyan A, Gonzalez-Ruiz C, et al. The management of complicated diverticulitis and the role of computed tomography. Am J Gastroenterol. 2005;100(4):910–7.
12. Skoldberg F, Granlund J, Discacciati A, Hjern F, Schmidt PT, Olen O. Incidence and lifetime risk of hospitalization and surgery for diverticular disease. Br J Surg. 2019;106:930–9.
13. Humes DJ, West J. Role of acute diverticulitis in the development of complicated colonic diverticular disease and 1-year mortality after diagnosis in the UK: population-based cohort study. Gut. 2012;61(1):95–100.
14. Binda GA, Mataloni F, Bruzzone M, Carabotti M, Cirocchi R, Nascimbeni R, et al. Trends in hospital admission for acute diverticulitis in Italy from 2008 to 2015. Tech Coloproctol. 2018;22(8):597–604.

15. Jamal Talabani A, Lydersen S, Endreseth BH, Edna TH. Major increase in admission- and incidence rates of acute colonic diverticulitis. Int J Color Dis. 2014;29(8):937–45.
16. Peery AF, Dellon ES, Lund J, Crockett SD, McGowan CE, Bulsiewicz WJ, et al. Burden of gastrointestinal disease in the United States: 2012 update. Gastroenterology. 2012;143(5):1179–87.e3.
17. Peery AF, Crockett SD, Murphy CC, Lund JL, Dellon ES, Williams JL, et al. Burden and cost of gastrointestinal, liver, and pancreatic diseases in the United States: update 2018. Gastroenterology. 2019;156(1):254–72.e11.
18. Klarenbeek BR, de Korte N, van der Peet DL, Cuesta MA. Review of current classifications for diverticular disease and a translation into clinical practice. Int J Color Dis. 2012;27(2):207–14.
19. Hansen O, Graupe F, Stock W. [Prognostic factors in perforating diverticulitis of the large intestine] Prognosefaktoren der perforierten Dickdarmdiverticulitis. Chirurg. 1998;69(4):443–9.
20. Kohler L, Sauerland S, Neugebauer E. Diagnosis and treatment of diverticular disease: results of a consensus development conference. The Scientific Committee of the European Association for Endoscopic Surgery. Surg Endosc. 1999;13(4):430–6.
21. Hinchey EJ, Schaal PG, Richards GK. Treatment of perforated diverticular disease of the colon. Adv Surg. 1978;12:85–109.
22. Wasvary H, Turfah F, Kadro O, Beauregard W. Same hospitalization resection for acute diverticulitis. Am Surg. 1999;65(7):632–5; discussion 6.
23. Vermeulen J, Lange JF. Treatment of perforated diverticulitis with generalized peritonitis: past, present, and future. World J Surg. 2010;34(3):587–93.
24. Azhar N, Johanssen A, Sundström T, et al. SCANDIV Study Group. Laparoscopic lavage vs primary resection for acute perforated diverticulitis: long-term outcomes from the Scandinavian Diverticulitis (SCANDIV) randomized clinical trial. JAMA Surg. 2021;156(2):121–7. https://doi.org/10.1001/jamasurg.2020.5618.
25. Schultz JK, Wallon C, Blecic L, et al. SCANDIV Study Group. One-year results of the SCANDIV randomized clinical trial of laparoscopic lavage versus primary resection for acute perforated diverticulitis. Br J Surg. 2017;104(10):1382–92. https://doi.org/10.1002/bjs.10567. Epub 2017 Jun 20.
26. Myers E, Hurley M, O'Sullivan GC, Kavanagh D, Wilson I, Winter DC. Laparoscopic peritoneal lavage for generalized peritonitis due to perforated diverticulitis. Br J Surg. 2008;95(1):97–101.
27. Bemelman WA. Perforated sigmoid diverticulitis: Hartmann's procedure or resection with primary anastomosis. Tech Coloproctol. 2018;22(10):739–40.
28. Horesh N, Emile SH, Khan SM, Freund MR, Garoufalia Z, Silva-Alvarenga E, Gefen R, Wexner SD. Meta-analysis of randomized clinical trials on long-term outcomes of surgical treatment of perforated diverticulitis. Ann Surg. 2023;278(5):e966–72. https://doi.org/10.1097/SLA.0000000000005909. Epub 2023 May 30.
29. Mayo WJ, Wilson LB, Giffin HZ. Acquired diverticulitis of the large intestine. Surg Gynec Obst. 1907;25:237.
30. Judd ES, Pollock LW. Diverticulitis of the colon. Ann Surg. 1924;80(3):425.
31. Lockhart-Mummery J. Late results in diverticulitis. Lancet. 1938;232(6016):1401–4.
32. Smithwick RH. Experiences with the surgical management of diverticulitis of the sigmoid. Ann Surg. 1942;115(6):969.
33. Hartmann H. Note sur un procede nouveau dextirpation des cancer de la partie terminale du colon. Bull Men Soc Chir Paris. 1923:1474–7.
34. Binda GA, Karas JR, Serventi A, Sokmen S, Amato A, Hydo L, et al. Primary anastomosis vs nonrestorative resection for perforated diverticulitis with peritonitis: a prematurely terminated randomized controlled trial. Color Dis. 2012;14(11):1403–10.
35. Bridoux V, Regimbeau JM, Ouaissi M, Mathonnet M, Mauvais F, Houivet E, et al. Hartmann's procedure or primary anastomosis for generalized peritonitis due to perforated diverticulitis: a prospective multicenter randomized trial (DIVERTI). J Am Coll Surg. 2017;225(6):798–805.
36. Oberkofler CE, Rickenbacher A, Raptis DA, Lehmann K, Villiger P, Buchli C, et al. A multicenter randomized clinical trial of primary anastomosis or Hartmann's procedure for perforated left colonic diverticulitis with purulent or fecal peritonitis. Ann Surg. 2012;256(5):819–26; discussion 26–7.
37. Lambrichts DPV, Vennix S, Musters GD, Mulder IM, Swank HA, Hoofwijk AGM, et al. Hartmann's procedure versus sigmoidectomy with primary anastomosis for perforated diverticulitis with purulent or faecal peritonitis (LADIES): a multicentre, parallel-group, randomised, open-label, superiority trial. Lancet Gastroenterol Hepatol. 2019;4:599–610.
38. O'Sullivan GC, Murphy D, O'Brien MG, Ireland A. Laparoscopic management of generalized peritonitis due to perforated colonic diverticula. Am J Surg. 1996;171(4):432–4.
39. Da AR, Guerriero S, Fiamingo P, Pariset S, Veroux M, Pilon F, et al. Laparoscopic colorrhaphy, irrigation and drainage in the treatment of complicated acute diverticulitis: initial experience. Chir Ital. 2004;56(1):95–8.
40. Faranda C, Barrat C, Catheline J-M, Champault GG. Two-stage laparoscopic management of generalized peritonitis due to perforated sigmoid diverticula: eighteen cases. Surg Laparosc Endosc Percutan Tech. 2000;10(3):135–8.
41. Taylor CJ, Layani L, Ghusn MA, White SI. Perforated diverticulitis managed by laparoscopic lavage. ANZ J Surg. 2006;76(11):962–5.

42. Toorenvliet B, Swank H, Schoones J, Hamming J, Bemelman W. Laparoscopic peritoneal lavage for perforated colonic diverticulitis: a systematic review. Color Dis. 2010;12(9):862–7.
43. Schultz JK, Yaqub S, Wallon C, Blecic L, Forsmo HM, Folkesson J, et al. Laparoscopic lavage vs primary resection for acute perforated diverticulitis: the SCANDIV randomized clinical trial. JAMA. 2015;314(13):1364–75.
44. Swank HA, Vermeulen J, Lange JF, Mulder IM, van der Hoeven JA, Stassen LP, et al. The ladies trial: laparoscopic peritoneal lavage or resection for purulent peritonitis and Hartmann's procedure or resection with primary anastomosis for purulent or faecal peritonitis in perforated diverticulitis (NTR2037). BMC Surg. 2010;10(1):29.
45. Thornell A, Angenete E, Gonzales E, Heath J, Jess P, Lackberg Z, et al. Treatment of acute diverticulitis laparoscopic lavage vs. resection (DILALA): study protocol for a randomised controlled trial. Trials. 2011;12:186.
46. Gregori M, Cassini D, Depalma N, Miccini M, Manoochehri F, Baldazzi GA. Laparoscopic lavage and drainage for Hinchey III diverticulitis: review of technical aspects. Updat Surg. 2018;71:237–46.
47. Franklin ME, Hernández MA. Perforated diverticulitis: laparoscopic lavage and drainage. In: Current common dilemmas in colorectal surgery. Springer; 2018. p. 121–8.
48. Ahmad G, Baker J, Finnerty J, Phillips K, Watson A. Laparoscopic entry techniques. Cochrane Database Syst Rev. 2019;1:CD006583.
49. Binda GA, Bonino MA, Siri G, Di Saverio S, Rossi G, Nascimbeni R, et al. Multicentre international trial of laparoscopic lavage for Hinchey III acute diverticulitis (LLO Study). Br J Surg. 2018;105(13):1835–43.
50. Franklin ME, Portillo G, Treviño JM, Gonzalez JJ, Glass JL. Long-term experience with the laparoscopic approach to perforated diverticulitis plus generalized peritonitis. World J Surg. 2008;32(7):1507–11.
51. Mazza D, Khoury-Helou A. Conservative laparoscopic treatment of diverticular peritonitis. J Chir. 2009;146(3):265–9.
52. Bretagnol F, Pautrat K, Mor C, Benchellal Z, Huten N, de Calan L. Emergency laparoscopic management of perforated sigmoid diverticulitis: a promising alternative to more radical procedures. J Am Coll Surg. 2008;206(4):654–7.
53. Rossi GL, Mentz R, Bertone S, Quintana GO, Bilbao S, Im VM, et al. Laparoscopic peritoneal lavage for Hinchey III diverticulitis: is it as effective as it is applicable? Dis Colon Rectum. 2014;57(12):1384–90.
54. White SI, Frenkiel B, Martin PJ. A ten-year audit of perforated sigmoid diverticulitis: highlighting the outcomes of laparoscopic lavage. Dis Colon Rectum. 2010;53(11):1537–41.
55. Horesh N, Zbar AP, Nevler A, Haim N, Gutman M, Zmora O. Early experience with laparoscopic lavage in acute complicated diverticulitis. Dig Surg. 2015;32(2):108–11.
56. Liang S, Russek K, Franklin ME. Damage control strategy for the management of perforated diverticulitis with generalized peritonitis: laparoscopic lavage and drainage vs. laparoscopic Hartmann's procedure. Surg Endosc. 2012;26(10):2835–42.
57. Schultz JK, Wallon C, Blecic L, Forsmo HM, Folkesson J, Buchwald P, et al. One-year results of the SCANDIV randomized clinical trial of laparoscopic lavage versus primary resection for acute perforated diverticulitis. Br J Surg. 2017;104(10):1382–92.
58. Vennix S, Musters GD, Mulder IM, Swank HA, Consten EC, Belgers EH, et al. Laparoscopic peritoneal lavage or sigmoidectomy for perforated diverticulitis with purulent peritonitis: a multicentre, parallel-group, randomised, open-label trial. Lancet. 2015;386(10000):1269–77.
59. Ceresoli M, Coccolini F, Montori G, Catena F, Sartelli M, Ansaloni L. Laparoscopic lavage versus resection in perforated diverticulitis with purulent peritonitis: a meta-analysis of randomized controlled trials. World J Emerg Surg. 2016;11(1):42.
60. Angenete E, Bock D, Rosenberg J, Haglind E. Laparoscopic lavage is superior to colon resection for perforated purulent diverticulitis—a meta-analysis. Int J Color Dis. 2017;32(2):163–9.
61. Cirocchi R, Di Saverio S, Weber D, Tabola R, Abraha I, Randolph J, et al. Laparoscopic lavage versus surgical resection for acute diverticulitis with generalised peritonitis: a systematic review and meta-analysis. Tech Coloproctol. 2017;21(2):93–110.
62. Galbraith N, Carter JV, Netz U, Yang D, Fry DE, McCafferty M, et al. Laparoscopic lavage in the management of perforated diverticulitis: a contemporary meta-analysis. J Gastrointest Surg. 2017;21(9):1491–9.
63. Marshall JR, Buchwald PL, Gandhi J, Schultz JK, Hider PN, Frizelle FA, et al. Laparoscopic lavage in the management of Hinchey grade III diverticulitis. Ann Surg. 2017;265(4):670–6.
64. Shaikh FM, Stewart PM, Walsh SR, Davies RJ. Laparoscopic peritoneal lavage or surgical resection for acute perforated sigmoid diverticulitis: a systematic review and meta-analysis. Int J Surg. 2017;38:130–7.
65. Acuna SA, Wood T, Chesney TR, Dossa F, Wexner SD, Quereshy FA, et al. Operative strategies for perforated diverticulitis: a systematic review and meta-analysis. Dis Colon Rectum. 2018;61(12):1442–53.
66. Penna M, Markar SR, Mackenzie H, Hompes R, Cunningham C. Laparoscopic lavage versus primary resection for acute perforated diverticulitis. Ann Surg. 2018;267(2):252–8.
67. Gralista P, Moris D, Vailas M, Angelou A, Petrou A, Felekouras E, et al. Laparoscopic approach in colonic diverticulitis: dispelling myths and misper-

ceptions. Surg Laparosc Endosc Percutan Tech. 2017;27(2):73–82.
68. Germer CT, Reibetanz J. Langzeitergebnisse der laparoskopischen Lavage vs. Sigmaresektion bei perforierter Sigmadivertikulitis: Ergebnisse einer Metaanalyse [Long-term results of laparoscopic lavage vs. sigmoid resection for perforated diverticulitis: results of a meta-analysis]. Chirurgie (Heidelb). 2023;94(11):963–4.https://doi.org/10.1007/s00104--023-01967-x. German. Epub 2023 Oct 12.
69. Cirocchi R, Popivanov G, Konaktchieva M, et al. The role of damage control surgery in the treatment of perforated colonic diverticulitis: a systematic review and meta-analysis. Int J Color Dis. 2021;36(5):867–79.https://doi.org/10.1007/s00384--020-03784-8. Epub 2020 Oct 22. PMID: 33089382.
70. Pan Z, Pan ZH, Pan RZ, Xie YX, Desai G. Is laparoscopic lavage safe in purulent diverticulitis versus colonic resection? A systematic review and meta-analysis. Int J Surg. 2019;71:182–9. https://doi.org/10.1016/j.ijsu.2019.10.007. Epub 2019 Oct 11.
71. Angenete E, Thornell A, Burcharth J, Pommergaard HC, Skullman S, Bisgaard T, et al. Laparoscopic lavage is feasible and safe for the treatment of perforated diverticulitis with purulent peritonitis: the first results from the randomized controlled trial DILALA. Ann Surg. 2016;263(1):117–22.
72. Thornell A, Angenete E, Bisgaard T, Bock D, Burcharth J, Heath J, et al. Laparoscopic lavage for perforated diverticulitis with purulent peritonitis: a randomized trial. Ann Intern Med. 2016;164(3):137–45.
73. Vennix S, van Dieren S, Opmeer BC, Lange JF, Bemelman WA. Cost analysis of laparoscopic lavage compared with sigmoid resection for perforated diverticulitis in the Ladies trial. Br J Surg. 2017;104(1):62–8.
74. Dindo D, Demartines N, Clavien P-A. Classification of surgical complications: a new proposal with evaluation in a cohort of 6336 patients and results of a survey. Ann Surg. 2004;240(2):205.
75. Kohl A, Rosenberg J, Bock D, Bisgaard T, Skullman S, Thornell A, et al. Two-year results of the randomized clinical trial DILALA comparing laparoscopic lavage with resection as treatment for perforated diverticulitis. Br J Surg. 2018;105(9):1128–34.
76. Hoek VT, Edomskis PP, Stark PW, et al. LADIES Trial Collaborators. Laparoscopic peritoneal lavage versus sigmoidectomy for perforated diverticulitis with purulent peritonitis: three-year follow-up of the randomised LOLA trial. Surg Endosc. 2022;36(10):7764–74. https://doi.org/10.1007/s00464-022-09326-3. Epub 2022 May 23.
77. Sneiders D, Lambrichts DPV, Swank HA, Blanken-Peeters C, Nienhuijs SW, Govaert M, et al. Long-term follow-up of a multicentre cohort study on laparoscopic peritoneal lavage for perforated diverticulitis. Color Dis. 2019;21:705–14.
78. Swank H, Mulder I, Hoofwijk A, Nienhuijs S, Lange J, Bemelman W, et al. Early experience with laparoscopic lavage for perforated diverticulitis. Br J Surg. 2013;100(5):704–10.
79. Gehrman J, Angenete E, Björholt I, Bock D, Rosenberg J, Haglind E. Health economic analysis of laparoscopic lavage versus Hartmann's procedure for diverticulitis in the randomized DILALA trial. Br J Surg. 2016;103(11):1539–47.
80. Vermeulen J, Gosselink MP, Busschbach JJ, Lange JF. Avoiding or reversing Hartmann's procedure provides improved quality of life after perforated diverticulitis. J Gastrointest Surg. 2010;14(4):651–7.
81. Azhar N, Johanssen A, Sundström T, et al. SCANDIV Study Group. Laparoscopic lavage vs primary resection for acute perforated diverticulitis: long-term outcomes from the Scandinavian Diverticulitis (SCANDIV) randomized clinical trial. JAMA Surg. 2021;156(2):121–7. https://doi.org/10.1001/jamasurg.2020.5618. Erratum in: JAMA Surg. 2021;156(9):894. https://doi.org/10.1001/jamasurg.2021.3556. PMID: 33355658.
82. Agresta F, Ansaloni L, Baiocchi GL, Bergamini C, Campanile FC, Carlucci M, et al. Laparoscopic approach to acute abdomen from the Consensus Development Conference of the Società Italiana di Chirurgia Endoscopica e nuove tecnologie (SICE), Associazione Chirurghi Ospedalieri Italiani (ACOI), Società Italiana di Chirurgia (SIC), Società Italiana di Chirurgia d'Urgenza e del Trauma (SICUT), Società Italiana di Chirurgia nell'Ospedalità Privata (SICOP), and the European Association for Endoscopic Surgery (EAES). Surg Endosc. 2012;26(8):2134–64.
83. Fozard JBJ, Armitage NC, Schofield JB, Jones OM. ACPGBI position statement on elective resection for diverticulitis. Color Dis. 2011;13:1–11.
84. Sartelli M, Viale P, Catena F, Ansaloni L, Moore E, Malangoni M, et al. 2013 WSES guidelines for management of intra-abdominal infections. World J Emerg Surg. 2013;8(1):3.
85. Sartelli M, Weber DG, Kluger Y, et al. 2020 update of the WSES guidelines for the management of acute colonic diverticulitis in the emergency setting. World J Emerg Surg. 2020;15(1):32. https://doi.org/10.1186/s13017-020-00313-4. PMID: 32381121; PMCID: PMC7206757.
86. Hall J, Hardiman K, Lee S, et al. Prepared on behalf of the Clinical Practice Guidelines Committee of the American Society of Colon and Rectal Surgeons. The American Society of Colon and Rectal Surgeons clinical practice guidelines for the treatment of left-sided colonic diverticulitis. Dis Colon Rectum. 2020;63(6):728–47. https://doi.org/10.1097/DCR.0000000000001679. PMID: 32384404.
87. Galetin T, Galetin A, Vestweber KH, Rink AD. Systematic review and comparison of national and international guidelines on diverticular disease. Int J Color Dis. 2018;33(3):261–72.
88. Sartelli M, Catena F, Ansaloni L, Coccolini F, Griffiths EA, Abu-Zidan FM, et al. WSES guidelines for the management of acute left sided colonic diver-

ticulitis in the emergency setting. World J Emerg Surg. 2016;11(1):37.
89. Schuster KM, Holena DN, Salim A, Savage S, Crandall M. American Association for the Surgery of Trauma emergency general surgery guideline summaries 2018: acute appendicitis, acute cholecystitis, acute diverticulitis, acute pancreatitis, and small bowel obstruction. Trauma Surg Acute Care Open. 2019;4(1):e000281.
90. Netherlands Society of Surgery. Guidelines of diagnostics and treatment of acute left-sided colonic diverticulitis. 2018.
91. Francis NK, Sylla P, Abou-Khalil M, Arolfo S, Berler D, Curtis NJ, et al. EAES and SAGES 2018 consensus conference on acute diverticulitis management: evidence-based recommendations for clinical practice. Surg Endosc. 2019;33(9):2726–41.
92. Schultz JK, Azhar N, Binda GA, Barbara G, Biondo S, Boermester MA, et al. European Society of Coloproctology: guidelines for the management of diverticular disease of the colon. Color Dis. 2020;22(Suppl 2):5–28.
93. Hall J, Hardiman K, Lee S, Lightner A, Stocchi L, Paquette IM, et al. The American Society of Colon and Rectal Surgeons clinical practice guidelines for the treatment of left-sided colonic diverticulitis. Dis Colon Rectum. 2020;63(6):728–47.
94. Greilsamer T, Abet E, Meurette G, Comy M, Hamy A, Lehur P-A, et al. Is the failure of laparoscopic peritoneal lavage predictable in Hinchey III diverticulitis management? Dis Colon Rectum. 2017;60(9):965–70.
95. Azhar N, Lambrichts D, Lange J, Yaqub S, Øresland T, Schultz J, Bemelman W, Buchwald P. Laparoscopic lavage for Hinchey III perforated diverticulitis: factors for treatment failure in two randomized clinical trials. Br J Surg. 2023;110(7):846–51. https://doi.org/10.1093/bjs/znad114. PMID: 37202860.
96. Radé F, Bretagnol F, Auguste M, Di Guisto C, Huten N, De Calan L. Determinants of outcome following laparoscopic peritoneal lavage for perforated diverticulitis. Br J Surg. 2014;101(12):1602–6.
97. Di Saverio S, Birindelli A, Catena F, Sartelli M, Segalini E, Masetti M, et al. The ladies trial: premature termination of the LOLA arm and increased adverse events incidence after laparoscopic lavage may be influenced by inter-hospital and inter-operator variability? Take-home messages from a center with laparoscopic colorectal expertise. Int J Surg. 2016;36(Pt A):118.
98. Harji DP, Marshall H, Gordon K, Twiddy M, Pullan A, Meads D, et al. Laparoscopic versus open colorectal surgery in the acute setting (LaCeS trial): a multicentre randomized feasibility trial. Br J Surg. 2020;107:1595–604.
99. Vennix S, Lips DJ, Di Saverio S, van Wagensveld BA, Brokelman WJ, Gerhards MF, et al. Acute laparoscopic and open sigmoidectomy for perforated diverticulitis: a propensity score-matched cohort. Surg Endosc. 2016;30(9):3889–96.

Technical Tips and Tricks in the Emergency Setting

13

Lawrence Lee and Maude Trepanier

Introduction

Operative management for acute diverticulitis poses particular challenges to the surgeon [1]. The inflamed colonic segment is difficult to manipulate, and normal planes are often obliterated, making the identification of the key structures difficult and thus prone to injury. Furthermore, there are increasing data to suggest that resection and primary anastomosis, with or without proximal diversion, are safe and feasible in select cases [2–4], adding additional complexity to the decision-making process. The surgeon must be aware of the important differences in the operative management between acute and elective cases. The objective of this chapter is to provide the reader with a standardized operative decision-making process and approach, as well as to provide insights into specific challenges that may be encountered in the emergency setting.

Supplementary Information The online version contains supplementary material available at https://doi.org/10.1007/978-3-032-21720-2_13.

L. Lee (✉)
Steinberg-Bernstein Centre for Minimally Invasive Surgery and Innovation, Department of Surgery, McGill University Health Centre, Montreal, QC, Canada

Colon and Rectal Surgery, Department of Surgery, McGill University Health Centre, Montreal, QC, Canada
e-mail: larry.lee@mail.mcgill.ca

M. Trepanier
Steinberg-Bernstein Centre for Minimally Invasive Surgery and Innovation, Department of Surgery, McGill University Health Centre, Montreal, QC, Canada
e-mail: maude.trepanier@mail.mcgill.ca

Operative Approach

Set-Up

The first decision that must be made is whether emergency surgery for acute diverticulitis should be approached via a laparoscopic or open approach. Evidence to support or refute the safety and effectiveness of laparoscopic surgery versus open surgical resection for the treatment of patients with acute diverticular disease is insufficient [5]. There are clear indications in which an open approach is prudent, especially for patients who are hemodynamically unstable or who have contraindications to laparoscopy, such as multiple previous laparotomies or severe pulmonary disease. The surgeon's skillset should also be considered in this decision, as experienced minimally invasive surgeons who perform a high volume of laparoscopic colectomies may have a lower threshold to consider laparoscopy versus those who primarily perform open surgery. Laparoscopic sigmoid resection is associated with decreased perioperative morbidity [6] but can be more difficult than for malignancy [7] and, therefore, may not be appropriate for surgeons

M. Boutros et al. (eds.), *Diverticulitis*, https://doi.org/10.1007/978-3-032-21720-2_13

who are early in their learning curve for minimally invasive left-sided colectomies [8, 9]. Hand-assisted laparoscopic resection may also be used, but this approach also has its own learning curve [10].

It is the authors' preference to attempt a laparoscopic approach whenever patient factors allow. For these cases, the patient is placed supine with split legs. The split leg positioning (Fig. 13.1) is preferred over the Lloyd-Davies position because of the decreased risk of lower extremity peripheral nerve injury. While the incidence of these injuries is low [10], they can result in significant functional impairments [11]. The split leg position enables access to the anus for potential anastomosis with the circular stapler and intra-operative endoscopy, if required. Extensive access to the anal canal is rarely required in this setting, eliminating the advantage of the Lloyd-Davies position. The patient is securely fastened to the operating room table with the arms tucked if a laparoscopic procedure is performed, or with the arms out in the case of a laparotomy. Steep Trendelenburg positioning is often required during the laparoscopic approach, and the patient may require additional support with a bean-bag wrapped around the patient's side and shoulders or with a Pink Pad® (Xodus Medical, New Kensington, PA). Additional support is usually not required during a laparotomy. A surgical pause with the World Health Organization (WHO) checklist is performed for all patients, and preoperative antibiotics and thromboprophylaxis are administered as necessary.

Laparoscopic Approach

Abdominal access is initially obtained using the open Hasson approach. A diagnostic laparoscopy is performed, and the abdomen is thoroughly explored to confirm the diagnosis of acute diverticulitis and assess the degree of contamination. If adequate working space can be obtained, additional trocars are placed under direct vision. Standard trocar positioning is shown in Fig. 13.2. The operator uses the right upper and lower quadrant trocars as the working ports, and the assistant stands to the operator's right to manipulate the camera and assist via the suprapubic port. The stepwise decision-making algorithm during the diagnostic laparoscopy is as follows:

1. *Is the diagnosis of acute diverticulitis confirmed?* The diagnostic accuracy of thin-slice computed tomography for acute diverticulitis is high. However, there may be diagnostic uncertainty based on radiologic imaging in approximately 10% of cases [12]. A long affected segment with pericolonic lymph nodes is highly suggestive of diverticulitis, but in the setting of perforation, it may be difficult to differentiate between diverticulitis and malignancy. Tactile feedback in these

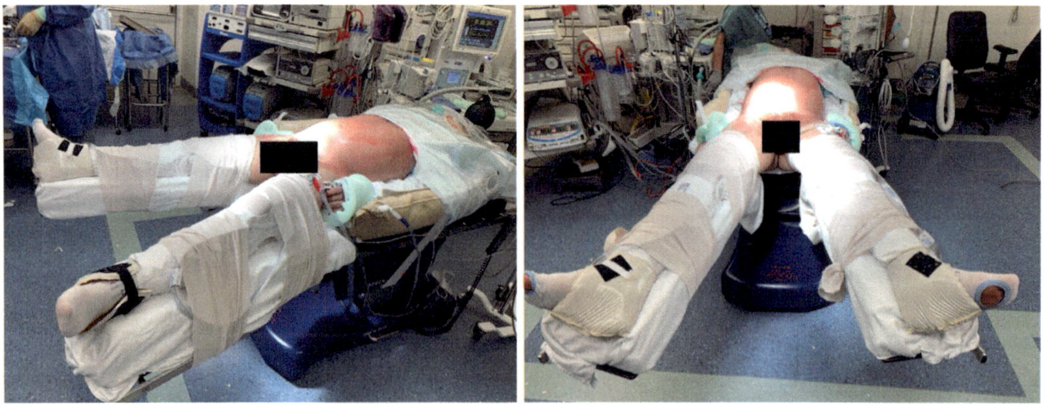

Fig. 13.1 Split leg positioning for left-sided resections. This decreases the risk of peripheral nerve injuries compared to the Lloyd-Davies (lithotomy) position while providing access to the anus for the introduction of a circular stapler

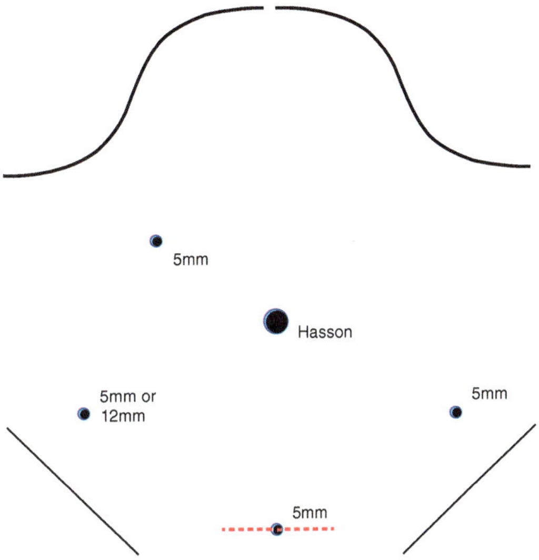

Fig. 13.2 Standard trocar placement for laparoscopic sigmoid resection. The suprapubic trocar is placed in the midline, two fingerbreadths above the pubic symphysis. The Pfannenstiel extraction incision is also made at this location (represented by the red dotted line). The right lower quadrant trocar is placed two fingerbreadths medial to the anterior superior iliac spine between the umbilical Hasson and the suprapubic trocars. The right upper quadrant trocar is placed one handbreadth diagonally above the umbilical trocar, between the right lower quadrant and umbilical trocars. The left lower quadrant trocar is placed as needed only and mirrors the right lower quadrant trocar

cases is essential, and if the surgeon has any doubt as to the diagnosis of acute diverticulitis, laparoscopy should be converted to hand-assist or an open procedure to allow for palpation and further assessment, as the extent of mesenteric resection is significantly different for these two conditions.

2. *Is there gross fecal contamination?* It is sometimes difficult to determine the degree of contamination based on preoperative imaging. During the diagnostic laparoscopy, the surgeon should assess whether the contamination is localized or diffuse, purulent or fecal, and whether adequate washout can be performed laparoscopically. In cases where there is diffuse fecal contamination, it is unlikely that a primary anastomosis will be feasible or that the abdomen can be sufficiently cleared of feces with laparoscopic suctions. In these cases, the procedure should be converted to a lower midline laparotomy to perform a Hartman's procedure and thoroughly irrigate the abdomen [13]. If the fecal contamination is relatively contained in the pelvis, the sigmoid mobilization and resection can be potentially completed through a suprapubic Pfannenstiel incision with or without hand-assisted laparoscopic guidance. A lower midline incision can also be used in these cases (discussed below).
3. *How inflamed is the affected segment of the sigmoid colon, and will it allow for safe laparoscopic handling?* It may be difficult to safely manipulate the affected segment laparoscopically due to tissue friability and inflammation. It is important that the surgeon be aware that the colon and its mesentery may tear easily and cause bleeding, which adds difficulty to the procedure. The affected segment can also be adherent to the retroperitoneal or anterior wall structures or surrounding bowel loops. It may be difficult to bluntly dissect the inflamed sigmoid colon off important structures if the tissues are very friable without fear of causing collateral damage. Furthermore, the proximal small bowel loops may be dilated and impede visualization. In these cases, conversion to hand-assisted laparoscopy or an open procedure may be prudent. The advantage of the hand-assist approach is that it allows for tactile feedback and easier bowel manipulation, while preserving the benefits of the minimally invasive approach. Furthermore, the hand-assist incision can be used for distal mobilization and/or transection, as well as specimen extraction. Blunt dissection using finger fracture can also be done during hand-assist. We usually create an 8–10 cm Pfannenstiel incision two fingerbreadths above the pubic symphysis for the hand port (GelPort®, Applied Medical, Rancho Santa Margarita, CA). There is debate whether a Pfannenstiel or a lower midline incision should be used for hand-assist. The Pfannenstiel incision is associated with fewer wound complications and is less painful than a lower midline [14]. The downside to a Pfannenstiel incision is that if a larger incision

or open access to the upper abdomen is required, this incision cannot be readily extended, and a midline laparotomy (which will "T" off the Pfannenstiel) may have to be created. Conversely, a lower midline incision can be readily extended if needed; however, exposure to the distal sigmoid and pelvis is limited with the smaller incision used for hand-assist, and it is ergonomically more challenging. If the surgeon does not have a lot of experience in hand-assist, a lower midline may be preferred due to the ease of extension.

4. *What are the proximal and distal resection margins?* The distal transection target is generally at the rectosigmoid junction and should include a small amount of the rectum. In cases where the inflammation may extend deep into the pelvis, the surgeon should avoid resecting more rectum than is absolutely necessary, as this may impede future attempts at restoring intestinal continuity. Proximally, the entire length of the hypertrophied colon should be resected. This is especially important if a primary anastomosis is under consideration, as both proximal and distal targets should be supple and non-inflamed. However, if technically difficult or in a damage-control setting, resection of the acutely inflamed segment is typically sufficient. The surgeon does not have to resect the entirety of the colon with diverticula, as often this can extend proximally up to the descending and transverse colon, and in some cases may even involve the whole colon to the ileocecal valve. It may be difficult to assess the degree of muscular hypertrophy during laparoscopy due to the lack of tactile feedback. The surgeon should decide whether proximal and distal intestinal transection should be performed laparoscopically with endoscopic staplers or open through a lower midline or Pfannenstiel incision.
5. *Is a primary anastomosis feasible?* There are increasing data to suggest that primary anastomosis in the setting of acute diverticulitis may be a viable option in select patients. Most recent evidence suggests that colonic resection with primary rectal anastomosis has better long-term outcomes than the Hartmann procedure for fecal peritonitis [15]. These patients should not have significant preoperative comorbidities or altered hemodynamics during the surgery. The contamination should be relatively contained and mild, and the proximal and distal targets should not be grossly inflamed. There have been several randomized trials that have compared resection and primary anastomosis with or without diverting ileostomy versus resection with end colostomy [3, 4, 16, 17]. In these trials, short-term morbidity and mortality were similar between the two groups, but there was a higher proportion of patients in the primary resection and anastomosis group who were stoma-free at 1 year [3, 4, 16]. These results suggest that resection and primary anastomosis are a feasible option in select patients. The use of this approach is increasing [18]. It is the authors' preference to perform this procedure whenever patient factors allow. However, in patients with significant comorbidities, altered hemodynamics, or gross contamination, resection with end colostomy remains the most prudent procedure. It is also important to consider that in cases where a Hartmann's procedure is performed, the major vessels, such as the left colic artery and inferior mesenteric vein, should be left intact so as to not make subsequent colostomy reversal more difficult.
6. *If a primary anastomosis is under consideration, is splenic flexure mobilization required to perform a tension-free anastomosis?* Sigmoid resection with subsequent primary anastomosis may require splenic flexure mobilization for adequate length to create a tension-free anastomosis [19]. This is especially important since the inferior mesentery artery (IMA) pedicle is often preserved in benign disease, thus limiting colonic reach. It is important to decide which vessel is the tethering point of the proximal margin. The left colic artery can usually be preserved in a colorectal anastomosis at the sacral promontory if the splenic flexure is fully mobilized [20]. However, if splenic flexure mobilization

is not adequate, the left colic artery is usually the tethering point after sigmoid resection for benign disease. A stepwise approach to vessel ligation is described below. It is our practice to mobilize the splenic flexure laparoscopically, even if the sigmoid mobilization is planned to be done open via a lower midline or Pfannenstiel incision, as this greatly reduces the total incision size.

The authors' favored approach is to perform the descending colon and splenic flexure mobilization laparoscopically, and then the remaining sigmoid dissection off of the lateral wall and retroperitoneum open through a Pfannenstiel incision. Mesenteric division, distal transection, and specimen extraction are done open through the same Pfannenstiel incision. This preserves the benefits of laparoscopy (mobilizing the descending colon and splenic flexure) while allowing for open visualization and tactile feedback of the most inflamed segment. Furthermore, abdominal washout can be done more effectively with large caliber open suctions, especially if there is some fecal contamination.

A lateral-to-medial approach is preferred for sigmoid and descending colon mobilization for diverticular disease. The base of the IMA usually does not need to be identified during resection for benign diverticular disease, as high ligation is rarely required in this context, especially if an end colostomy is planned. A medial-to-lateral approach in this context would require the surgeon to identify the correct plane of dissection between the colonic mesentery and the retroperitoneum above the superior rectal artery. This requires traversing through a potentially thickened and friable mesentery medially to reach the embryologic planes, which may result in bleeding that may further impede visualization. Energy devices can help avoid bleeding while going through the inflamed mesentery; however, this can be unsafe without first identifying the ureter, which may put it at risk for injury. Identification of the ureter from the medial to lateral approach is easiest and the least bloody if performed by incising the peritoneum at the level of the sacral promontory and lifting the superior rectal artery to expose the base of the inferior mesenteric artery and the retroperitoneum. However, this dissection exposes the sympathetic nerves to unnecessary potential injury, especially since an oncologic mesenteric resection is not required. A lateral-to-medial approach is advantageous as it addresses the most difficult part of the procedure for acute diverticulitis: dissection of an adherent and inflamed sigmoid off the retroperitoneum. If this is not feasible laparoscopically or with a hand-assist approach, then conversion to open surgery should be performed relatively quickly in order to avoid unnecessarily prolonged operative time. If the affected sigmoid segment can be safely dissected off the retroperitoneum, then the mesentery can be mobilized until the ureter is identified. This plane is usually bloodless and can be largely done with blunt dissection. This will avoid transection or thermal injuries to retroperitoneal structures during the lateral mobilization. Once the ureter is identified, the mesentery can be safely divided close to the bowel wall. Prior to mesenteric division, the lateral mobilization is continued proximally up the descending colon. The splenic flexure is selectively mobilized based on the decisions made during the diagnostic laparoscopy (see above). Mesenteric division is then performed intracorporeally with an energy device. Intracorporeal mesenteric division will facilitate specimen extraction.

The distal transection can then be done using an endoscopic stapling device. If a colostomy is planned, then a 12 mm trocar is placed at the site of the planned stoma. Once the distal margin is transected, the proximal staple line is grasped, the stoma aperture is created in standard fashion, and the bowel exteriorized. The proximal margin can then be divided, and the colostomy matured to the skin. This approach avoids any additional specimen extraction incisions. If intracorporeal stapling is not feasible, then a Pfannenstiel incision can be created two fingerbreadths above the pubic symphysis and the distal margin transected through the Pfannenstiel using an open stapler (Contour® Curved Cutter Stapler, Ethicon, Somerville, NJ). A wound protector device (Alexis wound protector, Applied Medical, Rancho Santa Margarita, CA) should be used to minimize the risk of surgical site infection [21], especially in the context of an inflamed or perforated sigmoid.

If a primary anastomosis is planned, then the 12 mm trocar is placed in the midline two fingerbreadths above the pubic symphysis at the intended Pfannenstiel specimen extraction site. A Pfannenstiel extraction incision is preferred as it allows for easier access to pelvic dissection and is the least morbid [14]. In cases when proximal diversion is performed after resection and primary anastomosis, the 12 mm trocar can be placed at the intended loop ileostomy site from which the specimen can also be extracted. This may require making the stoma aperture larger than one would normally create for an ileostomy, but the fascial incision can be partially closed afterwards if needed. Incision size should be at least as large as the anvil of the circular stapler, and often needs to be larger due to the size of the inflamed segment. A wound protector device should be used at the specimen extraction incision to minimize infection and the stapled end of the colon is exteriorized. The proximal margin is then transected extracorporeally and the anvil placed in an end-to-end or side-to-end configuration. There is no functional benefit of a side-to-end anastomosis for a colorectal anastomosis at the top of the rectum, however anastomotic leak rates may be lower [22]. The authors prefer a side-to-end configuration as this usually results in increased conduit mobility and less tension at the anastomosis. If this anastomosis is planned, it is important to make sure there is adequate distance from the circular stapler and the stapled end of the bowel. The spike of the anvil should be exited at the antimesenteric border away from the stapled end by at least 2 cm more than the radius of the circular stapler. For example, if a circular stapler of 29 mm diameter is to be used, then the spike of the anvil should be 3.5 cm away from the stapled end of the conduit (14 mm radius + 20 mm "pouch"). The exteriorized segment is then placed back into the abdomen and the anastomosis performed under direct vision. An air leak test should be performed with intraoperative flexible endoscopy, if available, as this allows for the inspection of the anastomosis and potential endoscopic intervention such as endoscopic clips for anastomotic bleeding, if needed. If flexible endoscopy is not available, then rigid sigmoidoscopy should be performed to insufflate the rectum and test the anastomosis.

Open Approach

While the laparoscopic approach may have potential short- and long-term benefits compared to the open approach, level I evidence is lacking [5]. One 2020 meta-analysis (including three randomized control trials) found that laparoscopic resection was superior to open surgery in terms of morbidity, while open surgery was superior in terms of severe complications [23]. Studies that favor laparoscopy report decreased morbidity and length of hospitalization, but are generally limited by small sample sizes and retrospective nature [24, 25]. If the surgeon is not an experienced laparoscopist or does not routinely perform laparoscopic colon resections, then the open approach is preferred in the acute setting. The open approach is also the default option in the setting of hemodynamic instability, multiple prior abdominal surgeries, or if contra-indications to laparoscopy are present. Cases that are begun laparoscopically but are found to have diffuse fecal or purulent peritonitis, or have significant bowel distension that prevents adequate working space, should be converted to a midline laparotomy with minimal delay.

The patient should be positioned supine with arms extended. Either split-leg or lithotomy can be used, but the authors prefer split-leg for the reasons described above. The operative team should ensure that antibiotics have been administered with appropriate timing to maximize blood levels for the beginning of the procedure (should be dosed within 2 h and at least 30 min prior to skin incision). A surgical pause and checklist should also be performed prior to starting the procedure. We begin with a lower midline laparotomy from the umbilicus to the pubis, as this generally provides adequate access to the lower abdomen and pelvis. The incision can be extended superiorly if additional exposure is required such as in the obese patient or if splenic flexure mobilization is required. A double-ring wound protector should be used to decrease the risk of surgical site infections and will also improve exposure. If a table-mounted retractor is required, the authors prefer a wishbone system instead of a full-ring system in case deeper pelvic retractors are required, as the full-ring will interfere with the placement of a handheld St. Mark's retractor. Once the midline laparotomy is performed, a thorough exploration of the abdominal cavity is required. Decision points 4 to 6 from the "Laparoscopic Approach" section above are then made.

We perform a lateral-to-medial mobilization of the sigmoid and descending colon using sharp dissection, making sure to stay in the avascular plane. There may be cases where the plane between the colon and the lateral wall/retroperitoneum is extremely difficult to correctly identify due to inflammation or fibrosis in the case of acute on chronic diverticulitis. In these cases, the finger fracture technique can be utilized to bluntly mobilize the colon. The risk in this procedure is entry into the retroperitoneum and injury to the structures contained within. Therefore, the surgeon should take extreme caution in these cases to identify the ureter and iliac vessels and ensure that these structures are not mobilized along with the phlegmonous or fibrotic colonic segment. Once mobilization is complete and the crucial structures identified, the proximal and distal resection margins are marked, and the intervening mesentery is divided. We prefer the use of a bipolar energy device for mesenteric division, but suture reinforcement may be necessary if the mesentery is extremely inflamed. The mesentery can be divided close to the bowel wall for these cases, and the left colic artery is usually preserved. The distal transection is then performed using a linear or transverse cutting stapler. In cases where an end colostomy is planned, the proximal margin is also transected using a linear stapler to minimize the size of the stoma aperture, and the specimen is sent off to pathology. The intended stoma site is then created, and the stapled proximal end of the descending colon is brought through the aperture and matured in standard fashion. In these cases, further division of the left colic artery is usually not required, except in rare cases (see the section "The Difficult Stoma", below).

If a primary anastomosis is intended, the surgeon must ensure that there is adequate mobilization to ensure a well-vascularized tension-free anastomosis. It is important to identify the vessel that most limits colonic reach. In the case of sigmoidectomy for benign disease, it is usually the left colic artery. However, ligation of the left colic may compromise the blood supply of the proximal segment. Therefore, the stepwise approach to gaining more reach is

1. Full lateral-to-medial mobilization of the descending colon up to the splenic flexure.
2. Splenic flexure mobilization.
3. Division of the inferior mesenteric vein at the base of the pancreas.
4. Division of the left colic artery at the bifurcation of the inferior mesenteric artery pedicle.

Generally, full lateral-to-medial with splenic flexure mobilization is adequate to obtain enough reach for a tension-free anastomosis. However, there are certain cases where reach is limited by a shortened or thickened mesentery (such as in obese patients). If this is the case, division of the inferior mesenteric vein and left colic artery is usually required and will almost always create enough length to perform a tension-free anastomosis at the sacral promontory [20, 26]. Similar to the laparoscopic approach, a side-to-end anastomosis is preferred by the authors as it usually results in less tension and is better vascularized; however, there is no functional benefit at this level. It is created in a similar manner, as described above. A proximal diversion with a loop ileostomy is then created if needed. An air leak test should always be performed. Drains are not routinely used in our practice.

Special Situations

Ureteric Stenting

Emergent operative intervention for acute diverticulitis poses important challenges. In particular, the acutely or chronically inflamed diverticular segment may be densely adherent to the retroperitoneum, making the identification of the ureter particularly difficult in certain cases. Ureteric injuries during colorectal surgery are associated with significant morbidity and mortality, and increased healthcare costs [27, 28]. Fortunately, these injuries are rare, but their incidence during surgery for diverticular disease is amongst the highest compared to other indications for colectomy. An analysis of over two million colorectal procedures from the National Surgical Quality Improvement Program (NSQIP) database reported an overall incidence of 0.3%. The specific incidence of ureteral injury during colectomy for diverticulitis was 2.9 per 1000 cases, with the highest being proctectomy for rectal cancer (7.1 per 1000 cases) and the lowest being colectomy for benign polyps (0.9 per 1000 cases) [27]. Another study found that surgery for diverticular disease was independently associated with ureteric injury, with an odds ratio of 2.1 (95% CI 1.6–2.7) compared to other indications [29]. It is unclear whether the risk is higher during laparoscopic colectomy. Certain studies have shown a protective effect for laparoscopy (24–26), whereas others have shown the opposite effect [30, 31].

Injuries to the ureter traditionally occur at three locations: the origin of the inferior mesenteric artery from the abdominal aorta, laterally at the pelvic brim, or in the pelvic sidewall near the lateral rectal ligaments [32]. Most commonly, the injuries are located in the middle or distal thirds of the ureter [33]. These can be direct trauma injuries with an immediate defect, or indirect thermal injuries that may present in a delayed fashion with leakage or stricture. It is essential that the ureter is properly identified prior to mesentery division and vessel ligation, especially near the inferior mesenteric artery pedicle and at the pelvic brim. Meticulous dissection in the embryologic planes between mesentery and retroperitoneum will decrease the risk of inadvertent ureteral injury; however, in the setting of diverticulitis this may be challenging. If the ureter cannot be identified during sigmoid mobilization, conversion to open surgery may be necessary during laparoscopic procedures. This allows for tactile feedback and potentially better visualization, especially in the setting of bleeding due to friable tissues or gross contamination/inflammation. Another potential option is to obtain an intraoperative consultation with a urologist, if available, for placement of a ureteric stent. This will allow for better delineation of the anatomic course of the ureter by allowing the surgeon to feel the stent in the retroperitoneum. Newer developments have allowed for the placement of a lighted ureteric stent, which may be useful during laparoscopic procedures [34]. Similarly, near-infrared immunofluorescence imaging with either indocyanine green (ICG) or methylene blue may also facilitate localization of the ureter [35, 36]. Video 13.1 demonstrates visualization of the anatomic course of the ureter using immunofluorescence imaging with ICG injected via cystoscopy.

If there is any concern of a ureteric injury intraoperatively, 10 mL of 10 mg/mL methylene blue or 5 mL of 8 mg/mL indigo carmine with 20 mg of furosemide can be administered intravenously. Leakage of blue dye into the peritoneal cavity will indicate a ureteric defect. This method will not identify thermal injuries that may cause delayed morbidity. If an injury is identified intraoperatively, it is prudent to obtain an intraoperative consultation with a urologist, if available, for evaluation and possible immediate repair. The specific management of ureteric injuries depends on the type of injury (laceration, transection, contusion, devascularization, or thermal injury), as well as the location of the injury. Thermal and contusion injuries can usually be managed with a placement of a ureteric ("double-J") stent for at least 4–6 weeks [32]. Laceration and transection injuries can usually be repaired by debridement and tension-free primary anastomosis over a ureteric stent in the middle third of the ureter, or by direct reimplantation into the bladder in the lower third of the ureter [33]. More complex repairs such as psoas hitch or Boari flap may be required if a tension-free anastomosis cannot be performed. Given the rarity of these procedures, urologic expertise is a necessity. If urologic expertise is not available, it is best to widely drain the injured ureteric segment and transfer the patient to another institution with the requisite expertise rather than attempting complex repairs. Imaging should be performed prior to stent removal to confirm the absence of a stricture or continued leak [37].

It is extremely important to diagnose these injuries intraoperatively, as missed injuries are a source of significant morbidity. These can present with vague abdominal symptoms such as pain, peritonitis, fever, and intra-abdominal collections. Serum creatinine levels may be elevated due to peritoneal absorption of creatinine. Diagnosis of delayed injuries can be made by percutaneous aspiration of the fluid collections demonstrating high fluid creatinine, by computed tomography with delayed intravenous contrast image sequences, or by laparotomy in the case of an unstable or peritonitic patient. These patients can be managed by percutaneous nephrostomy placement or ureteric stenting with delayed repair, or direct repair if possible. Repairs beyond 2 weeks after the index operation may be considerably more difficult, and most likely benefit from urinary diversion and delayed repair [38].

The surgeon's operative experience, as well as patient factors, should be taken into consideration in the decision to perform prophylactic ureteric stenting. There are certainly cases in which this is not feasible, especially in the emergent setting for a patient with altered hemodynamics or with diffuse peritonitis. If there is relative hemodynamic stability, then prophylactic ureteric stenting can be considered. Insertion of prophylactic stents usually takes approximately 20 min, but this additional operative time can be reduced if the catheters are placed simultaneously by the urologist as the abdominal team is working [39]. The role of prophylactic ureteric stenting is unclear, however. The available data suggest that ureteric stents do not decrease the incidence of ureteric injuries; however, there are no randomized trials. Most observational data are limited by the low overall incidence of ureteric injuries and by the fact that prophylactic stenting is usually performed in higher risk patients with diverticulitis or inflammatory bowel disease [40]. A recent systematic review did not identify a difference in the pooled incidence of ureteric injuries between stented and nonstented patients, but did show that prophylactic stents were used in higher risk patients [40].

The rationale behind prophylactic ureteric stenting is to be able to palpate the ureter if it is difficult to identify due to surrounding inflammatory changes or fibrosis. In the open setting, this tactile aid may be helpful to delineate the ureter's anatomic course. Prophylactic stenting may also facilitate intraoperative identification of ureteric injury [41]. However, there were no differences in intraoperative recognition of ureteric injuries in patients who received prophylactic stenting versus those without [40, 41]. Prophylactic stenting may decrease the need for conversion from laparoscopy to laparotomy if the ureter cannot be identified [42]. However, the lack of direct tactile feedback during laparoscopy can be overcome with the use of lighted stents [34, 43].

The potential complications of ureteric stents should also be taken into consideration. Ureteric stents can result in ureteral perforation, hematuria, acute kidney failure, and urinary tract infections [41]. There are also important cost considerations with prophylactic stenting. It is estimated that the added cost of prophylactic stenting ranges from 1500$ to 2500$. Chiu et al. [44] showed that the use of prophylactic stenting independently increased total hospital costs by $1983USD per patient. Other studies have shown similar cost implications [34, 45].

Problems Advancing the Circular Stapler Handle

There may be certain cases of resection and primary anastomosis in which the handle of the circular stapler cannot reach the top of the rectum. This may be caused by a variety of factors; most commonly, a segment of distal sigmoid is left in situ, or the rectal stump is too long. In this case, it is recommended to resect additional bowel so that the staple line of the rectal stump is on the top of the rectum. This shortens the stump and ensures a colorectal anastomosis (rather than a colosigmoid anastomosis), which will in turn decrease the risk of recurrent diverticulitis [46]. It is important however to ensure that adequate rectal length is preserved, as functional outcomes may be negatively impacted with a lower anastomosis than is required [47]. The authors routinely place the distal staple line immediately distal to where the tenia coli converge (signifying true anatomical rectum). If the stapler still cannot reach with an appropriate rectal stump length and staple line location, then a stapled with a longer handle can be attempted, if available. Alternatively, the circular anastomosis can be made on the anterior wall of the rectum at least 2 cm below the staple line. Care must be taken to ensure that there is adequate distance from the transverse staple line of the rectal stump and the circular anastomosis to prevent ischemia of the rectal wall in between staple lines. If the longer stapler is not available and the surgeon does not want to resect additional rectum due to concerns about impact on functional outcomes, a hand-sewn anastomosis may be required. In this case, the authors perform a side-to-end anastomosis with a two-layer closure using 3–0 polydiaxanone sutures. The incision on the proximal bowel should be performed at the anti-mesenteric border and should be made slightly smaller than the diameter of the rectum as it usually stretches with manipulation.

Other common reasons that may cause issues advancing the circular stapler are prominent valves of Houston or a tortuous rectum. If this is the case, then the authors mobilize the rectum in the avascular mesorectal plane posteriorly and laterally to be able to "straighten out" the rectum. During this dissection, the surgeon should err on the side of the mesorectum to avoid injury to the pelvic autonomic nerves, especially in benign disease. This mobilization is carried out until the anterior peritoneal reflection. It is rare to need to mobilize the extraperitoneal rectum. Cranial tension should be put on the rectal stump from the abdominal team while the stapler is advanced. These maneuvers usually facilitate the passage of the stapler. If there is still resistance, then sizers can be advanced up the rectal stump to "loosen" the valves of Houston prior to the stapler. The smallest sizer should be used first, with a sequential increase in sizer diameter until the size of the circular stapler is reached. Care must be taken in these cases to not cause trauma to the rectal mucosa, serosal tears, or full-thickness injuries during dilation.

The Difficult Stoma

There may be certain patients in whom creation of the end colostomy (in the case of a Hartmann's procedure) or a loop ileostomy (in the case of primary anastomosis with proximal diversion) can be challenging. These difficulties are classically encountered in obese patients with short and fatty mesenteries and thick abdominal walls, or in those with significant proximal bowel dilation. The surgeon should be cognizant of any potential stoma creation issues prior to making the stoma trephine. Ideally, the patient should be marked pre-operatively by a wound-care and ostomy professional, but this may not be feasible in the emergency setting. The upper abdomen usually has less subcutaneous adipose tissue and may be the preferred site in obese patients with thick abdominal walls. The first step is to ensure that the bowel used for stoma creation is free of any inflamed tissue, edema, or thickening. This may require additional resection in order to reach a disease-free bowel wall. The colonic appendages can also be resected to minimize the amount of surrounding tissues that need to be exteriorized; however, care must be taken to avoid mistaking epiploicae with mesentery. The stoma aperture may also have to be enlarged, but at the greater risk of future parastomal hernia. Placement of a wound protector in the stoma trephine can facilitate stoma creation in difficult situations [48]. The Alexis wound protector (Applied Medical, Rancho Santa Margarita, CA) is placed in the stoma aperture to compress the muscle, fascia, and subcutaneous tissues, allowing for the easier passage of the intended colostomy conduit. Once the segment of the colon is sufficiently exteriorized, the wound protector can then be cut and removed. This can be done regardless of laparoscopic or open approach. Another option is to exteriorize the colon in a two-step manner. First, skin and subcutaneous tissue flaps are mobilized off of the anterior rectus sheath until the stoma aperture is reached at its medial border [49]. A segment of bowel is first brought through the fascial opening. The segment should be long enough to traverse the subcutaneous tissues. Then, the loop of bowel above the fascial level is brought through the subcutaneous tissues and skin. The subcutaneous tissues should be tacked back onto the anterior rectus sheath so that there is no communication between the midline wound and the stoma site. This maneuver can only be done in the open setting.

Complete lateral mobilization of the left colon and splenic flexure may be necessary, with ligation of the left colic artery and inferior mesenteric vein on occasion, to obtain more length and facilitate exteriorization. An end-loop ostomy usually requires less reach than an end colostomy and should be considered. Ideally, the entire circumference is used to create the loop ostomy, but a "pseudo-loop" colostomy can be fashioned in which only the anti-mesenteric portion of the bowel wall is matured to the skin (akin to a blowhole colostomy) [50]. These stomas are not ideal and usually require later revision, but fortunately are rarely required (Fig. 13.3). Even with these maneuvers, it may be difficult to generate adequate reach for a well-perfused and protruding colostomy. In these cases, it may be more prudent to perform a primary anastomosis with proximal diverting loop ileostomy, as it is usually easier to form a loop ileostomy than a colostomy. The same maneuvers can be performed in cases of a difficult ileostomy. Finally, if none of these options will result in a viable stoma, an unprotected primary anastomosis may be necessary rather than creating an ostomy that is bound to fail and require further urgent operative intervention.

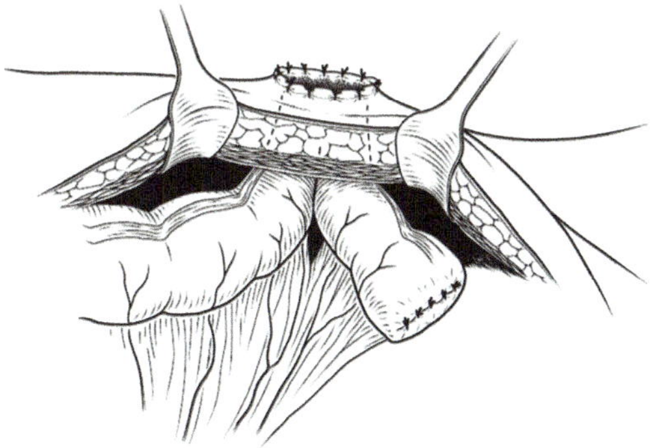

Fig. 13.3 Pseudoloop colostomy creation. From: Whitehead A, Cataldo PA. Technical Considerations in Stoma Creation. Clin Colon Rectal Surg. 2017 Jul;30(3):162–171. © Thieme Medical Publishers 2017. Open access

In the setting of a diverticular obstruction, it is ideal to fashion the stoma once the abdomen is closed to minimize the risk of surgical site infection from fecal spillage. However, an obstructed colon has reduced mobility and may require an oversized stoma aperture. It may be necessary to decompress the bowel prior to creating the stoma if it is felt that a stoma cannot be made otherwise. The abdominal cavity should be isolated as much as possible, usually with surgical towels. The staple line is then resected, and the bowel contents are emptied. Once decompressed, the bowel becomes more mobile, and the stoma aperture does not have to be large.

Conclusion

Surgery for acute diverticulitis in the emergency setting is associated with unique challenges. It is important for the surgeon to have a systematic approach when emergency surgical management is required, including operative approach, extent of resection, identification of critical structures, and whether or not to anastomose. Furthermore, the surgeon needs to have different techniques in their armamentarium if difficult scenarios are encountered, such as if the ureter cannot be identified or if there is difficulty in creating the stoma.

References

1. Roig JV, Sanchez-Guillen L, Garcia-Armengol JJ. Acute diverticulitis and surgical treatment. Minerva Chir. 2018;73(2):163–78.
2. Constantinides VA, Tekkis PP, Athanasiou T, Aziz O, Purkayastha S, Remzi FH, et al. Primary resection with anastomosis vs. Hartmann's procedure in nonelective surgery for acute colonic diver-

ticulitis: a systematic review. Dis Colon Rectum. 2006;49(7):966–81.
3. Oberkofler CE, Rickenbacher A, Raptis DA, Lehmann K, Villiger P, Buchli C, et al. A multicenter randomized clinical trial of primary anastomosis or Hartmann's procedure for perforated left colonic diverticulitis with purulent or fecal peritonitis. Ann Surg. 2012;256(5):819–26. discussion 26-7
4. Bridoux V, Regimbeau JM, Ouaissi M, Mathonnet M, Mauvais F, Houivet E, et al. Hartmann's procedure or primary anastomosis for generalized peritonitis due to perforated diverticulitis: a prospective multicenter randomized trial (DIVERTI). J Am Coll Surg. 2017;225(6):798–805.
5. Abraha I, Binda GA, Montedori A, Arezzo A, Cirocchi R. Laparoscopic versus open resection for sigmoid diverticulitis. Cochrane Database Syst Rev. 2017;11(11):CD009277. https://doi.org/10.1002/14651858.CD009277.pub2. PMID: 29178125; PMCID: PMC6486209
6. Klarenbeek BR, Veenhof AA, Bergamaschi R, van der Peet DL, van den Broek WT, de Lange ES, et al. Laparoscopic sigmoid resection for diverticulitis decreases major morbidity rates: a randomized control trial: short-term results of the Sigma Trial. Ann Surg. 2009;249(1):39–44.
7. Vargas HD, Ramirez RT, Hoffman GC, Hubbard GW, Gould RJ, Wohlgemuth SD, et al. Defining the role of laparoscopic-assisted sigmoid colectomy for diverticulitis. Dis Colon Rectum. 2000;43(12):1726–31.
8. Stam M, Draaisma WA, Pasker P, Consten E, Broeders I. Sigmoid resection for diverticulitis is more difficult than for malignancies. Int J Color Dis. 2017;32(6):891–6.
9. Celentano V. Laparoscopic sigmoid resection for diverticulitis is rarely a suitable case for the initial phase of the learning curve. Int J Color Dis. 2017;32(7):1095–6.
10. Pendlimari R, Holubar SD, Dozois EJ, Larson DW, Pemberton JH, Cima RR. Technical proficiency in hand-assisted laparoscopic colon and rectal surgery: determining how many cases are required to achieve mastery. Arch Surg. 2012;147(4):317–22.
11. Al-Temimi MH, Chandrasekaran B, Phelan MJ, Pigazzi A, Mills SD, Stamos MJ, et al. Incidence, risk factors, and trends of motor peripheral nerve injury after colorectal surgery: analysis of the National Surgical Quality Improvement Program Database. Dis Colon Rectum. 2017;60(3):318–25.
12. Sessa B, Galluzzo M, Ianniello S, Pinto A, Trinci M, Miele V. Acute perforated diverticulitis: assessment with multidetector computed tomography. Semin Ultrasound CT MR. 2016;37(1):37–48.
13. Vennix S, Boersema GS, Buskens CJ, Menon AG, Tanis PJ, Lange JF, Bemelman WA. Emergency laparoscopic sigmoidectomy for perforated diverticulitis with generalised peritonitis: a systematic review. Dig Surg. 2016;33(1):1–7. https://doi.org/10.1159/000441150. Epub 2015 Nov 10
14. Lee L, Abou-Khalil M, Liberman S, Boutros M, Fried GM, Feldman LS. Incidence of incisional hernia in the specimen extraction site for laparoscopic colorectal surgery: systematic review and meta-analysis. Surg Endosc. 2017;31(12):5083–93.
15. Horesh N, Emile SH, Khan SM, Freund MR, Garoufalia Z, Silva-Alvarenga E, Gefen R, Wexner SD. Meta-analysis of randomized clinical trials on long-term outcomes of surgical treatment of perforated diverticulitis. Ann Surg. 2023;278(5):e966–72. https://doi.org/10.1097/SLA.0000000000005909. Epub 2023 May 30
16. Lambrichts DPV, Vennix S, Musters GD, Mulder IM, Swank HA, Hoofwijk AGM, et al. Hartmann's procedure versus sigmoidectomy with primary anastomosis for perforated diverticulitis with purulent or faecal peritonitis (LADIES): a multicentre, parallel-group, randomised, open-label, superiority trial. Lancet Gastroenterol Hepatol. 2019;4(8):599–610.
17. Binda GA, Karas JR, Serventi A, Sokmen S, Amato A, Hydo L, et al. Primary anastomosis vs nonrestorative resection for perforated diverticulitis with peritonitis: a prematurely terminated randomized controlled trial. Color Dis. 2012;14(11):1403–10.
18. Cauley CE, Patel R, Bordeianou L. Use of primary anastomosis with diverting ileostomy in patients with acute diverticulitis requiring urgent operative intervention. Dis Colon Rectum. 2018;61(5):586–92.
19. Gachabayov M, Bergamaschi R, Boni L, Uranues S, Fingerhut A. Splenic flexure mobilization in sigmoid and rectal resections: a systematic review and meta-analysis of observational studies. Surg Technol Int. 2019;34:169–82.
20. Bonnet S, Berger A, Hentati N, Abid B, Chevallier JM, Wind P, et al. High tie versus low tie vascular ligation of the inferior mesenteric artery in colorectal cancer surgery: impact on the gain in colon length and implications on the feasibility of anastomoses. Dis Colon Rectum. 2012;55(5):515–21.
21. Zhang L, Elsolh B, Patel SV. Wound protectors in reducing surgical site infections in lower gastrointestinal surgery: an updated meta-analysis. Surg Endosc. 2018;32(3):1111–22.
22. Brown CJ, Fenech DS, McLeod RS. Reconstructive techniques after rectal resection for rectal cancer. Cochrane Database Syst Rev. 2008;2008(2):CD006040.
23. Lin H, Zhuang Z, Huang X, Li Y. The role of emergency laparoscopic surgery for complicated diverticular disease: a systematic review and meta-analysis. Medicine (Baltimore). 2020;99(40):e22421. https://doi.org/10.1097/MD.0000000000022421. PMID: 33019419; PMCID: PMC7535780
24. Vennix S, Lips DJ, Di Saverio S, van Wagensveld BA, Brokelman WJ, Gerhards MF, et al. Acute laparoscopic and open sigmoidectomy for perforated diverticulitis: a propensity score-matched cohort. Surg Endosc. 2016;30(9):3889–96.
25. Vennix S, Boersema GS, Buskens CJ, Menon AG, Tanis PJ, Lange JF, et al. Emergency laparoscopic

sigmoidectomy for perforated diverticulitis with generalised peritonitis: a systematic review. Dig Surg. 2016;33(1):1–7.
26. Thum-umnuaysuk S, Boonyapibal A, Geng YY, Pattana-Arun J. Lengthening of the colon for low rectal anastomosis in a cadaveric study: how much can we gain? Tech Coloproctol. 2013;17(4):377–81.
27. Halabi WJ, Jafari MD, Nguyen VQ, Carmichael JC, Mills S, Pigazzi A, et al. Ureteral injuries in colorectal surgery: an analysis of trends, outcomes, and risk factors over a 10-year period in the United States. Dis Colon Rectum. 2014;57(2):179–86.
28. Zafar SN, Ahaghotu CA, Libuit L, Ortega G, Coleman PW, Cornwell EE 3rd, et al. Ureteral injury after laparoscopic versus open colectomy. JSLS. 2014;18(3):e2014.00158.
29. Coakley KM, Kasten KR, Sims SM, Prasad T, Heniford BT, Davis BR. Prophylactic ureteral catheters for colectomy: a National Surgical Quality Improvement Program-Based Analysis. Dis Colon Rectum. 2018;61(1):84–8.
30. Andersen P, Andersen LM, Iversen LH. Iatrogenic ureteral injury in colorectal cancer surgery: a nationwide study comparing laparoscopic and open approaches. Surg Endosc. 2015;29(6):1406–12.
31. Palaniappa NC, Telem DA, Ranasinghe NE, Divino CM. Incidence of iatrogenic ureteral injury after laparoscopic colectomy. Arch Surg. 2012;147(3):267–71.
32. Delacroix SE Jr, Winters JC. Urinary tract injuries: recognition and management. Clin Colon Rectal Surg. 2010;23(3):221.
33. Selzman AA, Spirnak JP. Iatrogenic ureteral injuries: a 20-year experience in treating 165 injuries. J Urol. 1996;155(3):878–81.
34. Chahin F, Dwivedi AJ, Paramesh A, Chau W, Agrawal S, Chahin C, et al. The implications of lighted ureteral stenting in laparoscopic colectomy. JSLS. 2002;6(1):49–52.
35. Slooter MD, Janssen A, Bemelman WA, Tanis PJ, Hompes R. Currently available and experimental dyes for intraoperative near-infrared fluorescence imaging of the ureters: a systematic review. Tech Coloproctol. 2019;23(4):305–13.
36. Soriano CR, Cheng RR, Corman JM, Moonka R, Simianu VV, Kaplan JA. Feasibility of injected indocyanine green for ureteral identification during robotic left-sided colorectal resections. Am J Surg. 2022;223(1):14–20. https://doi.org/10.1016/j.amjsurg.2021.07.012. Epub 2021 Jul 19
37. Brandes S, Coburn M, Armenakas N, McAninch J. Diagnosis and management of ureteric injury: an evidence-based analysis. BJU Int. 2004;94(3):277–89.
38. Althumairi AA, Efron JE. Genitourinary considerations in Reoperative and complex colorectal surgery. Clin Colon Rectal Surg. 2016;29(2):145–51.
39. Pokala N, Delaney CP, Kiran RP, Bast J, Angermeier K, Fazio VW. A randomized controlled trial comparing simultaneous intra-operative vs sequential prophylactic ureteric catheter insertion in re-operative and complicated colorectal surgery. Int J Color Dis. 2007;22(6):683–7.
40. Croghan SM, Zaborowski A, Mohan HM, Mulvin D, McGuire BB, Murphy M, et al. The sentinel stent? A systematic review of the role of prophylactic ureteric stenting prior to colorectal resections. Int J Color Dis. 2019;34(7):1161–78.
41. da Silva G, Boutros M, Wexner SD. Role of prophylactic ureteric stents in colorectal surgery. Asian J Endosc Surg. 2012;5(3):105–10.
42. Tsujinaka S, Wexner SD, DaSilva G, Sands DR, Weiss EG, Nogueras JJ, et al. Prophylactic ureteric catheters in laparoscopic colorectal surgery. Tech Coloproctol. 2008;12(1):45–50.
43. Senagore AJ, Luchtefeld M. An initial experience with lighted ureteral catheters during laparoscopic colectomy. J Laparoendosc Surg. 1994;4(6):399–403.
44. Chiu AS, Jean RA, Gorecka J, Davis KA, Pei KY. Trends of ureteral stent usage in surgery for diverticulitis. J Surg Res. 2018;222(203–11):e3.
45. Bothwell WN, Bleicher RJ, Dent TL. Prophylactic ureteral catheterization in colon surgery. A five-year review. Dis Colon Rectum. 1994;37(4):330–4.
46. Thaler K, Baig MK, Berho M, Weiss EG, Nogueras JJ, Arnaud JP, et al. Determinants of recurrence after sigmoid resection for uncomplicated diverticulitis. Dis Colon Rectum. 2003;46(3):385–8.
47. Ziv Y, Gimelfarb Y, Igov I. Post anterior rectal resection syndrome–a retrospective multicentre study. Color Dis. 2013;15(6):e317–22.
48. Meagher AP, Owen G, Gett R. Multimedia article. An improved technique for end stoma creation in obese patients. Dis Colon Rectum. 2009;52(3):531–3.
49. Beck SJ. Stoma issues in the obese patient. Clin Colon Rectal Surg. 2011;24(4):259–62.
50. Whitehead A, Cataldo PA. Technical considerations in stoma creation. Clin Colon Rectal Surg. 2017;30(3):162–71.

Management After an Acute Episode of Diverticulitis

14

Rohin Mittal and Tan Arulampalam

Introduction

Colonic diverticulosis is common in the Western world, with one-half of the population affected by the sixth decade of life and two-thirds by the ninth decade [1]. Most people remain asymptomatic, and only approximately 5% will go on to develop diverticulitis [2, 3]. Diverticulitis is mild or uncomplicated in most patients and often resolves with nonoperative management. A minority of patients develop complicated diverticulitis, characterized by a pericolic or pelvic abscess, colonic perforation, fistula, or stricture. These patients may require radiological intervention or surgery. There is a vast amount of literature available on the management of acute diverticulitis, both for complicated and uncomplicated disease. There are also many consensus statements available for the management of these patients, with detailed insight on questions such as the use of antibiotics, the need for radiological interventions, the role of laparoscopy, as well as the indications for resection, with or without a stoma [3–9].

While these guidelines help in decision--making during an acute attack of diverticulitis, the management of a patient after recovery from an episode of diverticulitis often remains unclear. The literature is limited and consists mostly of low-quality evidence, with very few guidelines to aid in management. Furthermore, guidelines that do cover these subjects largely focus on the role of elective surgery or the surgical management of recurrent diverticulitis, which applies to a minority of these patients. Guidelines for lifestyle changes, dietary modifications, and pharmacotherapy to reduce the risk of recurrence are often lacking. In this chapter, we will review the natural history of diverticulitis, identify patients likely to benefit from elective surgery, and look into important factors that play a role in reducing recurrence.

Natural History of Diverticular Disease

Acute diverticulitis develops in approximately 5% of patients with diverticular disease [2, 3]. An acute episode may be uncomplicated or complicated. Complicated diverticulitis is defined as diverticulitis with a pericolic abscess, perforation, fistula, or stricture. The management of uncomplicated diverticulitis typically included antibiotics and bowel rest. However, more recent evidence does not support antibiotics to be typical management of uncomplicated diverticulitis. Complicated diverticular disease may be treated by radiological drainage, laparoscopy, or

R. Mittal
Department of Surgery Unit 2 (Colorectal Surgery), Christian Medical College and Hospital, Vellore, Tamil Nadu, India

T. Arulampalam (✉)
School of Medicine, Anglia Ruskin University, Chelmsford, UK

M. Boutros et al. (eds.), *Diverticulitis*, https://doi.org/10.1007/978-3-032-21720-2_14

laparotomy with or without resection. The management of acute diverticulitis has been covered elsewhere in the book.

The majority (85%) of patients who develop diverticulitis will have acute uncomplicated diverticulitis [7] and will recover with nonoperative management. Recurrence remains one of the most important clinical outcomes in this subgroup of patients. It has been historically believed that diverticulitis has a high recurrence rate, with significant morbidity and mortality which increases with every recurrent episode. Parks, in his series in 1975, quoted a recurrence rate of 40% with a 60% complication rate [10]. He also quoted mortality of 4.7% on first admission and 7.8% at subsequent admissions for diverticulitis [11]. Other older studies have quoted recurrence rates as high as 62% [12]. It is based on these data, historically, that routine elective colectomy was offered to patients who had recurrent acute diverticulitis.

However, more recent studies have found recurrence and morbidity to be much lower than previously quoted. Large studies have quoted a recurrence rate between 13% and 47% [13–18]. Broderick-villa et al. [13] studied 3165 patients with acute diverticulitis, and only 13.3% of patients treated nonoperatively developed a recurrence. Interestingly, studies that have required a CT scan as part of the diagnostic criteria for recurrence have reported a lower recurrence rate (of around 15%) compared to studies that included cases of recurrence diagnosed on clinical grounds alone.

The historical belief that recurrences were more severe and had higher mortality has been proven incorrect by many modern studies. In a retrospective cohort of 271 patients, Pittet et al. concluded that recurrent diverticulitis was not associated with higher rates of complications or treatment failure [19]. They also concluded that patients presenting with recurrence had lower rates of surgery at admission, with no difference in mortality. Most recurrences were uncomplicated, with only 2–5% of patients developing complicated diverticulitis during the second or subsequent episodes [14, 15, 20]. Furthermore, patients are at the highest risk for recurrence during the first year of follow-up, with the risk reducing to as low as 3% thereafter [20].

Many risk factors for recurrence have been identified. A high C-reactive protein (CRP) (>240 mg/L) at the index episode has been shown to be a predictor for recurrence, with a 22% recurrence rate at 6 months [15]. Other risk factors include a family history of diverticular disease, multiple previous episodes, retroperitoneal abscess, higher comorbidity index, >5 cm of colonic involvement, as well as male sex [1, 14, 15]. Young age (<50 years) has been shown in many studies to be associated with an increased recurrence rate. These recurrences are, however, not of increased severity [1, 15, 21]. Conversely, a meta-analysis showed a correlated between older age and recurrence [22].

Additional risk factors for developing complicated diverticulitis include smoking, nonsteroidal anti-inflammatory drug use, renal failure, organ transplant, and steroid use [21]. Table 14.1 lists the common risk factors for the recurrence of diverticulitis.

Table 14.1 Risk factors for recurrence after acute diverticulitis

	Risk factors for recurrence after acute diverticulitis
1.	CRP >240 mg/L at index presentation
2.	Retroperitoneal abscess
3.	>3 previous episodes
4.	> 5 cm of colonic involvement
5.	High comorbidity index
6.	Male sex
7.	Positive family history
8.	Age

Elective Surgery After Diverticulitis

Based on our current understanding of the natural history and patterns of recurrence of acute diverticulitis, the recommendation to offer elective surgery to everyone after a single attack of complicated diverticulitis or recurrent attacks of uncomplicated diverticulitis no longer holds. As we have seen, most patients will continue to be asymptomatic after a single attack, and among patients who do present with recurrence, most will have uncomplicated disease. Decision analysis models have shown that surgical treatment of diverticulitis after the third [23] or fourth [24] attack, in both younger and older patients, is not associated with increased mortality or colostomy rate, and is cost-saving to the healthcare system. Furthermore, the suggestion that a decline in surgical treatment may lead to a higher incidence of complicated diverticulitis has been proven to be false. Ricciardi et al. [25] followed 685,390 diverticulitis discharges over 15 years and reported a decline in the rates of surgical treatment for diverticulitis without a corresponding increase in free perforation. Therefore, the decision to operate should be individualized to the patient, based on symptoms and other associated factors, rather than just the number of attacks (Table 14.2). The risk of operative therapy, the overall medical condition of the patient, and the effect of symptoms on quality of life, as well as postoperative complications, should be balanced before making any decision on surgical treatment. The patient needs to be involved in every step, and the risks and benefits discussed. This approach is recommended by most current guidelines [3, 5, 7] and is discussed in more depth in Chap. 17.

Table 14.2 Factors influencing decision on elective colectomy

	Factors influencing decision on elective colectomy
1.	Recurrent attacks causing substantial morbidity
2.	Complicated diverticulitis
3.	Immunocompromised state
4.	Smoldering diverticulitis with persistent symptoms
5.	Symptomatic fistula or stricture
6.	Suspected cancer
7.	Limited access to medical care

Role of Colonoscopy After an Acute Episode of Diverticulitis

Colorectal cancer may present with symptoms mimicking an acute episode of diverticulitis, and diverticular disease may co-exist with colorectal cancer. This has been the basis for recommending a routine colonoscopy after the resolution of an acute attack of diverticulitis. Most current international guidelines, including the American Gastroenterology Association (AGA), Association of Coloproctology of Great Britain and Ireland (ACPGBI), as well as the American Society of Colon and Rectal Surgeons (ASCRS), recommend a routine colonoscopy after resolution of an acute episode of diverticulitis to rule out an underlying colorectal cancer [3, 4, 6–9, 26].

Before the widespread availability of CT scans, a diagnosis of diverticulitis was often made clinically or following a contrast enema. Among all patients who were diagnosed with diverticulitis clinically, approximately one-third had their diagnosis changed after cross-sectional imaging [27]. Furthermore, a contrast enema detects a concomitant malignancy in only one--half of patients [28]. Therefore, in such a scenario, a colonoscopy both confirms the diagnosis and rules out colorectal cancer.

With the increasing use of CT scans in the diagnosis of acute diverticulitis, the role of routine colonoscopy after recovery has been questioned. Modern CT scans have a sensitivity and specificity approaching 99% for the diagnosis of diverticulitis and its complications [29]. Improvements in quality and resolution of CT scanning, as well as multiplanar reconstructions, have greatly improved the evaluation of the disease.

Colonoscopy, while having a high detection rate for colorectal malignancies, is labor intensive and places a significant burden on the healthcare system. Colonoscopy is also associated with a small but real risk of morbidity and mortality. The risk of perforation with a routine colonoscopy has been reported as 0.1–0.2% [30]. In addition, there is associated patient discomfort and technical difficulties due to the presence of adhesions, luminal narrowing, and colonic spasm.

A recent systematic review and meta-analysis including 11 studies from 7 countries and 1970 patients estimated an overall risk of colorectal cancer after an episode of diverticulitis to be 1.6%. However, the risk of colorectal cancer after an episode of complicated diverticulitis was estimated to be 10.8%, while that after an episode of uncomplicated diverticulitis to be 0.7% [30]. An updated 2019 meta-analysis reports the pooled risk to be 1.3% for uncomplicated versus 7.9% for complicated diverticulitis [31]. The authors concluded that the risk of colonic malignancy was low after an acute episode of uncomplicated colonic diverticulitis and that a routine colonoscopy may not be necessary for these patients. However, patients with complicated diverticulitis had a significantly higher risk of colorectal cancer and should undergo routine colonoscopy.

Another systematic review looking at only uncomplicated diverticulitis (9 studies, 2490 patients) also concluded that routine colonoscopy after an attack of diverticulitis, in the absence of any other signs of colorectal cancer, was not necessary [32]. There have been two more systematic reviews on the same topic and both have also arrived at the same conclusion [33, 34].

All of the above studies have found the incidence of colorectal cancer in patients with uncomplicated diverticulitis to be between 0.7% and 1%. This is very similar to the rate of colorectal cancer detection following screening of asymptomatic individuals (0.78–1.1%) [35, 36]. This implies that the risk of developing colorectal neoplasia in patients recovering from uncomplicated diverticulitis is similar to that of the general population. The latest meta-analysis reported a pooled rate of 1.9%, almost twice that of colorectal cancer detected in asymptomatic individuals during screening. The statements that a colonoscopy after an acute attack of diverticulitis needs to be revised. If the patient was up to date with their screening colonoscopy, then perhaps a colonoscopy may not be needed after acute diverticulitis. Otherwise, colonoscopy would have an important role [31]. These patients, therefore, should be offered a colonoscopy if they fulfill the criteria for screening as per local and national guidelines. A routine colonoscopy after recovery is not indicated.

In addition to malignant lesions, colonoscopy may also be important for the detection of undiagnosed adenomas. A recent meta-analysis revealed an adenoma detection rate of 19% (15–23%) in patients with resolved diverticulitis. When age was taken into consideration, there was no difference in the rate of advanced adenoma detection in patients with diverticulitis compared to asymptomatic individuals [30]. Other studies have also shown similar adenoma detection rates [33], including advanced adenomas, among patients with resolved diverticulitis compared to the general screening population [32].

Among patients who warrant an interval colonoscopy, the optimal timing for endoscopy after an attack of acute diverticulitis is not known. Most guidelines recommend an interval of about 6–8 weeks after resolution of an acute attack before proceeding with colonoscopy. Studies have shown that in uncomplicated diverticulitis, in the absence of pericolic air, a colonoscopy may be performed early, even at the index admission [37, 38]. However, the fear of perforation precludes early colonoscopy in complicated diverticulitis, and the optimal timing for colonoscopy in this subgroup of patients is unknown. In patients where conventional colonoscopy is contraindicated or has failed, a CT colonography is a good option to assess the colon.

Recommendations for selective colonoscopy apply only to patients who have had a CT scan, with no suspicion of colorectal cancer on the scan. If the initial CT scan revealed any findings suspicious for malignancy, these patients must undergo a colonoscopy. High-risk features on CT scan include, but are not limited to, suspicion of cancer by a radiologist, bowel wall thickening exceeding 15 mm, no diverticula observed, and the presence of previously undiagnosed metastatic disease [39]. Some of these features are

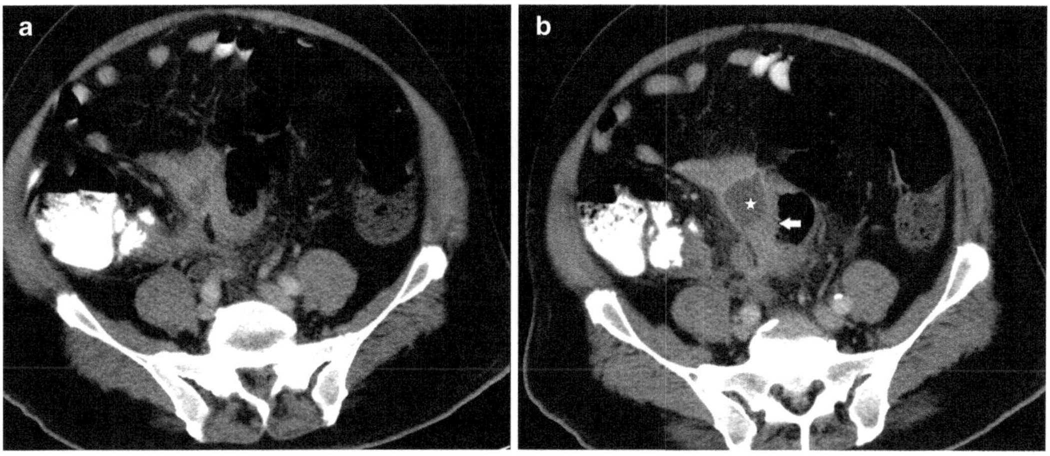

Fig. 14.1 CT scan in a patient with acute complicated diverticulitis. A: Bowel wall thickening with pericolic inflammation and B: pericolic abscess (star) and bowel wall thickening with perforation (arrow). These features are radiologically indistinguishable from a perforated colonic malignancy

shown in Figs. 14.1 and 14.2. The report of the initial CT scan is also, to some degree, operator dependent, with the experience of the radiologist playing an important role. Despite best efforts, some malignancies may be missed.

Patients with smoldering diverticulitis may also warrant an interval colonoscopy. Even with uncomplicated diverticulitis in the absence of high-risk features on CT scan, persistent symptoms that fail to completely resolve with treatment should raise the concern for an underlying colonic lesion. In an observational study from Israel, Lahat et al. [40] studied 306 patients with diverticulitis, 23 of whom had persistent disease (defined as symptoms persisting beyond 1 week despite optimal treatment, or early recurrence of symptoms within 2 months). They performed an early interval colonoscopy in all of the patients, and reported positive findings (neoplasm or foreign body) in four (17.4%) patients. Despite there not being a large body of evidence on this subject, it is important to consider alternative diagnoses when the patient has an unexpected and/or prolonged course of disease.

Many other factors, such as age, personal history, family history, and examination findings, need to be considered before making a decision on colonoscopy [30]. An important nationwide cohort study showed that patients with diverticular disease have higher odds of colon cancer (OR = 1.71) compared to those without diverticular disease [41].

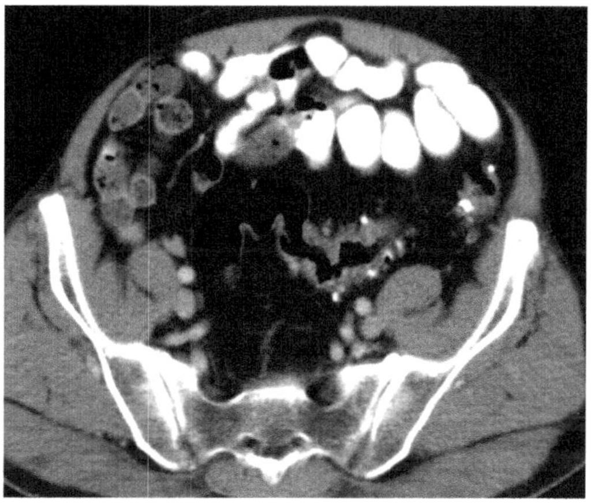

Fig. 14.2 CT scan in a case of uncomplicated diverticulitis. Diverticula are visible along with colonic thickening and pericolic stranding. Although uncomplicated, the colonic thickening in this case mandates colonoscopy to rule out colonic malignancy

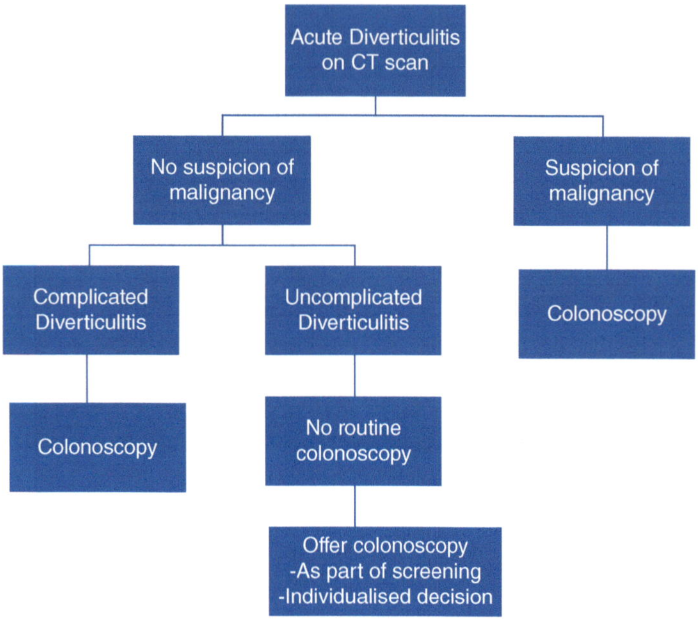

Fig. 14.3 Flowchart for recommending colonoscopy after acute diverticulitis

Figure 14.3 shows a flowchart for recommending a colonoscopy in individuals after an acute attack of diverticulitis.

Prevention of Recurrence After an Acute Attack

There are many lifestyle and dietary changes, as well as some drugs that may decrease the risk of recurrent diverticulitis. We will have a brief look at some of these factors.

Role of Fiber

Dietary fiber intake provides many health benefits, including reduced risk of developing diabetes, hypertension, coronary artery disease, stroke, obesity, as well as certain gastrointestinal disorders. It has other added benefits such as improving blood glucose control in diabetes, lowering of blood pressure in hypertension, as well as improving serum lipid concentrations and immune function [42]. The recommended daily intake for fiber is dependent on the recommended daily calorie intake. In the United States, the current recommended daily intake for fiber is 14 g/1000 kcal [43]. However, it has been shown that most people only consume about half that amount [44].

Dietary fiber deficiency causes increased luminal pressure in the colon, contributing to diverticula formation and diverticulitis [45]. Fiber deficiency also changes the colonic microflora, with a decrease in healthy flora and an increase in pathogenic bacteria. This change in the microflora may lead to chronic inflammation and symptomatic diverticulitis [46]. A high fiber diet also decreases contact time between bowel contents and the diverticulum, thus lowering inflammation rates [47]. A high fiber diet, therefore, has been recommended for both primary prevention of diverticulitis as well as the prevention of recurrences. Most international guidelines recommend a high fiber diet for the prevention of recurrence [3, 7], while others are equivocal on its use [5].

While commonly recommended, the body of evidence for a high fiber diet in the prevention of diverticulitis or its recurrence is very little, and the impact of diet on the incidence of diverticulitis is conflicting [48]. While some studies do recommend a high fiber diet [49], they suffer from poor quality and methodological errors. A systematic review in 2012 failed to identify a single trial that addressed the modification of dietary fiber intake to reduce the risk of recurrence of diverticulitis [50]. A more recent systematic review published in 2018 identified three studies addressing this question. Two of the three studies did not have a low fiber control group, and therefore no pooled analysis could be performed. However, the authors made a strong recommendation for long-term high fiber dietary intake. While this was based on very low-quality evidence, the authors noted that they found no evidence to the contrary (supporting a low fiber diet) and that a high fiber diet should be recommended as a standard diet for all adults as per national dietary guidelines [47]. Another recent meta-analysis, including 19 studies comparing a high fiber diet to various other interventions, also concluded that high fiber, both dietary and supplemental, could be beneficial in the treatment of symptomatic uncomplicated diverticular disease.

A high fiber diet is defined as a diet that meets the recommended daily fiber intake, as per national guidelines (e.g., 14 g/1000 kcal in the USA). Sustaining a diet modification to maintain this amount of dietary fiber can be difficult, especially when not supported by the food environment [47]. People from a low socioeconomic background may require additional support to achieve high dietary fiber, as they may have a poorer quality of diet at baseline, and may not have the resources to access dietary support services [51]. Additionally, patients may not be aware of what constitutes a high fiber diet and how it may be achieved [52]. It is therefore important that patients are referred to dietary support services so that they can be supported to achieve a high fiber diet [47].

Role of Nuts and Popcorn

Physicians have traditionally advised patients with diverticular disease to avoid nuts, seeds, and popcorn. These high-residue foods were believed to obstruct or traumatize the diverticular lumen, leading to diverticulitis. This practice was, however, not backed by literature. In a large cohort study by Strate et al. [53], 47,228 people with diverticulosis were followed up for 18 years. This study found that nuts and popcorn consumption had an inverse association with the risk of diverticulitis, while corn consumption did not have any association with diverticulitis. Therefore, the avoidance of nuts and popcorn is not required in patients with diverticular disease.

Role of Probiotics

Probiotics have been useful in the treatment of conditions like irritable bowel syndrome, which shares some of its pathophysiology with diverticular disease. Changes in the colonic microflora in both of these conditions lead to low-grade inflammation, visceral hypersensitivity, and abnormal colonic motility, which are responsible for many of the symptoms [54, 55]. Probiotics modify the gut microbial balance, inhibit colonic bacterial overgrowth and metabolism of pathogens, and potentially have anti-inflammatory effects, and are therefore an attractive choice for use in diverticular disease [56, 57].

Literature on the use of probiotics for the prevention of recurrence in diverticular disease is scanty, with very few high-quality studies. Most studies have used a probiotic in conjunction with a drug, and different strains of probiotics have been used in different studies. No placebo-controlled trials on the use of probiotics in the prevention of recurrence of diverticulitis have been conducted. Small trials that have used probiotics as an adjunct to either a high fiber diet [58, 59] or mesalamine [60] have found the combination to be more effective than the drug alone. However, the lack of a placebo arm makes these results less reliable. In a study by Stollman et al. [61], a combination of mesalamine and probiotics was compared to mesalamine alone or a placebo, and no differences in outcomes were found between the three groups.

A recent systematic review on the use of probiotics was inconclusive about its use in diverticulitis. Eight of the 11 included studies assessed the effect of probiotics along with another drug, and most of the studies used different probiotics, either single species or in combination. The authors concluded that there remained a paucity of evidence for the use of probiotics in diverticulitis, with scant high-quality data. No definite conclusion could be drawn, and further research was recommended [62]. A more recent systematic review that included 13 studies (3 double-blind randomized placebo-controlled, 6 open randomized, and 4 non-randomized) provided an updated measure of evidence on the efficacy of probiotics in a different phase of diverticular disease. Although the majority of the included studies are still preliminary, current data show a possible clinical application of certain probiotic strains in all stages of diverticular disease [63].

The AGA guidelines advise against the use of probiotics in patients with a history of uncomplicated diverticulitis, due to lack of high-quality evidence, as well as the uncertainties of the role of the gut microbiome in the pathophysiology of diverticular disease [7].

Role of Mesalamine

There has been some suggestion that the pathophysiology of diverticular disease involves chronic low-grade inflammation of the colon [64]. Thus, the suggestion that mesalamine (5-aminosalicylic acid; 5-ASA), a drug used to control inflammation in ulcerative colitis, may be useful in diverticular disease to prevent recurrence. Mesalamine is both immunomodulatory and anti-inflammatory; therefore, it was proposed as a medication to reduce the frequency of recurrent attacks [65]. The use of mesalamine, however, is not without risk. Adverse effects include headache, malaise, diarrhea, cramping, as well as pancreatitis, pneumonitis, pericarditis, and interstitial nephritis [66].

There have been many trials comparing mesalamine to placebo or another drug in preventing the recurrence of acute diverticular disease. Mesalamine has been used in different doses as well as cyclically. A recent Cochrane review by Carter et al. [67] in 2017 included 7 studies and 1805 participants. Three of these studies tested mesalamine against placebo, one against a combination with probiotics, one against a combination with antibiotics, and one against no intervention. While two trials were in favor of the use of mesalamine to reduce recurrence, five others were not. The overall conclusion was that mesalamine offered no advantage compared to placebo. The authors noted that the effect of 5-ASA on the prevention of recurrence was uncertain, although the quality of the evidence was very low. There were no differences in adverse effects in the two groups either. In another systematic review by Iannone et al. [68] in 2018, 13 RCTs with 3028 participants were included. Diverticulitis recurrence was studied in 9 of these trials, including 2414 participants. There was no difference in recurrence rates between mesalamine and control interventions (RR 0.83 95% CI 0.58-1.19). However, in the subgroup of symptomatic recurrent diverticular disease, mesalamine could reduce recurrences but not symptoms. The AGA recommends against the use of mesalamine to prevent recurrence after acute uncomplicated diverticulitis [7, 38]. The ASCRS guidelines state that mesalamine, rifaximin, and probiotics are not typically recommended to reduce the risk of diverticulitis recurrence but may be effective in reducing chronic symptoms [9].

Role of Rifaximin

Rifaximin is a nonabsorbable oral antibiotic that has a broad spectrum of action against Gram-positive and -negative bacteria, aerobes, and anaerobes. It has been studied by some authors in the prevention of symptoms and recurrence in diverticular disease. The proposed mechanism of action is through a reduction in intestinal bacterial overgrowth [69]. Rifaximin and high fiber may have a synergistic effect due to the reduced proliferation of gut microflora as well as expansion in fecal mass [70]. Data from a few retrospective observational studies have pointed to a benefit of using cyclical rifaximin therapy in the prevention of recurrence of diverticular disease [71, 72].

There have been four prospective randomized trials evaluating the role of rifaximin in the prevention of symptoms or recurrence in diverticular disease. Each of these trials used cyclical rifaximin at a dose of 400 mg twice daily for 7 days a month in addition to a high fiber diet as standard treatment. Three of these trials were open labeled [73–75] and only one was double-blinded and placebo controlled [76]. While the three open-label trials showed rifaximin to be beneficial in reducing symptoms, the placebo-controlled trial failed to show any benefit or reduction in recurrence rate at 1 year with the use of rifaximin. A recent meta-analysis looked at these four trials and revealed a pooled rate difference of 29% in favor of rifaximin for reducing symptoms [77]. At 1 year, the number needed to treat for primary prevention of complications was 59, which was statistically, but not clinically, significant. The authors, therefore, concluded that the evidence for the use of rifaximin over standard fiber supplementation was poor [77]. Similarly, the AGA guidelines do not recommend routine use of rifaximin to prevent recurrence after an attack of acute diverticulitis [7].

Role of Nonsteroidal Anti-inflammatory Drugs and Aspirin

Nonsteroidal anti-inflammatory drugs (NSAIDs) have been increasingly recognized as risk factors for colonic disease, including diverticulitis [78]. These drugs disrupt mucosal integrity through impaired prostaglandin synthesis and also by direct topical injury [79]. The use of NSAIDs has been found to be a risk factor for developing diverticulitis and even perforation in many case-control and cohort studies [80, 81]. In a recent systematic review of risk factors for diverticulitis, NSAID use was one of the predictors for severe diverticulitis [82]. Most of these publications have studied NSAIDs as a whole, including both aspirin and non-aspirin NSAIDs.

The differentiation between aspirin and non-aspirin NSAIDs is clinically important because of the widespread beneficial use of aspirin, especially in cardiovascular conditions. Morris et al. [83] in their case-control study analyzed the effects of aspirin and non-aspirin NSAIDs separately. They concluded that the consumption of non-aspirin NSAIDs was significantly associated with perforated diverticular disease, but a similar association was not seen with aspirin. In another large cohort study, the use of aspirin was associated with a very low increase in diverticulitis, whereas the use of non-aspirin NSAIDs was associated with a significant increase in the risk of recurrent diverticulitis [84]. It would, therefore, appear that non-aspirin NSAIDs, but not aspirin, should be avoided to prevent recurrences. In keeping with these findings, the AGA recommends avoidance of non-aspirin NSAIDs but not aspirin [7].

Role of Physical Activity and Exercise

Physical activity and exercise have a beneficial role in many chronic diseases, including gastrointestinal disorders. Physical activity has a number of potential benefits on the colon, including reduced risk of colon cancer as well as diverticular disease [85, 86]. This is through increased colonic transit rate and decreased transit time, decreased colonic pressures, and enhanced immune function with reduced inflammation [86]. Results from a large cohort study including 47,288 patients followed up for 18 years suggested that there was a significant inverse relationship between physical activity and the risk of diverticulitis and diverticular bleeding. Vigorous physical activity (defined as 6 metabolic equivalents or more), and more specifically running, was associated with reduced risk of diverticulitis (RR 0.66 95%CI 0.51-0.86) and diverticular bleeding (RR 0.6195% CI 0.41-0.90). However, non-vigorous physical activity, as well as time spent in sedentary activity, was not associated with these outcomes [86]. These findings were further confirmed in a study by Williams et al., where the authors showed an inverse association between vigorous physical activity and incident diverticular disease in runners [87]. The decrease

Table 14.3 Interventions aimed at preventing recurrence after acute diverticulitis

Prevention of recurrence of acute diverticulitis	
High fiber diet	Recommended
Nuts, popcorn, and seeds	Do not restrict
NSAIDs	Avoid
Aspirin	May be used
Probiotics	Not beneficial
Mesalamine	Not beneficial
Rifaximin	Not beneficial
Physical activity and exercise	Recommended

in risk for diverticulitis was proportional to the distance run per week. Another Swedish study concluded that exercise <30 min/day was associated with a 42% increase in risk for diverticular disease [88]. A systematic review, which included five cohort studies, also concluded that a higher level of physical activity may reduce the risk of diverticulitis [89]. It is therefore important that all patients be advised about the role of physical activity in reducing recurrences and be encouraged to adopt a healthy lifestyle. Table 14.3 lists some of the common recommendations to prevent recurrence after an acute episode of diverticulitis.

References

1. Buchs NC, Mortensen NJ, Ris F, Morel P, Gervaz P. Natural history of uncomplicated sigmoid diverticulitis. World J Gastrointest Surg. 2015;7:313–8.
2. Heise CP. Epidemiology and pathogenesis of diverticular disease. J Gastrointest Surg Off J Soc Surg Aliment Tract. 2008;12:1309–11.
3. Feingold D, Steele SR, Lee S, et al. Practice parameters for the treatment of sigmoid diverticulitis. Dis Colon Rectum. 2014;57:284–94.
4. Deery SE, Hodin RA. Management of diverticulitis in 2017. J Gastrointest Surg Off J Soc Surg Aliment Tract. 2017;21:1732–41.
5. Sartelli M, Catena F, Ansaloni L, et al. WSES guidelines for the management of acute left sided colonic diverticulitis in the emergency setting. World J Emerg Surg. 2016;11:37.
6. Fozard JBJ, Armitage NC, Schofield JB, Jones OM. Association of coloproctology of Great Britain and Ireland. ACPGBI position statement on elective resection for diverticulitis. Color Dis. 2021;13(Suppl 3):1–11.
7. Stollman N, Smalley W, Hirano I, AGA Institute Clinical Guidelines Committee. American Gastroenterological Association Institute guideline on the management of acute diverticulitis. Gastroenterology. 2015;149:1944–9.
8. Sartelli M, Weber DG, Kluger Y, et al. 2020 update of the WSES guidelines for the management of acute colonic diverticulitis in the emergency setting. World J Emerg Surg. 2020;15:32. https://doi.org/10.1186/s13017-020-00313-4.
9. Hall J, Hardiman K, Lee S, et al. Prepared on behalf of the clinical practice guidelines Committee of the American Society of colon and Rectal surgeons. The American Society of Colon and Rectal Surgeons clinical practice guidelines for the treatment of left-sided colonic diverticulitis. Dis Colon Rectum. 2020 Jun;63(6):728–47. https://doi.org/10.1097/DCR.0000000000001679.
10. Parks TG. Natural history of diverticular disease of the colon. Clin Gastroenterol. 1975;4:53–69.
11. Parks TG. Natural history of diverticular disease of the colon. A review of 521 cases. Br Med J. 1969;4:639–42.
12. Stollman NH, Raskin JB. Diagnosis and management of diverticular disease of the colon in adults. Ad Hoc practice parameters Committee of the American College of gastroenterology. Am J Gastroenterol. 1999;94:3110–21.
13. Broderick-Villa G, Burchette RJ, Collins JC, Abbas MA, Haigh PI. Hospitalization for acute diverticulitis does not mandate routine elective colectomy. Arch Surg. 2005;140:576–81. discussion 581-583
14. Hall JF, Roberts PL, Ricciardi R, et al. Long-term follow-up after an initial episode of diverticulitis: what are the predictors of recurrence? Dis Colon Rectum. 2011;54:283–8.
15. Buchs NC, Konrad-Mugnier B, Jannot A-S, Poletti P-A, Ambrosetti P, Gervaz P. Assessment of recurrence and complications following uncomplicated diverticulitis. Br J Surg. 2013;100:976–9. discussion 979
16. Binda GA, Serventi A, Altomare DF. Multicentre observational study of the natural history of left-sided acute diverticulitis (Br J Surg 2012; 99: 276–285) (Br J Surg 2012; 99: 285–286). Br J Surg. 2012;99:738.
17. Mueller MH, Glatzle J, Kasparek MS, et al. Long-term outcome of conservative treatment in patients with diverticulitis of the sigmoid colon. Eur J Gastroenterol Hepatol. 2005;17:649–54.
18. Mäkelä JT, Kiviniemi HO, Laitinen ST. Spectrum of disease and outcome among patients with acute diverticulitis. Dig Surg. 2010;27:190–6.
19. Pittet O, Kotzampassakis N, Schmidt S, Denys A, Demartines N, Calmes J-M. Recurrent left colonic diverticulitis episodes: more severe than the initial diverticulitis? World J Surg. 2009;33:547–52.
20. Eglinton T, Nguyen T, Raniga S, Dixon L, Dobbs B, Frizelle FA. Patterns of recurrence in patients with acute diverticulitis. Br J Surg. 2010;97:952–7.
21. Vennix S, Morton DG, Hahnloser D, Lange JF, Bemelman WA. Research Committee of the European

Society of Coloproctocology. Systematic review of evidence and consensus on diverticulitis: an analysis of national and international guidelines. Color Dis. 2014;16:866–78.
22. Kang G, Son S, Shin YM, Pyo JS. Recurrence of uncomplicated diverticulitis: a meta-analysis. Medicina (Kaunas). 2022;58(6):758. https://doi.org/10.3390/medicina58060758. PMID: 35744021; PMCID: PMC9228700
23. Richards RJ, Hammitt JK. Timing of prophylactic surgery in prevention of diverticulitis recurrence: a cost-effectiveness analysis. Dig Dis Sci. 2002;47:1903–8.
24. Salem L, Veenstra DL, Sullivan SD, Flum DR. The timing of elective colectomy in diverticulitis: a decision analysis. J Am Coll Surg. 2004;199:904–12.
25. Ricciardi R, Baxter NN, Read TE, Marcello PW, Hall J, Roberts PL. Is the decline in the surgical treatment for diverticulitis associated with an increase in complicated diverticulitis? Dis Colon Rectum. 2009;52:1558–63.
26. Fozard JB, Armitage NC, Schofield JB, Jones OM. Association of coloproctology of Great Britain and Ireland. ACPGBI position statement on elective resection for diverticulitis. Color Dis. 2011;13(Suppl 3):1–11. https://doi.org/10.1111/j.1463-1318.2010.02531.x.
27. Toorenvliet BR, Bakker RFR, Breslau PJ, Merkus JWS, Hamming JF. Colonic diverticulitis: a prospective analysis of diagnostic accuracy and clinical decision-making. Color Dis. 2010;12:179–86.
28. Schnyder P, Moss AA, Thoeni RF, Margulis AR. A double-blind study of radiologic accuracy in diverticulitis, diverticulosis, and carcinoma of the sigmoid colon. J Clin Gastroenterol. 1979;1:55–66.
29. Rao PM, Rhea JT, Novelline RA, et al. Helical CT with only colonic contrast material for diagnosing diverticulitis: prospective evaluation of 150 patients. Am J Roentgenol. 1998;170:1445–9.
30. Sharma PV, Eglinton T, Hider P, Frizelle F. Systematic review and meta-analysis of the role of routine colonic evaluation after radiologically confirmed acute diverticulitis. Ann Surg. 2014;259:263–72.
31. Meyer J, Orci LA, Combescure C, et al. Risk of colorectal cancer in patients with acute diverticulitis: a systematic review and meta-analysis of observational studies. Clin Gastroenterol Hepatol. 2019;17(8):1448–1456.e17. https://doi.org/10.1016/j.cgh.2018.07.031. Epub 2018 Jul 26
32. de Vries HS, Boerma D, Timmer R, van Ramshorst B, Dieleman LA, van Westreenen HL. Routine colonoscopy is not required in uncomplicated diverticulitis: a systematic review. Surg Endosc. 2014;28:2039–47.
33. Daniels L, Unlü C, de Wijkerslooth TR, Dekker E, Boermeester MA. Routine colonoscopy after left-sided acute uncomplicated diverticulitis: a systematic review. Gastrointest Endosc. 2014;79:378–89. quiz 498–498.e5
34. Sai VF, Velayos F, Neuhaus J, Westphalen AC. Colonoscopy after CT diagnosis of diverticulitis to exclude colon cancer: a systematic literature review. Radiology. 2012;263:383–90.
35. Niv Y, Hazazi R, Levi Z, Fraser G. Screening colonoscopy for colorectal cancer in asymptomatic people: a meta-analysis. Dig Dis Sci. 2008;53:3049–54.
36. Pox CP, Altenhofen L, Brenner H, Theilmeier A, Von Stillfried D, Schmiegel W. Efficacy of a nationwide screening colonoscopy program for colorectal cancer. Gastroenterology. 2012;142:1460–1467.e2.
37. Lahat A, Yanai H, Menachem Y, Avidan B, Bar-Meir S. The feasibility and risk of early colonoscopy in acute diverticulitis: a prospective controlled study. Endoscopy. 2007;39:521–4.
38. Peery AF, Shaukat A, Strate LL. AGA clinical practice update on medical management of colonic diverticulitis: expert review. Gastroenterology. 2021;160(3):906–911.e1. https://doi.org/10.1053/j.gastro.2020.09.059. Epub 2020 Dec 3. PMID: 33279517; PMCID: PMC7878331
39. Sallinen V, Mentula P, Leppäniemi A. Risk of colon cancer after computed tomography-diagnosed acute diverticulitis: is routine colonoscopy necessary? Surg Endosc. 2014;8:961–6.
40. Lahat A, Yanai H, Sakhnini E, Menachem Y, Bar-Meir S. Role of colonoscopy in patients with persistent acute diverticulitis. World J Gastroenterol. 2008;14(17):2763–6. https://doi.org/10.3748/wjg.14.2763. PMID: 18461662; PMCID: PMC2709057
41. Ma W, Walker MM, Thuresson M, et al. Cancer risk in patients with diverticular disease: a nationwide cohort study. J Natl Cancer Inst. 2023;115(1):62–70. https://doi.org/10.1093/jnci/djac190. PMID: 36200887; PMCID: PMC9830486
42. Anderson JW, Baird P, Davis RH, Ferreri S, Knudtson M, Koraym A, Waters V, Williams CL. Health benefits of dietary fiber. Nutr Rev. 2009;67:188–205.
43. Appendix 7. Nutritional goals for age-sex groups based on dietary reference intakes and dietary guidelines recommendations – 2015–2020 Dietary guidelines – health.gov. https://health.gov/dietaryguidelines/2015/guidelines/appendix-7/. Accessed 22 Jun 2019.
44. Park Y, Hunter DJ, Spiegelman D, et al. Dietary fiber intake and risk of colorectal cancer: a pooled analysis of prospective cohort studies. JAMA. 2005;294:2849–57.
45. Commane DM, Arasaradnam RP, Mills S, Mathers JC, Bradburn M. Diet, ageing and genetic factors in the pathogenesis of diverticular disease. World J Gastroenterol. 2009;15:2479–88.
46. Tursi A, Papagrigoriadis S. Review article: the current and evolving treatment of colonic diverticular disease. Aliment Pharmacol Ther. 2009;30:532–46.
47. Dahl C, Crichton M, Jenkins J, et al. Evidence for dietary fibre modification in the recovery and prevention of reoccurrence of acute, uncomplicated diverticulitis: a systematic literature review. Nutrients. 2018;10(2):137. https://doi.org/10.3390/nu10020137.
48. Tursi A. Dietary pattern and colonic diverticulosis. Curr Opin Clin Nutr Metab Care. 2017;20:409–13.

49. Aune D, Sen A, Norat T, Riboli E. Dietary fibre intake and the risk of diverticular disease: a systematic review and meta-analysis of prospective studies. Eur J Nutr. 2019;59(2):421–32. https://doi.org/10.1007/s00394-019-01967-w.
50. Unlü C, Daniels L, Vrouenraets BC, Boermeester MA. Systematic review of medical therapy to prevent recurrent diverticulitis. Int J Color Dis. 2012;27:1131–6.
51. Darmon N, Drewnowski A. Does social class predict diet quality? Am J Clin Nutr. 2008;87:1107–17.
52. Parmenter K, Waller J, Wardle J. Demographic variation in nutrition knowledge in England. Health Educ Res. 2000;15:163–74.
53. Strate LL, Liu YL, Syngal S, Aldoori WH, Giovannucci EL. Nut, corn, and popcorn consumption and the incidence of diverticular disease. JAMA. 2008;300:907–14.
54. Gill HS. Probiotics to enhance anti-infective defences in the gastrointestinal tract. Best Pract Res Clin Gastroenterol. 2003;17:755–73.
55. Sullivan Å, Nord CE. Probiotics and gastrointestinal diseases. J Intern Med. 2005;257:78–92.
56. White J. Probiotics and their use in diverticulitis. J Clin Gastroenterol. 2006;40(Suppl 3):S160–2. https://doi.org/10.1097/01.mcg.0000225504.67547.d9.
57. Sheth A, Floch M. Probiotics and diverticular disease. Nutr Clin Pract Off Publ Am Soc Parenter Enter Nutr. 2009;24:41–4.
58. Annibale B, Maconi G, Lahner E, De Giorgi F, Cuomo R. Efficacy of Lactobacillus paracasei sub. paracasei F19 on abdominal symptoms in patients with symptomatic uncomplicated diverticular disease: a pilot study. Minerva Gastroenterol Dietol. 2011;57:13–22.
59. Dughera L, Serra AM, Battaglia E, Tibaudi D, Navino M, Emanuelli G. Acute recurrent diverticulitis is prevented by oral administration of a polybacterial lysate suspension. Minerva Gastroenterol Dietol. 2004;50:149–53.
60. Tursi A, Brandimarte G, Elisei W, et al. Randomised clinical trial: mesalazine and/or probiotics in maintaining remission of symptomatic uncomplicated diverticular disease–a double-blind, randomised, placebo-controlled study. Aliment Pharmacol Ther. 2013;38:741–51.
61. Stollman N, Magowan S, Shanahan F, Quigley EMM, DIVA Investigator Group. A randomized controlled study of mesalamine after acute diverticulitis: results of the DIVA trial. J Clin Gastroenterol. 2013;47:621–9.
62. Lahner E, Bellisario C, Hassan C, Zullo A, Esposito G, Annibale B. Probiotics in the treatment of diverticular disease. A Systematic Review. J Gastrointest Liver Dis. 2016;25:79–86.
63. Ojetti V, Petruzziello C, Cardone S, et al. The use of probiotics in different phases of diverticular disease. Rev Recent Clin Trials. 2018;13(2):89–96. https://doi.org/10.2174/1574887113666180402143140.
64. Floch MH. A hypothesis: is diverticulitis a type of inflammatory bowel disease? J Clin Gastroenterol. 2006;40(Suppl 3):S121–5.
65. Tursi A, Brandimarte G, Daffinà R. Long-term treatment with mesalazine and rifaximin versus rifaximin alone for patients with recurrent attacks of acute diverticulitis of colon. Dig Liver Dis. 2002;34:510–5.
66. Ransford R, a. J, Langman MJS. Sulphasalazine and mesalazine: serious adverse reactions re-evaluated on the basis of suspected adverse reaction reports to the committee on safety of medicines. Gut. 2002;51:536–9.
67. Carter F, Alsayb M, Marshall JK, Yuan Y. Mesalamine (5-ASA) for the prevention of recurrent diverticulitis. Cochrane Database Syst Rev. 2017;10:CD009839.
68. Iannone A, Ruospo M, Wong G, et al. Mesalazine for people with diverticular disease: a systematic review of randomized controlled trials. Can J Gastroenterol Hepatol. 2018;2018:5437135.
69. Corazza GR, Ventrucci M, Strocchi A, et al. Treatment of small intestine bacterial overgrowth with rifaximin, a non-absorbable rifamycin. J Int Med Res. 1988;16:312–6.
70. Di Stefano M, Malservisi S, Veneto G, Ferrieri A, Corazza GR. Rifaximin versus chlortetracycline in the short-term treatment of small intestinal bacterial overgrowth. Aliment Pharmacol Ther. 2000;14:551–6.
71. Di Mario F, Miraglia C, Cambiè G, et al. Long-term efficacy of rifaximin to manage the symptomatic uncomplicated diverticular disease of the colon. J Investig Med. 2019;67:767–70.
72. Festa V, Spila Alegiani S, et al. Retrospective comparison of long-term ten-day/month rifaximin or mesalazine in prevention of relapse in acute diverticulitis. Eur Rev Med Pharmacol Sci. 2017;21:1397–404.
73. Papi C, Ciaco A, Koch M, Capurso L. Efficacy of rifaximin on symptoms of uncomplicated diverticular disease of the colon. A pilot multicentre open trial. Diverticular Disease Study Group. Ital J Gastroenterol. 1992;24:452–6.
74. Latella G, Pimpo MT, Sottili S, et al. Rifaximin improves symptoms of acquired uncomplicated diverticular disease of the colon. Int J Color Dis. 2003;8:55–62.
75. Colecchia A, Vestito A, Pasqui F, et al. Efficacy of long term cyclic administration of the poorly absorbed antibiotic Rifaximin in symptomatic, uncomplicated colonic diverticular disease. World J Gastroenterol. 2007;13:264–9.
76. Papi C, Ciaco A, Koch M, Capurso L. Efficacy of rifaximin in the treatment of symptomatic diverticular disease of the colon. A multicentre double-blind placebo-controlled trial. Aliment Pharmacol Ther. 1995;9:33–9.
77. Bianchi M, Festa V, Moretti A, et al. Meta-analysis: long-term therapy with rifaximin in the management of uncomplicated diverticular disease. Aliment Pharmacol Ther. 2011;33:902–10.
78. Laine L, Curtis SP, Langman M, et al. Lower gastrointestinal events in a double-blind trial of the

cyclo-oxygenase-2 selective inhibitor etoricoxib and the traditional nonsteroidal anti-inflammatory drug diclofenac. Gastroenterology. 2008;135:1517–25.
79. Lanas A, Sopeña F. Nonsteroidal anti-inflammatory drugs and lower gastrointestinal complications. Gastroenterol Clin N Am. 2009;38:333–52.
80. Campbell K, Steele RJC. Non-steroidal anti-inflammatory drugs and complicated diverticular disease: a case—control study. Br J Surg. 1991;78:190–1.
81. Mpofu S, Mpofu CMA, Hutchinson D, Maier AE, Dodd SR, Moots RJ. Steroids, non-steroidal anti-inflammatory drugs, and sigmoid diverticular abscess perforation in rheumatic conditions. Ann Rheum Dis. 2004;63:588–90.
82. Tan JPL, Barazanchi AWH, Singh PP, Hill AG, Maccormick AD. Predictors of acute diverticulitis severity: a systematic review. Int J Surg. 2016;26:43–52.
83. Morris CR, Harvey IM, Stebbings WSL, Speakman CTM, Kennedy HJ, Hart AR. Anti-inflammatory drugs, analgesics and the risk of perforated colonic diverticular disease. Br J Surg. 2003;90:1267–72.
84. Strate LL, Liu YL, Huang ES, Giovannucci EL, Chan AT. Use of aspirin or nonsteroidal anti-inflammatory drugs increases risk for diverticulitis and diverticular bleeding. Gastroenterology. 2011;140:1427–33.
85. Colditz GA, Cannuscio CC, Frazier AL. Physical activity and reduced risk of colon cancer: implications for prevention. Cancer Causes Control. 1997;8:649–67.
86. Strate LL, Liu YL, Aldoori WH, Giovannucci EL. Physical activity decreases diverticular complications. Am J Gastroenterol. 2009;104:1221–30.
87. Williams PT. Incident diverticular disease is inversely related to vigorous physical activity. Med Sci Sports Exerc. 2009;41:1042–7.
88. Hjern F, Wolk A, Håkansson N. Obesity, physical inactivity, and colonic diverticular disease requiring hospitalization in women: a prospective cohort study. Am J Gastroenterol. 2012;107:296–302.
89. Aune D, Sen A, Leitzmann MF, Norat T, Tonstad S, Vatten LJ. Body mass index and physical activity and the risk of diverticular disease: a systematic review and meta-analysis of prospective studies. Eur J Nutr. 2017;56:2423–38.

Risk Factors for Recurrent Diverticulitis

15

Sarah E. Koller, Andreas M. Kaiser, Sebastiano Biondo, Thomas Golda, and Neyla Boukhili

Diverticulitis: A Wide Spectrum of Disease

Diverticulitis refers to segmental colonic inflammation superimposed onto and complicating existing diverticular disease. Though one diverticulum suffices, multiple diverticula are typically involved. Infection is commonly considered a critical component of the pathophysiology. Diverticulitis has a wide range of clinical and subclinical presentations [1]. While this condition is generally straightforward to treat, it may result in significant morbidity and may represent a life-threatening event in a fraction of patients [2]. The severity of the disease process depends on an array of insufficiently characterized factors that sway the balance between aggressive and protective forces. Variability is seen both with regard to the index episode of diverticulitis, as well as in the number and severity of subsequent attacks (i.e., recurrences). These range from a single recurrent episode to greater than ten recurrences throughout the patient's life. A disease flare-up shortly following an acute episode may reflect persistent or inadequately cleared diverticulitis, whereas true recurrence is seen when a new attack occurs after a variable interval of quiescence. The observed variability is multifactorial and reflects variations in the treatment of the individual episodes, to a significant degree.

This variability in diverticulitis disease presentation and management makes it an interesting albeit challenging disease to manage and study. In contrast to patients suffering from cancer, diverticulitis patients are not well captured and followed in major national databases. Research efforts aim at pinning down the characteristics that influence both the severity of the index episode and the likelihood of recurrent attacks with their associated risk. Robust evidence would allow surgeons to better predict the risk for recurrent diverticulitis and provide patients with accurate recommendations in determining the role of surgery compared to nonoperative management in preserving or restoring quality of life.

S. E. Koller
Department of Surgery, Division of Colorectal Surgery, Keck School of Medicine of the University of Southern California, Los Angeles, CA, USA
e-mail: Sarah.koller@med.usc.edu

A. M. Kaiser
Department of Surgery, Division of Colorectal Surgery, City of Hope National Medical Center, Duarte, CA, USA
e-mail: akaiser@coh.org

S. Biondo · T. Golda
Colorectal Unit, Department of General and Digestive Surgery, Bellvitge University Hospital, University of Barcelona, Barcelona, Spain
e-mail: tgolda@bellvitgehospital.cat

N. Boukhili (✉)
Department of Surgery, McGill University, Montreal, QC, Canada
e-mail: neyla.boukhili@mail.mcgill.ca

M. Boutros et al. (eds.), *Diverticulitis*, https://doi.org/10.1007/978-3-032-21720-2_15

Disease Severity at Presentation

Disease severity grade for each diverticulitis patient must be known in order to reliably assess short- and long-term prognoses, to optimize treatment strategies, and to accurately compare patient cohorts. Since the original 1978 Hinchey classification based on clinical and operative findings, a number of scoring systems have been suggested to characterize the severity of acute diverticulitis [3]. Cross-sectional imaging, most commonly computed tomography (CT), has invariably been recognized as a crucial assessment tool for the acute episode, but it may have been underutilized to define the risk for recurrent or smoldering diverticulitis [4, 5]. The Ambrosetti classification is CT-based and distinguishes mild from severe diverticulitis in the acute setting, where severe disease is defined by the presence of extraluminal air, contrast, or abscess (see Chap. 6) [6]. The modified Hinchey classification builds on the original categories but provides additional subclasses for acute and chronic presentations (see Chap. 6) [4, 7].

The optimal treatment strategies are comparably intuitive for the mildest and the most severe of presentations [1]. Of all patients with acute diverticulitis, approximately two-thirds experience a mild or uncomplicated episode [8]. *Uncomplicated diverticulitis* refers to inflammation limited to the colon without systemic illness. Abdominal contrast-infused CT scans typically demonstrate wall thickening of the affected colon segment with associated increased density (stranding) of the pericolic fat. The infection resulting from diverticular microperforation neither extends to the peritoneum, nor does it cause other extraluminal sequelae. In contrast, 25–30% of patients show evidence of severe or *complicated diverticulitis* (Table 15.1), which may involve disease extension beyond the colon [9]. In the American Society of Colon and Rectal Surgeons Practice Parameters for the Treatment of Sigmoid Diverticulitis, complicated diverticulitis is defined as diverticulitis associated with peritonitis, abscess formation, fistula, obstruction, or stricture [2, 10]. The term "perforated diverticulitis" should be avoided because it is nonspecific and leaves room for ambiguity, as even uncomplicated disease may include microperforation. It is therefore better to refer to the specific extent of the "perforation" as abscess formation or free (macro-)perforation with purulent or feculent peritonitis [1, 2].

Table 15.1 Complicated diverticulitis (25–30% of cases)

Acuity category	Details
Highly acute	Perforation, feculent Perforation, nonfeculent
Acute/intermediate	Abscess formation
Intermediate/low	Multiple episodes of otherwise uncomplicated diverticulitis Multiple episodes of complicated diverticulitis Smoldering diverticulitis
Chronic (or subacute)	Fistulization (bladder, vagina, cutaneous) Stricture formation with/without clinical signs of obstruction

Challenges in Evaluating Recurrence Risk

From a surgical perspective, recurrent diverticulitis is a complex entity that carries several important questions:

- What criteria define a recurrent attack?
- What is the absolute risk of a recurrent attack?
- Can the risk of recurrence be individually predicted?
- Can this risk be reduced with nonsurgical measures?
- Is each subsequent attack more severe than the last?
- Is the safety of surgical intervention impacted by the number and frequency of episodes?
- What is the risk of a temporary or permanent stoma?
- Which approach is best suited to return patients to their functional baseline without symptoms?
- How do the cost of the nonsurgical and surgical approaches compare?

Unfortunately, the tools to study these important questions are remarkably limited. The quality of most available evidence is poor and stems from retrospective analyses of institutional or larger national databases. Such studies lack standardization and reflect the sum of referral and selection bias as well as individualized judgment rather than decision-making based on randomized trials.

Defining Recurrence

Similar to the index episode of diverticulitis, recurrent diverticulitis should be diagnosed based on the patient's history, symptomatology, and clinical presentation. However, it is highly desirable to confirm the diagnosis with cross-sectional imaging [4, 11]. Up to one-third of patients with CT-proven uncomplicated diverticulitis present with nonspecific abdominal symptoms alone; conversely, "characteristic" abdominal symptoms may be reflective of underlying malignancy, inflammatory bowel disease, or to other intestinal conditions such as constipation or irritable bowel syndrome in the absence of inflammatory parameters or characteristic CT findings [11–13]. Surgery should not be considered for the latter two alternate diagnoses as the primary symptoms may persist [14].

Defining the Risk of Recurrence

In defining predictive and prognostic factors influencing the risk of recurrence, both extrinsic and intrinsic parameters must be considered (Tables 15.2 and 15.3). The most important factor to consider is arguably the management modality used for the index episode. A key factor to consider is whether the diseased bowel segment was excised as well as the timing of the resection. This crucial element is currently poorly defined and studied in the available literature. When the diseased segment is left in situ and persistently contains disease-triggering activity, a higher recurrence rate is inevitable.

Table 15.2 Risk factors for recurrent diverticulitis

	Risk factor
Overall incidence	Family history of diverticulitis Male sex? Smoking
Perforated diverticulitis/ emergent surgery	Obesity Medications: NSAIDS Opiates Steroids Immunosuppressants Chemotherapy Diabetes Collagen-vascular disease Immunocompromised status

Table 15.3 Reported ranges of recurrent attacks after preceding event

Preceding circumstances	Incidence of recurrence
Uncomplicated at index episode	
Overall recurrence	13–19%
Complicated recurrence	2–4%
Complicated at index episode	
Overall recurrence	20–61%
Complicated recurrence	48–63%
After image-guided drain placement	42–74%
After surgery	
Surgical resection	5–8%
Laparoscopic peritoneal lavage/drainage	>28% (within 30 days)

Patient-Related Factors Influencing the Risk of Recurrence

Factors that have been associated with a higher incidence of diverticulitis on index episode, such as a Western diet, red meat consumption, obesity, smoking, family history as well as NSAID, steroid, and opiate use, continue to apply for recurrent episodes (Table 15.2) [11]. Several genetic and ethnic parameters have been associated with diverticulitis, which prompts the question of "nature versus nurture" to remain of epidemiological interest; however, these parameters have not been sufficiently studied in the context of recurrence [15, 16]. It is important to note that historically, "constipation" was touted as the sole culprit in the development of diverticulitis in older patients but is insufficient to explain the undisputable rising incidence of diverticulitis in younger patients. As for popcorn and peanuts, they are nothing but myth [17, 18]. Several drugs, such as NSAIDs, opiates, and steroids, have been associated with an increased risk of a primary episode of diverticulitis, but only steroids resulted in an increased risk of recurrence [19–21].

Smoking

Two studies investigating smoking and diverticular disease had conflicting results [22, 23]. However, these studies were investigating the role of smoking in the development of symptomatic diverticular disease rather than as a risk factor for recurrent AD. Conversely, a large English population-based cohort study with 65,162 National Health Service hospital admissions identified smoking as a risk factor for recurrent AD [24]. Two other studies appeared to show an increase in the risk of recurrent diverticulitis, with an apparent dose-dependent effect [24–26]. In conclusion, results of smoking habits are somewhat conflicting, and while more data is needed, there is some evidence to support smoking as a dose-dependent risk factor in the development of recurrent diverticulitis.

Obesity

Similarly, obesity, and dyslipidemia have been associated with an increased risk of recurrent diverticulitis. In a retrospective study from the United Kingdom including 65,162 patients admitted for acute diverticulitis over a 5-year period in the National Health Service hospitals, smoking (RR 1.26, $p < 0.001$), obesity (RR 1.38, $p < 0.001$), and dyslipidemia (RR 1.29, $p < 0.001$) all correlated with an increased risk of recurrence [24]. Obesity and sedentary lifestyle also lead to an increased risk of requiring urgent or emergent surgery, though it remains to be determined whether this is related to masking of clinical signs or different disease behavior [27]. Morbid [body mass index (BMI) ≥ 35 and super-obesity (BMI ≥ 40)] present undeniable technical challenges and result in a known higher incidence of general and specific postoperative complications after any type of major surgery. Obesity should therefore not be the sole criterion for surgical indication, and the decision should heavily rely on clinical, serological, and imaging parameters [25].

Family History

Family history and genetic predisposition of diverticulitis were investigated in very few studies. One epidemiological study with 672 patients found an influence on recurrence, suggesting a genetic or an environmental component influencing the disease; however, this study did not mention the number of patients with positive family history [28]. In a retrospective cohort study with prospective telephone survey follow-up of 433 patients with left-sided diverticulitis managed nonoperatively, patients with a positive family history not only had a higher cumulative incidence of recurrences (HR, 2.93; 95% CI, 1.96–4.39), but also of complicated recurrences (HR, 8.30; 95% CI, 3.64–18.9) [29]. Furthermore, twin studies have demonstrated a genetic component of diverticulitis; however, the specific pathways are yet to be elucidated [15, 16]. Family history is a risk factor for both primary and recurrent diverticulitis, and it appears to translate into more complicated recurrences.

Sex

Thirteen retrospective studies, including 438,903 individuals, analyzed the impact of gender on the recurrence of AD [24, 30]. Four studies presented a slightly increased risk in females and one study presented a protective tendency in males [31]. Nine studies showed no effect of gender on the risk of recurrence [30, 32–34]. Overall, reports of gender impact on the incidence of recurrent diverticulitis have been inconsistent, with male gender swaying the risk in some, and female gender in other studies [24, 35, 36]. With such conflicting evidence, no clear conclusion can be drawn regarding the impact of sex on the risk of recurrent diverticulitis.

Age

The concept that younger patients with diverticulitis follow a more severe course requiring surgery earlier has sparked some controversy in recent years [34, 37, 38]. Twenty-three studies including 452,085 patients investigated the association of age and recurrence: two prospective studies, one study containing both prospective and retrospective data and 19 retrospective studies [24, 30].

The two prospective cohort studies found no significant influence of age on recurrence (age ≤ 45 years: 24%; age 45–70 years: 17%; age > 70: 20%) [37, 39]. Similarly, the distribution of complicated recurrences was similar among the different age groups as well. A study on retrospectively and prospectively collected data found an association of age younger than 40 years with a higher risk of recurrence on multivariate analysis [40].

Among the retrospective studies, 11 studies had results indicating a relationship between age and recurrence risk. Age younger than 50 years has been shown to be significantly associated with increased recurrence risk [24, 30]. However, there was no effect of age on the recurrence risk in the additional nine included studies [21, 34, 41–44]. Overall, many of the retrospective studies lack an imaging-proven diagnosis, which may provoke confusion of different diseases with comparable symptoms. Another confounding variable seems to be the huge variability in the duration of follow-up [45].

In a recent meta-analysis of 23,078 patients from eight studies, patients under the age of 50 years were more likely to have a recurrent attack [34]. However, the recurrence rates were highly variable (13.3% to 36%) depending on the population under study and the duration of follow-up. Additionally, all studies focused primarily on recurrences diagnosed and managed in a hospital setting, whereas there are no estimates of recurrent diverticulitis managed in the primary care setting [46].

Overall, younger patients seem to have a similar absolute risk of recurrence, albeit a higher lifetime risk [47, 48]. Younger patients may also be more willing to undergo surgery due to the lower relative surgical risk and their longer life expectancy with consequent increased potential for future episodes. However, most studies have not documented a greater likelihood of perforation or increased morbidity among young patients who develop recurrent disease. Considering all the existing data, there is no evidence that younger patients should be treated differently from older patients [37, 44, 47–50].

In summary, data on the impact of younger versus older age on the risk of recurrence or complications also show substantial variability, but as a whole do not support the notion of increased risk, higher severity, or worse short- or long-term clinical outcomes except that younger patients have a longer lifetime span in which recurrent attacks could occur [2, 4, 44, 51]. The American Society of Colon and Rectal Surgeons (ASCRS) and the European Society of Coloproctology stipulate that young age does not increase the rate of recurrence [10, 52].

Immunosuppression

There are conflicting results for immunosuppression leading to increased recurrence risk.

Immunosuppressed patients, such as those with solid organ transplants, collagen vascular diseases, steroid use, malnutrition, and chronic renal failure, were found in one retrospective study to have a fivefold greater risk of complicated recurrence and perforation compared with nonimmunosuppressed patients (36% vs 7%) [53]. Immunosuppressed status may not only mask the severity of an attack but also increase both surgical and medical morbidity and mortality [25, 54, 55]. Due to conflicting and inconclusive evidence at present, no strong recommendation for elective surgery is possible in immunocompromised patients.

Disease-Related Factors Influencing the Risk of Recurrence

Number of Prior Episodes

Numerous studies have demonstrated that the best predictor of recurrence of diverticulitis is the number of prior episodes [30, 32]. Of all people with a single initial episode of diverticulitis, the lifetime risk of having at least one additional episode is approximately 20%. The risk of recurrence in the first year is around 8%, and each subsequent episode increases the risk of yet another recurrence. For example, a second episode of diverticulitis raises the risk of recurrence to 18% and 55% at 1 and 10 years, respectively; and after a third episode, the risk of recurrence goes up to 40% at 3 years [11].

Time to Recurrence and Smoldering Diverticulitis

Recurrence rates within the first year after a first episode of AD were highest compared to future years, and were reported with a frequency between 10.0% and 82.0% [24, 43, 56]. Two studies showed a reduction in the proportion of recurrences at 2 years after disease remission; our own study showed a reduction in the recurrence rate from 66% during the first year to 16% while another study demonstrated a reduction in recurrence from 64% to 36% [42, 57]. In summary, recurrence risk is higher within the first year after remission.

Similarities seem to exist for the pathophysiology between diverticulitis, irritable bowel syndrome, and inflammatory bowel disease [58, 59]. Although the mechanisms of inflammation are unknown, recurrent or smoldering diverticulitis displays histological and chemical similarities (higher levels of histamine, TNF-α and matrix metalloproteinases to inflammatory bowel disease and irritable bowel syndrome [60–62]. Persistent low-grade inflammation following an episode of AD, even in the presence of uncomplicated AD, may also explain its recurrence. After a 24-month follow-up period, one study found endoscopic inflammation still detected in 27.6% of patients and active histological inflammation in 36.6%. This was shown to be a predictor of diverticulitis recurrence ($p = 0.0004$) [62]. Thus, inflammation persistence may play a role as a risk factor for disease recurrence. Uncomplicated diverticulitis may also not just be a benign self-limiting disease. Up to 30% of patients without further episodes have ongoing abdominal symptoms labeled "smouldering" diverticulitis (see Chap. 9). Some authors state that this is a different and not comparable entity [59, 63].

The argument has been made that episodes occurring within 60 days should be labeled as persistent disease rather than recurrence, in which case some numbers and rates found in the current literature would drastically change if this definition were to be applied universally [64]. The rationale behind some authors defining them as separate episodes is that such a distinction can be considered clinically irrelevant if the patients, by all parameters, have recovered, and the subsequent episode was significant enough to require re-hospitalization and surgical intervention [65].

Severity of Index Episode

CT Findings

Evidence of complicated diverticulitis is of prognostic significance as it is predictive of subsequent disease manifestations and complications. While the literature, including our own data, shows that complicated episodes of diverticulitis increase the risk of developing additional and potentially more complicated episodes, there remains a lack of specificity. As previously stated, the best tool to assess the severity of an episode of diverticulitis is the analysis of CT findings. In one study of 107 patients with non-surgically treated first episode of diverticulitis, 48% of the patients with severe diverticulitis (see Chap. 6) as opposed to 16% of patients with mild diverticulitis experienced a complicated subsequent outcome, defined as one of the following: recurrent diverticulitis, persistence of symptoms, colonic stenosis, residual abscess, or colovesical fistula [35]. From our own data, we found that of all patients with recurrences after complicated diverticulitis, disease aggravation and renewed complications were noted in 42% and 63%, respectively, and 26% of these recurrences required an urgent operation for peritonitis or uncontrolled sepsis [66]. An area for further research would be the development of a radiographic composite score weighing the risk of surgery against the benefit of preventing subsequent complications from recurrent episodes and allow for better patient counseling regarding elective colectomy.

Inflammatory Extension

Two studies with 943 individuals evaluated the impact of inflammatory extension within the colon on AD recurrence [28, 67]. Intestinal inflammation involving more than 5 cm measured by CT scan during the primary episode was associated with an increased risk of recurrence (multivariate HR 1.7, 95% CI 1.3–2.3) [28]. Inflammatory extension in patients with a primary and recurrent diverticulitis did not differ significantly [67]. In summary, an inflamed segment >5 cm may lead to an increased risk of AD recurrence.

Uncomplicated Episodes

Most patients with uncomplicated diverticulitis are unlikely to develop a recurrence. However, non-specific symptoms may persist in more than a third of patients [12]. In one study, the overall recurrence rate after an initial episode of uncomplicated diverticulitis was 16% after a median follow-up of 24 months, and 87% of recurrences were of similar severity [39]. Eglinton et al. [56] found a 19% risk of recurrence and a 5% risk of developing complicated disease after a first episode of uncomplicated diverticulitis. A meta-analysis of studies evaluating long-term outcomes after an episode of uncomplicated diverticulitis demonstrated a pooled recurrence rate of approximately 13% over a period of up to 24 months [68]. When patients with uncomplicated diverticulitis develop recurrent episodes, they are unlikely to experience mortality or to require emergency surgery [69–72]. Studies have demonstrated a 2–4% risk of developing a complicated recurrence after successful nonoperative treatment of uncomplicated diverticulitis, with 1.4% requiring emergency surgery upon representation [39, 73].

Complicated Episodes

In comparison to uncomplicated diverticulitis, complicated diverticulitis seems to recur more frequently, over a shorter time period and with a greater complication rate. Several studies show that the presence of a diverticular abscess on imaging is a strong predictor of recurrent complicated diverticulitis. Ville et al. [21] estimated a hazard ratio of 6.2 in such a setting. As for timing, another study showed that complicated diverticulitis tended to recur within 12 months of the first episode [56]. In an analysis of 107 patients with diverticular abscess, during a median follow-up of 110 months, the overall recurrence rate was 20%, and the median time to recurrence was 4 ± 11.7 months [74]. Other reports showed recurrence rates of 25–30% for all patients presenting with diverticulitis complicated by abscess, with a median time until recurrence of 23 months [75, 76].

Diverticular Abscesses: A Unique Entity with a High Risk of Recurrence

It is estimated that 10–25% of patients with an acute episode of diverticulitis have complicated disease [77, 78]. The most common form of complicated diverticulitis is the development of a diverticular abscess [11]. Diverticular abscesses are particularly concerning because they may lead to long-term complications such as smoldering disease, recurrence, fistula, or stricture [1, 10]. Current practice guidelines lack nuanced recommendations when it comes to patients with complicated diverticulitis, particularly in those with diverticular abscesses. Many aspects of the disease behavior have not been sufficiently elucidated. It remains unclear why some patients experience abscess resolution without interventional radiology or surgery, while others do not. Patients who do not require immediate operation but may potentially benefit from elective intervention are not well defined. The management for this group of patients often seems to be a matter of surgeon or institutional culture; some patients are subjected to a mandatory operation during the index hospitalization, while others are offered elective surgery as either absolute or optional recommendation [79, 80]. In our recent meta-analysis of patients who underwent successful nonoperative management of diverticulitis with abscess, we pointed out this variability: 364 patients had no plans for elective resection in contrast to 375 patients who underwent planned surgery at an average of 2–7 months [71, 80]. It is incumbent upon surgeons to consider both the patient and disease characteristics in order to make an informed decision about how to manage both the acute episode and the long-term sequelae.

Impact of Acute Abscess Management on Recurrence

In a 2005 study of 73 patients with mesocolic and pelvic abscesses, 18 (25%) underwent surgery on index hospitalization. Of the remaining 55 patients, 34% required an operation 2 months to 9 years later [81]. In 2014, our systematic review and meta-analysis studying patients with acute diverticulitis and abscess formation (modified Hinchey grades IB and II) identified 1051 patients in 22 studies of substantial heterogeneity regarding the immediate management and the institutional philosophy about the role of surgery [80]. The overall recurrence rate was 28%; and only 28% of all patients had neither surgery nor did they have a recurrence. In fact, 30% of patients underwent a surgery during the index hospitalization. Among patients awaiting elective resection and those for whom no surgery was planned, the recurrence rates were 39% and 18%, respectively [80].

We subsequently performed a retrospective analysis of 210 patients with diverticulitis complicated by an abscess at our partner public hospital, which mostly serves an indigenous patient population [66]. Due to logistical issues as well as resource limitations, elective resection after seemingly successful medical management of diverticular abscesses was only offered on a very limited basis. Limited access to other institutions in this patient population allowed for studying the natural course of diverticular abscesses after discharge with an emphasis on recurrent attacks and a subsequent need for urgent surgery. The study found an astonishingly high recurrence rate of 61% over an average time period of 5.3 months, including 42% experiencing more than one episode, 46% experiencing a more severe recurrence than the index episode, and 63% of patients presenting with diverticulitis-related complications [66]. Furthermore, 26% of recurrences required urgent operation for peritonitis or uncontrolled sepsis [66]. The observed recurrence rates were not only significantly higher than reported in the literature, but they were also at odds with the notion that the first episode of diverticulitis is typically the worst [54, 82].

Small Abscesses

While clearer understanding and guidelines around management of larger abscesses are nearing, patients with smaller abscesses represent a particular challenge in selecting treatment modalities. There seem to be three distinct groups of patients with small diverticular abscesses: (a) those who recover completely, and not the other hand those whose infection (b) smolders, or (c) ultimately flares up and develops into a larger abscess or another type of complication, such as fistulization, requiring intervention. We do not currently have sufficient evidence to characterize the risk of diverticulitis recurrence specifically in patients with small abscesses.

Complicated Diverticulitis with Macroperforation

In patients with acute diverticulitis and free intraperitoneal air from a ruptured abscess (modified Hinchey class III), nonoperative management in the acute setting is the exception rather than the norm. It can, however, be successful; one group reported the immediate success rate of avoiding an emergency intervention was 95% for 131 patients [83]. However, the evidence suggests that a significant number of patients with complicated diverticulitis will eventually require an urgent surgery, even if initially successfully treated nonoperatively. Another study followed 70 patients who had complicated diverticulitis on index admission; 7 of 44 patients (16%) who were initially treated nonoperatively required urgent surgery [84]. The data analysis is currently limited to determining whether the patients who ultimately required surgery did so because of persistence of the insufficiently treated primary disease or otherwise due to a recurrent episode.

Management-Related Factors Influencing the Risk of Recurrence

Secondary Prophylaxis

Pharmacological and other measures including probiotics, 5-aminosalicylic acid (5-ASA)/mesalazine, and probiotics, among others, have generally failed to demonstrate a significant advantage in reducing the risk of recurrent diverticulitis (see Chap. 8) [85].

Treatment of Uncomplicated Diverticulitis

Treatment of uncomplicated diverticulitis without antibiotics has gained substantial interest since the landmark "Antibiotics Vs. Observation in uncomplicated Diverticulitis" (AVOD) trial in 2012 [86]. The issue remains a focus of ongoing research. Based on the data available to date, the omission of antibiotics for uncomplicated diverticulitis neither aggravates the immediate recovery nor increases the risk of recurrent attacks; however, for unclear reasons as of yet, there may be an increased incidence of subsequent elective surgeries [86–89].

Percutaneous Drain Placement

Percutaneous drain placement has become an important management tool for septic abdominal emergencies. In the context of complicated diverticulitis, the immediate success rate of a percutaneous drain placement ranges between 54–95% and correlates with the size and location of the abscess [4, 81, 90, 91]. Success is defined as the ability to safely access and drain the abscess and achieve resolution of associated signs of sepsis. Commonly, larger abscesses, those >3–5 cm, are more likely to be amenable to drain placement [4, 81, 90, 91]. However, increasing abscess size and distance from the originating bowel segment are also indicative of more severe disease [66, 80, 92]. Our most recent study noted a 94% immediate success rate with percutaneous drainage of diverticular abscesses; however, patients experienced a 71% recurrence rate, 74% of which were complicated [66]. It is therefore recommended to consider and discuss with such patients that even after successful CT-guided drainage; the incidence of future recurrences or complications is high, and drainage may best serve as a bridge to elective surgery rather than as a definitive treatment.

Surgical Intervention

Recurrence After Surgical Resection

Surgical resection for diverticulitis aims at removing the diseased colon segment as well as the high-pressure zone of the rectosigmoid junction. However, it by no means intends to remove all diverticula-bearing colon segments, and there is a risk of developing subsequent diverticulitis even after resection. Nonetheless, when proper diverticulitis surgery is performed (e.g. resection all the way down to the rectosigmoid junction), the risk is substantially reduced and estimated to be around 4–8% [74, 93]. This represents a significant risk reduction when compared with the spontaneous course and a greater than 50% (up to almost 100%) risk in patients with a track record of recurrences or a history of significant disease complications. It should be noted that failure to resect the high-pressure zone has been associated with an up to fourfold risk increase of diverticulitis recurrence postoperatively, which approaches that of patients managed nonoperatively.

In some patients, recurrent diverticulitis after a sigmoidectomy may in fact represent a smoldering anastomotic leak or organ space surgical site infection, rather than true diverticulitis. It is thus important to thoroughly evaluate the patient's symptoms with a critical index of suspicion.

Recurrence After Nonresective Surgery (Laparoscopic Lavage)

The early hype about nonresective surgical intervention has not been able to stand the test of time even if proponents continue to aggressively emphasize the positive effect of laparoscopic lavage [94–97]. The objective evidence suggests that preservation of the diseased colon segment fails to achieve source control. Hence, the risk of nonresolution or recurrent activity is substantially higher than acceptable, and there is a non-negligible risk of missing a perforated cancer [95–98]. The reintervention rate within 30 days was 28.3% after lavage compared to 8% after surgical resection [99]. Sufficiently robust data on the long-term incidence of recurrent attacks is not yet available (see Chap. 12).

Impact of Knowledge About Recurrences

Specific and reliable knowledge of recurrence risk (Table 15.3), and the nature of those recurrences, after successful nonoperative management, is the key element in the debate regarding the need for elective colectomy—whether it be for management of disease sequelae or prophylactic intention [77]. Patients with acceptable operative risk who present with several risk factors for developing diverticulitis, recurrences, or disease complications should be considered for elective surgery to allow for optimal perioperative management.

There is currently no straightforward or standardized way to predict into which group a given patient will fall. An approach that may help in making more evidence-based recommendations would be to implement routine radiographic reimaging after resolution of the acute episode in a set interval, for example, at 6–12 weeks. Persistent findings on CT in the absence of active clinical signs should raise concern. Such findings may include fluid collections or persistent wall thickening of the bowel, indirect signs of strictures or extraluminal pockets of air [100]. It could be beneficial to dedicate further research on studying how CT findings can help us predict recurrences and the nature of those recurrences.

Conclusion

Management of diverticulitis is complex and often multimodal. The goals of care should distinguish between simply overcoming the acute episode and taking prophylactic steps to limit recurrent attacks. Most patients can avoid a surgical intervention at the time of an acute attack. However, there exists a constellation of risk factors that are associated with substantially increased incidence of recurrent and potentially more severe subsequent episodes. More specifically, the presence of a complicated disease such as an abscess is of prognostic and predictive significance and associated with a high risk of recurrence. Further research will have to identify discrete parameters that allow distinction of patients who will likely remain recurrence-free from those who should be considered for surgical resection.

References

1. Kaiser AM. Chapter 4. Diseases and problems. McGraw-hill manual: colorectal surgery. New York, NY: The McGraw-Hill Companies; 2009.
2. Feingold D, Steele SR, Lee S, et al. Practice parameters for the treatment of sigmoid diverticulitis. Dis Colon Rectum. 2014;57:284–94.
3. Hinchey EJ, Schaal PG, Richards GK. Treatment of perforated diverticular disease of the colon. Adv Surg. 1978;12:85–109.
4. Kaiser AM, Jiang JK, Lake JP, et al. The management of complicated diverticulitis and the role of computed tomography. Am J Gastroenterol. 2005;100:910–7.
5. Radé F, Bretagnol F, Auguste M, Di Guisto C, Huten N, de Calan L. Determinants of outcome following laparoscopic peritoneal lavage for perforated diverticulitis. Br J Surg. 2014;101:1602–6. discussion 6
6. Ambrosetti P, Jenny A, Becker C, Terrier TF, Morel P. Acute left colonic diverticulitis–compared performance of computed tomography and water-soluble contrast enema: prospective evaluation of 420 patients. Dis Colon Rectum. 2000;43:1363–7.
7. Wasvary H, Turfah F, Kadro O, Beauregard W. Same hospitalization resection for acute diverticulitis. Am Surg. 1999;65:632–5. discussion 6
8. Li D, Baxter NN, McLeod RS, Moineddin R, Wilton AS, Nathens AB. Evolving practice patterns in the management of acute colonic diverticulitis: a population-based analysis. Dis Colon Rectum. 2014;57:1397–405.
9. Sartelli M, Catena F, Ansaloni L, et al. WSES guidelines for the management of acute left sided colonic

diverticulitis in the emergency setting. World J Emerg Surg. 2016;11:37.
10. Hall J, Hardiman K, Lee S, et al. The American Society of Colon and Rectal Surgeons clinical practice guidelines for the treatment of left-sided colonic diverticulitis. Dis Colon Rectum. 2020;63:728–47.
11. Strate LL, Morris AM. Epidemiology, pathophysiology, and treatment of diverticulitis. Gastroenterology. 2019;156:1282–98.e1.
12. van Dijk ST, Daniels L, de Korte N, et al. Quality of life and persistent symptoms after uncomplicated acute diverticulitis. Dis Colon Rectum. 2019;62:608–14.
13. Egger B, Peter MK, Candinas D. Persistent symptoms after elective sigmoid resection for diverticulitis. Dis Colon Rectum. 2008;51:1044–8.
14. Levack MM, Savitt LR, Berger DL, et al. Sigmoidectomy syndrome? Patients' perspectives on the functional outcomes following surgery for diverticulitis. Dis Colon Rectum. 2012;55:10–7.
15. Franks I. Genetics: genetic susceptibility has a role in the development of diverticular disease. Nat Rev Gastroenterol Hepatol. 2012;9:246.
16. Granlund J, Svensson T, Olén O, et al. The genetic influence on diverticular disease–a twin study. Aliment Pharmacol Ther. 2012;35:1103–7.
17. Strate LL, Liu YL, Syngal S, Aldoori WH, Giovannucci EL. Nut, corn, and popcorn consumption and the incidence of diverticular disease. JAMA. 2008;300:907–14.
18. Elisei W, Tursi A. The pathophysiology of colonic diverticulosis: inflammation versus constipation? Inflamm Intest Dis. 2018;3:55–60.
19. Strate LL, Liu YL, Huang ES, Giovannucci EL, Chan AT. Use of aspirin or nonsteroidal anti-inflammatory drugs increases risk for diverticulitis and diverticular bleeding. Gastroenterology. 2011;140:1427–33.
20. Humes DJ, Fleming KM, Spiller RC, West J. Concurrent drug use and the risk of perforated colonic diverticular disease: a population-based case-control study. Gut. 2011;60:219–24.
21. Sallinen V, Mali J, Leppäniemi A, Mentula P. Assessment of risk for recurrent diverticulitis: a proposal of risk score for complicated recurrence. Medicine (Baltimore). 2015;94:e557.
22. Rosemar A, Angerås U, Rosengren A. Body mass index and diverticular disease: a 28-year follow-up study in men. Dis Colon Rectum. 2008;51:450–5.
23. Aldoori WH, Giovannucci EL, Rimm EB, Wing AL, Trichopoulos DV, Willett WC. A prospective study of alcohol, smoking, caffeine, and the risk of symptomatic diverticular disease in men. Ann Epidemiol. 1995;5:221–8.
24. El-Sayed C, Radley S, Mytton J, Evison F, Ward ST. Risk of recurrent disease and surgery following an admission for acute diverticulitis. Dis Colon Rectum. 2018;61:382–9.
25. Papagrigoriadis S. When should we operate for recurrent diverticulitis? J Clin Gastroenterol. 2016;50(Suppl 1):S80–2.
26. El-Gazzaz G, Zutshi M, Hull T. A retrospective review of chronic anal fistulae treated by anal fistulae plug. Color Dis. 2010;12:442–7.
27. Bailey MB, Davenport DL, Procter L, McKenzie S, Vargas HD. Morbid obesity and diverticulitis: results from the ACS NSQIP dataset. J Am Coll Surg. 2013;217:874–80.e1.
28. Hall JF, Roberts PL, Ricciardi R, et al. Long-term follow-up after an initial episode of diverticulitis: what are the predictors of recurrence? Dis Colon Rectum. 2011;54:283–8.
29. Almalki T, Garfinkle R, Kmiotek E, et al. Family history is associated with recurrent diverticulitis after an episode of diverticulitis managed nonoperatively. Dis Colon Rectum. 2020;63:944–54.
30. Hupfeld L, Burcharth J, Pommergaard HC, Rosenberg J. Risk factors for recurrence after acute colonic diverticulitis: a systematic review. Int J Color Dis. 2017;32:611–22.
31. Bharucha AE, Parthasarathy G, Ditah I, et al. Temporal trends in the incidence and natural history of diverticulitis: a population-based study. Am J Gastroenterol. 2015;110:1589–96.
32. Broderick-Villa G, Burchette RJ, Collins JC, Abbas MA, Haigh PI. Hospitalization for acute diverticulitis does not mandate routine elective colectomy. Arch Surg. 2005;140:576–81. discussion 81-3
33. Parente F, Bargiggia S, Prada A, et al. Intermittent treatment with mesalazine in the prevention of diverticulitis recurrence: a randomised multicentre pilot double-blind placebo-controlled study of 24-month duration. Int J Color Dis. 2013;28:1423–31.
34. van de Wall BJ, Draaisma WA, Consten EC, van der Kaaij RT, Wiezer MJ, Broeders IA. Does the presence of abscesses in diverticular disease prelude surgery? J Gastrointest Surg. 2013;17:540–7.
35. Ambrosetti P, Robert J, Witzig JA, et al. Prognostic factors from computed tomography in acute left colonic diverticulitis. Br J Surg. 1992;79:117–9.
36. Alexandersson BT, Stefánsson T. Incidence and recurrence rate of sigmoid diverticulitis in patients requiring admission to hospital in Iceland from 1985 to 2014: nationwide population-based register study. BJS Open. 2020;4:1217–26.
37. Lopez-Borao J, Kreisler E, Millan M, et al. Impact of age on recurrence and severity of left colonic diverticulitis. Color Dis. 2012;14:e407–12.
38. Katz LH, Guy DD, Lahat A, Gafter-Gvili A, Bar-Meir S. Diverticulitis in the young is not more aggressive than in the elderly, but it tends to recur more often: systematic review and meta-analysis. J Gastroenterol Hepatol. 2013;28:1274–81.
39. Buchs NC, Konrad-Mugnier B, Jannot AS, Poletti PA, Ambrosetti P, Gervaz P. Assessment of recurrence and complications following uncomplicated diverticulitis. Br J Surg. 2013;100:976–9. discussion 9
40. Binda GA, Arezzo A, Serventi A, et al. Multicentre observational study of the natural history of left-sided acute diverticulitis. Br J Surg. 2012;99:276–85.

41. Mueller MH, Glatzle J, Kasparek MS, et al. Long-term outcome of conservative treatment in patients with diverticulitis of the sigmoid colon. Eur J Gastroenterol Hepatol. 2005;17:649–54.
42. Ünlü Ç, van de Wall BJ, Gerhards MF, et al. Influence of age on clinical outcome of acute diverticulitis. J Gastrointest Surg. 2013;17:1651–6.
43. Reisman Y, Ziv Y, Kravrovitc D, Negri M, Wolloch Y, Halevy A. Diverticulitis: the effect of age and location on the course of disease. Int J Color Dis. 1999;14:250–4.
44. Hjern F, Josephson T, Altman D, Holmström B, Johansson C. Outcome of younger patients with acute diverticulitis. Br J Surg. 2008;95:758–64.
45. van Dijk ST, Rottier SJ, van Geloven AAW, Boermeester MA. Conservative treatment of acute colonic diverticulitis. Curr Infect Dis Rep. 2017;19:44.
46. Humes DJ, Spiller RC. Review article: the pathogenesis and management of acute colonic diverticulitis. Aliment Pharmacol Ther. 2014;39:359–70.
47. Faria GR, Almeida AB, Moreira H, Pinto-de-Sousa J, Correia-da-Silva P, Pimenta AP. Acute diverticulitis in younger patients: any rationale for a different approach? World J Gastroenterol. 2011;17:207–12.
48. Lahat A, Menachem Y, Avidan B, et al. Diverticulitis in the young patient–is it different ? World J Gastroenterol. 2006;12:2932–5.
49. Ritz JP, Lehmann KS, Stroux A, Buhr HJ, Holmer C. Sigmoid diverticulitis in young patients–a more aggressive disease than in older patients? J Gastrointest Surg. 2011;15:667–74.
50. Biondo S, Parés D, Martí Ragué J, Kreisler E, Fraccalvieri D, Jaurrieta E. Acute colonic diverticulitis in patients under 50 years of age. Br J Surg. 2002;89:1137–41.
51. Nelson RS, Velasco A, Mukesh BN. Management of diverticulitis in younger patients. Dis Colon Rectum. 2006;49:1341–5.
52. Schultz JK, Azhar N, Binda GA, et al. European Society of Coloproctology: guidelines for the management of diverticular disease of the colon. Color Dis. 2020;22(Suppl 2):5–28.
53. Klarenbeek BR, Samuels M, van der Wal MA, van der Peet DL, Meijerink WJ, Cuesta MA. Indications for elective sigmoid resection in diverticular disease. Ann Surg. 2010;251:670–4.
54. Chapman J, Davies M, Wolff B, et al. Complicated diverticulitis: is it time to rethink the rules? Ann Surg. 2005;242:576–81. discussion 81-3
55. Hwang SS, Cannom RR, Abbas MA, Etzioni D. Diverticulitis in transplant patients and patients on chronic corticosteroid therapy: a systematic review. Dis Colon Rectum. 2010;53:1699–707.
56. Eglinton T, Nguyen T, Raniga S, Dixon L, Dobbs B, Frizelle FA. Patterns of recurrence in patients with acute diverticulitis. Br J Surg. 2010;97:952–7.
57. Biondo S, Borao JL, Kreisler E, et al. Recurrence and virulence of colonic diverticulitis in immunocompromised patients. Am J Surg. 2012;204:172–9.
58. Morris AM, Regenbogen SE, Hardiman KM, Hendren S. Sigmoid diverticulitis: a systematic review. JAMA. 2014;311:287–97.
59. Lembcke B. The gastroenterologist's view. Dig Dis. 2012;30:122–8.
60. Altadill A, Eiró N, González LO, et al. Comparative analysis of the expression of metalloproteases and their inhibitors in resected crohn's disease and complicated diverticular disease. Inflamm Bowel Dis. 2012;18:120–30.
61. Tursi A, Elisei W, Brandimarte G, et al. Mucosal expression of basic fibroblastic growth factor, Syndecan 1 and tumor necrosis factor-alpha in diverticular disease of the colon: a case-control study. Neurogastroenterol Motil. 2012;24:836–e396.
62. Haboubi NY, Alqudah M. Pathology and pathogenesis of diverticular disease and patterns of colonic mucosal changes overlying the diverticula. Dig Dis. 2012;30:29–34.
63. Boostrom SY, Wolff BG, Cima RR, Merchea A, Dozois EJ, Larson DW. Uncomplicated diverticulitis, more complicated than we thought. J Gastrointest Surg. 2012;16:1744–9.
64. Garfinkle R, Boutros M. Recurrent versus persistent diverticulitis: an important distinction. Dis Colon Rectum. 2016;59:e437.
65. Kaiser AM. The author replies. Dis Colon Rectum. 2016;59:e437–8.
66. Devaraj B, Liu W, Tatum J, Cologne K, Kaiser AM. Medically treated diverticular abscess associated with high risk of recurrence and disease complications. Dis Colon Rectum. 2016;59:208–15.
67. Pittet O, Kotzampassakis N, Schmidt S, Denys A, Demartines N, Calmes JM. Recurrent left colonic diverticulitis episodes: more severe than the initial diverticulitis? World J Surg. 2009;33:547–52.
68. Balasubramanian I, Fleming C, Mohan HM, Schmidt K, Haglind E, Winter DC. Out-patient management of mild or uncomplicated diverticulitis: a systematic review. Dig Surg. 2017;34:151–60.
69. Mäkelä J, Vuolio S, Kiviniemi H, Laitinen S. Natural history of diverticular disease: when to operate? Dis Colon Rectum. 1998;41:1523–8.
70. Chapman JR, Dozois EJ, Wolff BG, Gullerud RE, Larson DR. Diverticulitis: a progressive disease? Do multiple recurrences predict less favorable outcomes? Ann Surg. 2006;243:876–30. discussion 80-3
71. Chautems RC, Ambrosetti P, Ludwig A, Mermillod B, Morel P, Soravia C. Long-term follow-up after first acute episode of sigmoid diverticulitis: is surgery mandatory?: a prospective study of 118 patients. Dis Colon Rectum. 2002;45:962–6.
72. Haglund U, Hellberg R, Johnsén C, Hultén L. Complicated diverticular disease of the sigmoid colon. An analysis of short and long term outcome in 392 patients. Ann Chir Gynaecol. 1979;68:41–6.
73. Daniels L, Ünlü Ç, de Korte N, et al. Randomized clinical trial of observational versus antibiotic treatment for a first episode of CT-proven

uncomplicated acute diverticulitis. Br J Surg. 2017;104:52–61.
74. Buchwald P, Dixon L, Wakeman CJ, Eglinton TW, Frizelle FA. Hinchey I and II diverticular abscesses: long-term outcome of conservative treatment. ANZ J Surg. 2017;87:1011–4.
75. Garfinkle R, Kugler A, Pelsser V, et al. Diverticular abscess managed with long-term definitive non-operative intent is safe. Dis Colon Rectum. 2016;59:648–55.
76. Gregersen R, Mortensen LQ, Burcharth J, Pommergaard HC, Rosenberg J. Treatment of patients with acute colonic diverticulitis complicated by abscess formation: a systematic review. Int J Surg. 2016;35:201–8.
77. Bendl RF, Bergamaschi R. Do patients mandate resection after a first episode of acute diverticulitis of the colon with a complication? Adv Surg. 2017;51:179–91.
78. Beckham H, Whitlow CB. The medical and nonoperative treatment of diverticulitis. Clin Colon Rectal Surg. 2009;22:156–60.
79. Alvarez JA, Baldonedo RF, Bear IG, et al. Presentation, management and outcome of acute sigmoid diverticulitis requiring hospitalization. Dig Surg. 2007;24:471–6.
80. Lamb MN, Kaiser AM. Elective resection versus observation after nonoperative management of complicated diverticulitis with abscess: a systematic review and meta-analysis. Dis Colon Rectum. 2014;57:1430–40.
81. Ambrosetti P, Chautems R, Soravia C, Peiris-Waser N, Terrier F. Long-term outcome of mesocolic and pelvic diverticular abscesses of the left colon: a prospective study of 73 cases. Dis Colon Rectum. 2005;48:787–91.
82. Kaiser AM. Complicated diverticulitis: it is not yet time to rethink the rules! Ann Surg. 2006;243:707–8. author reply 8-9
83. Dharmarajan S, Hunt SR, Birnbaum EH, Fleshman JW, Mutch MG. The efficacy of nonoperative management of acute complicated diverticulitis. Dis Colon Rectum. 2011;54:663–71.
84. Suarez Alecha J, Amoza Pais S, Batlle Marin X, Oronoz Martinez B, Balen Ribera E, Yarnoz IC. Safety of nonoperative management after acute diverticulitis. Ann Coloproctol. 2014;30:216–21.
85. Unlü C, Daniels L, Vrouenraets BC, Boermeester MA. Systematic review of medical therapy to prevent recurrent diverticulitis. Int J Color Dis. 2012;27:1131–6.
86. Chabok A, Påhlman L, Hjern F, Haapaniemi S, Smedh K. Randomized clinical trial of antibiotics in acute uncomplicated diverticulitis. Br J Surg. 2012;99:532–9.
87. Shabanzadeh DM, Wille-Jørgensen P. Antibiotics for uncomplicated diverticulitis. Cochrane Database Syst Rev. 2012;11:Cd009092.
88. Mege D, Yeo H. Meta-analyses of current strategies to treat uncomplicated diverticulitis. Dis Colon Rectum. 2019;62:371–8.
89. Peery AF. It's actually a little complicated: antibiotics for uncomplicated diverticulitis. Am J Gastroenterol. 2018;113:949–50.
90. Siewert B, Tye G, Kruskal J, et al. Impact of CT-guided drainage in the treatment of diverticular abscesses: size matters. AJR Am J Roentgenol. 2006;186:680–6.
91. Nelson RS, Ewing BM, Wengert TJ, Thorson AG. Clinical outcomes of complicated diverticulitis managed nonoperatively. Am J Surg. 2008;196:969–72. discussion 73-4
92. Gaertner WB, Willis DJ, Madoff RD, et al. Percutaneous drainage of colonic diverticular abscess: is colon resection necessary? Dis Colon Rectum. 2013;56:622–6.
93. You K, Bendl R, Taut C, Sullivan R, Gachabayov M, Bergamaschi R. Randomized clinical trial of elective resection versus observation in diverticulitis with extraluminal air or abscess initially managed conservatively. Br J Surg. 2018;105:971–9.
94. Galbraith N, Carter JV, Netz U, et al. Laparoscopic lavage in the management of perforated diverticulitis: a contemporary meta-analysis. J Gastrointest Surg. 2017;21:1491–9.
95. Vennix S, Musters GD, Mulder IM, et al. Laparoscopic peritoneal lavage or sigmoidectomy for perforated diverticulitis with purulent peritonitis: a multicentre, parallel-group, randomised, open-label trial. Lancet. 2015;386:1269–77.
96. Schultz JK, Yaqub S, Wallon C, et al. Laparoscopic lavage vs primary resection for acute perforated diverticulitis: the SCANDIV randomized clinical trial. JAMA. 2015;314:1364–75.
97. Sneiders D, Lambrichts DPV, Swank HA, et al. Long-term follow-up of a multicentre cohort study on laparoscopic peritoneal lavage for perforated diverticulitis. Color Dis. 2019;21:705–14.
98. Penna M, Markar SR, Mackenzie H, Hompes R, Cunningham C. Laparoscopic lavage versus primary resection for acute perforated diverticulitis: review and meta-analysis. Ann Surg. 2018;267:252–8.
99. Marshall JR, Buchwald PL, Gandhi J, et al. Laparoscopic lavage in the management of Hinchey Grade III diverticulitis: a systematic review. Ann Surg. 2017;265:670–6.
100. van Dijk ST, Daniels L, Nio CY, Somers I, van Geloven AAW, Boermeester MA. Predictive factors on CT imaging for progression of uncomplicated into complicated acute diverticulitis. Int J Color Dis. 2017;32:1693–8.

16 Symptomatic Uncomplicated Diverticular Disease or Irritable Bowel Syndrome: How Can You Tell?

Mythili P. Pathipati and Kyle Staller

Introduction

Diverticular disease is one of the most common gastrointestinal conditions in the world. Prevalence increases with age and a country's level of industrialization. In the United States, an estimated 5% of patients below age 40 have diverticula, with rates of diverticulosis rising to greater than 50% in patients above age 60 [1]. The condition accounts for more than 2.5 million clinic visits in the United States, 1 million inpatient days, and $2 billion in spending annually [1, 2].

There are several different manifestations of diverticular disease (Fig. 16.1). A large majority (~75–90%) of patients with diverticula are asymptomatic [3]. Among those who do have symptoms, problems include diverticulitis, diverticular bleeding, and segmental colitis.

One of the most common causes of persistent symptoms in diverticular disease is symptomatic uncomplicated diverticular disease (SUDD); however, SUDD remains poorly characterized. In this chapter, we review the literature on SUDD, including its definition, pathogenesis, risk factors, and epidemiology. In addition, SUDD shares considerable overlap with irritable bowel syndrome (IBS). We will therefore review the similarities and differences between the conditions and consider shared treatment modalities.

M. P. Pathipati
Department of Gastroenterology, Palo Alto Medical Foundation/Sutter Health, Palo Alto, CA, USA

K. Staller (✉)
Division of Gastroenterology, Massachusetts General Hospital, Boston, MA, USA
e-mail: KSTALLER@mgh.harvard.edu

Symptomatic Uncomplicated Diverticular Disease (SUDD)

Definition

Diverticulosis refers to sac-like protrusions of the colonic wall. In many cases of diverticular disease, there is an obvious association between the physical structure and an associated pathology such as inflammation, bleeding, among others. SUDD, by contrast, is a clinical diagnosis based on abdominal symptoms in the presence of diverticula.

Formal definitions of SUDD vary, including definitions from guideline bodies [4, 5]. The Italian Consensus Conference on Diverticular Disease defines SUDD as a "syndrome characterized by recurrent abdominal symptoms such as abdominal pain and bloating resembling or overlapping IBS symptoms, attributed to diverticula in the absence of macroscopically evident alterations other than the presence of diverticula" [6]. Meanwhile, the Italian Society of Colon and Rectal Surgery defines SUDD as simply "mild, recurring abdominal pain attributed to diverticula" [7]. SUDD is not discussed in US guidelines

M. Boutros et al. (eds.), *Diverticulitis*, https://doi.org/10.1007/978-3-032-21720-2_16

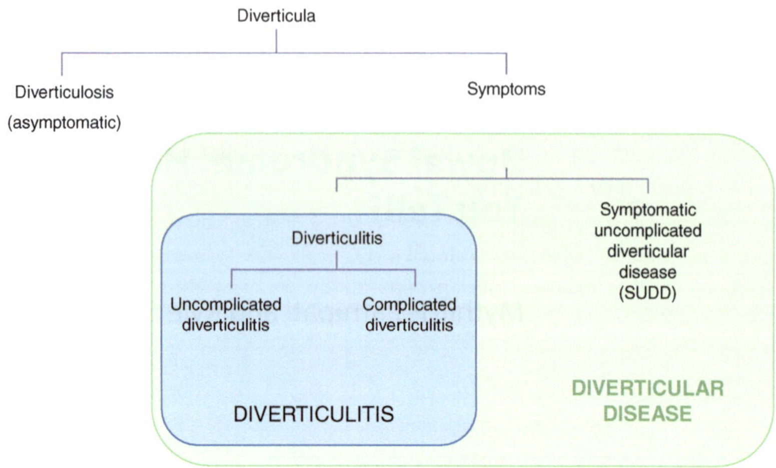

Fig. 16.1 Classification of diverticular disease [4]. (Copyright: © 2017 Acta Bio Medica Society of Medicine and Natural Sciences of Parma. This work is licensed under a Creative Commons Attribution 4.0 International License)

due to the limited quality of evidence on the condition.

Other authors have offered their own definitions. Peery et al. [8] noted that one common description of SUDD is "chronic gastrointestinal symptoms attributed to colonic diverticulosis in the absence of overt inflammation." Tursi and Elisei [9] offer specific clinical characteristics to distinguish SUDD from IBS, namely location (left lower abdomen) and duration (>24 h of symptoms).

In our practice, we may entertain a diagnosis of SUDD in patients with diverticulosis plus symptoms of abdominal pain or loose stools in the prior 3 months. Common themes across definitions include the following:

1. Presence of diverticula
2. Abdominal symptoms, including pain, bloating, or changes in bowel habits
3. Lack of macroscopic evidence for other pathology

Pathophysiology

The lack of consensus on a definition of SUDD speaks to an underlying lack of understanding of its pathogenesis. The connection between uncomplicated diverticula and symptoms remains unclear.

Several theories have been put forward. One hypothesis is that symptoms arise from visceral hypersensitivity. Humes et al. [10] conducted barostat-mediated rectal distention testing on asymptomatic and symptomatic patients with diverticula and found that symptomatic patients reported a lower threshold to pain and higher overall pain ratings. Similarly, Clemens et al. [11] found that SUDD patients had a higher sensitivity to colonic distention than asymptomatic controls despite no differences in wall compliance.

Multiple researchers have proposed low-grade inflammation as a mechanism for visceral hypersensitivity in SUDD. In their study, Humes et al. [10] found that there was low-grade inflammation and upregulation of tachykinins on staining of biopsied tissue. Horgan et al. [12] found that 76% of symptomatic patients who underwent surgical resection showed signs of peridiverticular inflammation. Tursi et al. [13] found that fecal calprotectin levels, which correlate with inflammatory infiltrate, are elevated in acute uncomplicated diverticulitis and SUDD, but not in asymptomatic diverticulosis, patients with IBS, or healthy controls. Of note, there is also some ambiguity in differentiating SUDD from segmental colitis associated with diverticulitis (SCAD) when considering the role of inflammation (*See* Chap. 4 *for further details*).

In spite of these findings, the association between low-grade inflammation and SUDD remains controversial. For instance, Peery et al. [8] found that diverticulosis, whether symptomatic or not, was not associated with mucosal inflammation in a prospective study of 619 patients undergoing a screening colonoscopy with biopsy. The authors went on to question whether SUDD was a real clinical entity or simply a variant of IBS. Jarbink-Sehgal et al. [14] found a similar result in a case-control study of 254 subjects who underwent colonoscopy and reported no association between inflammation and symptoms in patients with diverticulosis.

Another proposed explanation for SUDD is abnormal colonic motility. Bassotti et al. [15] found that patients with diverticulosis have a reduced number of colonic interstitial cells of Cajal, which act as pacemakers for intestinal smooth muscle. While the specific mechanism is not established, the authors suggest that symptomatic diverticulosis may therefore relate to slowed colonic transit. A related study of 24-h colonic manometry in 12 patients with SUDD compared to 20 healthy controls found that patients with SUDD had an increased duration of rhythmic, low-frequency, contractile activity, most notably in areas with diverticula. The authors concluded that the rhythmic contractions were associated with the pain seen in SUDD patients [16].

Yet another possibility is that SUDD arises due to increased nerve fiber sprouting. Barbaro et al. found that patients with diverticulosis had a higher density of nerve fibers in the diverticular regions than healthy controls. Moreover, patients with SUDD had a higher density of GAP43+ fibers (i.e., nerve fibers undergoing sprouting) in diverticular regions compared to patients with asymptomatic diverticulosis. The authors suggested that symptoms may therefore relate specifically to nerve fiber growth [17].

There are many other possible pathophysiologic explanations, including genetic variants, and altered gut microbiota [18, 19]. However, these theories have limited evidence to date which mostly consists of small, retrospective studies. Further prospective investigation is needed to elucidate the true underlying mechanism of SUDD, which very well may be multifactorial and include several of the proposed theories above.

Risk Factors

While the clinical risk factors for diverticular disease are well established (e.g., age, fiber, meat, and alcohol intake, obesity, medications, medical comorbidities, and others) [18], few studies have specifically evaluated the risk factors that differentiate asymptomatic diverticulosis from SUDD.

Humes et al. [10] offered some insight into this question in their questionnaire-based study of 136 patients with known diverticula. At a mean follow-up of 7 years, the two variables that significantly predicted risk of recurrent abdominal pain (consistent with SUDD) were an episode of acute diverticulitis (OR 3.98, CI 1.39–11.36) and an anxiety score >7 on the Hospital Anxiety and Depression Scale (OR 2.53, CI 1.09–5.86).

The authors argue that the association with diverticulitis provides evidence that an inflammatory process contributes to SUDD. With that said, they also note that there appears to be an important psychological component to recurrent symptoms and recommend psychological screening prior to determining treatment for SUDD patients.

Given the lack of macroscopic pathology in SUDD, there is a growing sense that it may represent a Disorder of Gut-Brain Interaction (also known as a functional gastrointestinal disease). Follow-up studies have validated a relationship between somatic symptoms and SUDD. For example, Spiller et al. [20] reported that among 296 patients with diverticulosis who completed a Patient Health Questionnaire-12 somatic symptom score, patients with SUDD were more than twice as likely to have evidence of somatization compared to those with asymptomatic diverticulosis.

Few studies explored SUDD prevalence, and the results are contrasting. In an Italian case–control study including 5451 patients with colonic diverticula, Tursi et al. [21] found a prevalence of SUDD in 6.8% of patients. Interestingly, abdominal pain was recorded in almost 21% of patients, diarrhea in 5.3%, and constipation in 9.8% among patients with colonic diverticulosis.

Epidemiology

Epidemiologic data on SUDD is limited. However, the prevalence of SUDD has paralleled that of diverticulosis, and as a result, certain patterns have emerged. SUDD is more common in older patients (particularly those >60 years old) and in developed nations. Specific estimates of prevalence are widely variable depending on the age and demographics of any given study sample [22].

The gender distribution of diverticular disease appears to be age-stratified. More specifically, it is more common in males under the age of 50 but more common in females over 50. Overall, there appears to be a roughly even gender balance in diverticular disease [18].

There is likely a race-based element to diverticular disease as well. For instance, the location of diverticula varies by ethnicity, with Asians more likely to have right-sided diverticula while other ethnic groups have predominantly left-sided diverticula [23]. Another study found that African Americans were more likely to have right-sided diverticula than white Americans [24]. However, it is not known how these variations correlate with SUDD.

Irritable Bowel Syndrome

Definition

Similar to SUDD, IBS is a clinical diagnosis. The Rome IV diagnostic criteria for IBS include recurrent abdominal pain, on average, at least 1 day/week in the last 3 months, and two or more of the following criteria [25]:

1. Related to defecation
2. Associated with a change in frequency of stool
3. Associated with a change in the form (appearance) of stool

IBS can be further categorized into subtypes based on predominant bowel habits on days with abnormal bowel movements and include IBS with predominant constipation (IBS-C), IBS with predominant diarrhea (IBS-D), IBS with mixed bowel habits (IBS-M), and unsubtyped IBS (IBS-U). Categorization into subtypes is based on the Bristol Stool Form Scale (BSFS).

Pathophysiology

The pathophysiology of IBS is not clear, and several of the mechanisms suggested overlap with those linked to SUDD. A considerable body of research focuses on intestinal motility as the cause of IBS. For example, Chey et al. [26] found that patients with IBS-D had an elevated motility index and a higher number of high-amplitude propagating contractions than healthy controls. Agrawal et al. [27] evaluated IBS-C patients and found that they had delayed transit compared to healthy controls. Other studies have evaluated the role of irregular small bowel contractions [28].

Visceral hypersensitivity is another possible explanation. Several studies have demonstrated that patients with IBS experience pain with rectal distention at a lower threshold than controls [29, 30]. In addition, the pain associated with distention occurred independently of contractile activity [30].

Third, intestinal inflammation may contribute to symptoms of IBS. Studies have demonstrated higher levels of intestinal lymphocytes [31], mast cells [32], and cytokines [33] in IBS patients compared to controls.

There is a long list of other possible explanations for IBS, reflecting many of the same factors that may play a role in SUDD. These include microbiota, genetic changes, dietary issues, and more. Once again, the evidence for each of these mechanisms is limited. However, altogether, there is a much more established and accepted body of evidence for the pathophysiology of IBS compared to SUDD.

Risk Factors

Several clinical risk factors are associated with IBS including smoking, alcohol consumption, and younger age [34]. Food sensitivities, including food allergies and gluten intolerance, may correlate with a greater likelihood of IBS as well, although evidence is mixed [35].

There is a well-established relationship between gastrointestinal infection and IBS. A meta-analysis of 18 studies also found that the odds of developing IBS were six times more likely following an acute GI infection, implying an inflammatory process at work [36].

Several studies suggest that psychosocial function plays a role in IBS as well. For example, IBS patients showed greater changes in colonic motility, visceral perception, intestinal secretion, autonomic nervous system tone, and hypothalamic-pituitary axis function in response to stressors than healthy controls [37]. In a prospective study, psychosocial problems (including anxiety, sleep disorders, and somatic symptoms) independently predicted the development of IBS [38]. In our experience in a tertiary care center, we have found that ~50% of IBS patients have either a psychiatric or functional comorbidity.

Epidemiology

IBS affects an estimated 10–25% of the global community, with pooled estimates placing the prevalence around 11%. The lowest rates are in South Asia, while the highest are in South America [39].

IBS occurs in all age groups, although it more commonly begins in younger patients. Approximately 50% of patients with IBS report the onset of symptoms before the age of 35 and it is uncommon for patients to receive a diagnosis of IBS after age 50 [40].

IBS is more common in women than in men. Overall prevalence is estimated to be ~67% higher in women, which corresponds to an absolute difference in prevalence of 5% (8.9% for men and 14.0% for women) [40].

Overlap Between SUDD and IBS

There are striking similarities between SUDD and IBS. Both conditions have similar clinical presentations, namely abdominal symptoms and changes in bowel habits. Both have a poorly characterized pathophysiology but appear connected to motility abnormalities, visceral hypersensitivity, and possibly inflammation. Both also share clinical risk factors including associations with inflammatory processes (diverticulitis in SUDD, gastroenteritis in IBS) and psychosocial abnormalities. The similarities between the two conditions have raised a question as to whether SUDD is a distinct pathologic process or simply identifies patients who have IBS as well as asymptomatic diverticula.

At the same time, there are differences (Table 16.1). Patients with SUDD more often report pain localized to the left lower quadrant, while IBS patients report more generalized pain. IBS episodes also tend to be shorter, less severe, and are more likely to be associated with defecation.

While these differences are clinically observed and reported anecdotally, there is no consensus on clinical criteria to distinguish the two conditions. As a result, perhaps the most important distinguishing feature between SUDD and IBS is their respective epidemiology. SUDD generally occurs in older patients and does not have the same female predominance that is present in IBS.

Further research is needed to elucidate the differences, should they truly exist, between SUDD and IBS. This includes systematic evaluation of differences in clinical presentation and additional research on their underlying mechanisms.

Distinguishing Between SUDD and Smoldering Diverticulitis

Smoldering diverticulitis refers to persistent, low-grade inflammation following an episode of acute diverticulitis. Differentiating between this and SUDD is clinically challenging, as both may present with chronic abdominopelvic pain after a CT-proven episode of diverticulitis. In patients

Table 16.1 Comparison of SUDD and IBS

Factor	SUDD	IBS
Demographics	Older with minimal gender skew	Young and female
Typical age of onset	Above 50	Between ages 30 and 50
Symptoms	Abdominal symptoms	Abdominal symptoms, altered bowel habits
Medical risk factors	Diverticulitis	GI infection
Psychological risk factors	Anxiety, somatization	Anxiety, somatization
Specialty care	Surgeons	Gastroenterologists

IBS irritable bowel syndrome, *SUDD* symptomatic uncomplicated diverticular disease

with persistent symptoms after acute diverticulitis, ongoing inflammation or complications (strictures, fistulae, malignancy) should be excluded with both CT imaging and colonoscopy (this can be done 6–8 weeks after the acute episode). There is no established time interval that defines the transition from resolving diverticulitis to SUDD. Most recurrences of diverticulitis occur within the first year, but chronic symptoms can persist even after apparent radiologic and clinical resolution. The decision to label symptoms as SUDD versus ongoing inflammation is based on clinical judgment, supported by negative imaging and endoscopic findings.

Implications for Treatment

The classification of SUDD and IBS is important insofar as it shapes how physicians manage the two conditions. Clinicians have historically followed different paradigms for SUDD and IBS. Treatment of SUDD largely follows a gut modulation paradigm. In other words, treatments target structural causes of gastrointestinal distress. These include probiotics and rifaximin to address microbiota abnormalities, fiber to improve stool passage and reduce straining, mesalazine to reduce inflammation, and in cases with complications like recurrent diverticulitis, surgery to remove the diverticula.

However, there is minimal evidence to support the use of these therapies. Recent systematic reviews have cast doubt on the quality of evidence supporting the use of probiotics [41], fiber [42], and mesalamine for SUDD [43]. International guidelines offer an array of changing and conflicting recommendations [44, 45]. For instance, Italian guidelines reported a lack of evidence to support the use of mesalamine in SUDD while German guidelines recommended mesalamine as an appropriate treatment option. Danish and Polish guidelines support the use of fiber supplements but Italian guidelines state that they have limited use in isolation. There is currently a consensus between Italian, Danish, and Polish guidelines on the use of cyclic rifaximin in combination with fiber supplements.

By contrast, treatment of IBS addresses both gut and neuromodulation. This includes a combination of motility agents (laxatives for IBS-C, antidiarrheals for IBS-D), dietary changes (including fiber, low FODMAP diet) and probiotics, and neuromodulators to address visceral hypersensitivity. Common neuromodulators include tricyclic antidepressants (TCAs) and selective serotonin reuptake inhibitors (SSRIs), while cognitive behavioral therapy (CBT) and gut-directed hypnotherapy likely serve a similar role and may be used alone or in combination with pharmacotherapy. TCAs, in particular, show a strong effect in reducing IBS symptoms, possibly due to their effects on slowing intestinal transit time. SSRIs and CBT also contribute to significant improvements in IBS symptoms, although the effect is not as strong [46, 47].

Conclusion

While SUDD and IBS may be distinct pathologic entities, we believe that there is minimal difference from the clinician's point of view. There is little evidence to suggest that diverticula are a structural cause of symptoms in SUDD and existing approaches to treatment have had mixed results. However, there is growing evidence that psychosocial factors contribute to SUDD. We therefore recommend use of both gut and neuromodulation strategies in the treatment of both conditions.

References

1. Weizman AV, Nguyen GC. Diverticular disease: epidemiology and management. Can J Gastroenterol. 2011;25(7):385. https://www.ncbi.nlm.nih.gov/pmc/articles/PMC3174080/. Accessed June 24, 2019.
2. Papa A, Papa V. The economic burden of diverticular disease. J Clin Gastroenterol. 2016;50:S2–3. https://doi.org/10.1097/MCG.0000000000000598.
3. Cremon C, Bellacosa L, Barbaro MR, Cogliandro RF, Stanghellini V, Barbara G. Diagnostic challenges of symptomatic uncomplicated diverticular disease. Minerva Gastroenterol Dietol. 2017;63(2):119–29. https://doi.org/10.23736/S1121-421X.17.02370-4.
4. Maconi G. Diagnosis of symptomatic uncomplicated diverticular disease and the role of Rifaximin in management. Acta Biomed. 2017;88(1):25–32. https://doi.org/10.23750/abm.v88i1.6360.
5. Calini G, Abd El Aziz MA, Paolini L, Abdalla S, Rottoli M, Mari G, Larson DW. Symptomatic uncomplicated diverticular disease (SUDD): practical guidance and challenges for clinical management. Clin Exp Gastroenterol. 2023;16:29–43. https://doi.org/10.2147/CEG.S340929. PMID: 37013200; PMCID: PMC10066719.
6. Cuomo R, Barbara G, Pace F, et al. Italian consensus conference for colonic diverticulosis and diverticular disease. United Eur Gastroenterol J. 2014;2(5):413. https://doi.org/10.1177/2050640614547068.
7. Binda GA, Cuomo R, Laghi A, et al. Practice parameters for the treatment of colonic diverticular disease: Italian Society of Colon and Rectal Surgery (SICCR) guidelines. Tech Coloproctol. 2015;19(10):615–26. https://doi.org/10.1007/s10151-015-1370-x.
8. Peery AF, Keku TO, Addamo C, et al. Colonic diverticula are not associated with mucosal inflammation or chronic gastrointestinal symptoms. Clin Gastroenterol Hepatol. 2018;16(6):884–891.e1. https://doi.org/10.1016/j.cgh.2017.05.051.
9. Tursi A, Elisei W. Role of inflammation in the pathogenesis of diverticular disease. Mediat Inflamm. 2019;2019:8328490. https://doi.org/10.1155/2019/8328490.
10. Humes DJ, Simpson J, Smith J, et al. Visceral hypersensitivity in symptomatic diverticular disease and the role of neuropeptides and low grade inflammation. Neurogastroenterol Motil. 2012;24(4):318-e163. https://doi.org/10.1111/j.1365-2982.2011.01863.x.
11. Clemens CHM, Samsom M, Roelofs J, van Berge Henegouwen GP, Smout AJPM. Colorectal visceral perception in diverticular disease. Gut. 2004;53(5):717–22. https://doi.org/10.1136/gut.2003.018093.
12. Horgan AF, McConnell EJ, Wolff BG, The S, Paterson C. Atypical diverticular disease: surgical results. Dis Colon Rectum. 2001;44(9):1315–8. http://www.ncbi.nlm.nih.gov/pubmed/11584207. Accessed June 24, 2019.
13. Tursi A, Brandimarte G, Elisei W, Giorgetti GM, Inchingolo CD, Aiello F. Faecal calprotectin in colonic diverticular disease: a case–control study. Int J Color Dis. 2009;24(1):49–55. https://doi.org/10.1007/s00384-008-0595-9.
14. Järbrink-Sehgal ME, Rassam L, Jasim A, et al. Diverticulosis, symptoms and colonic inflammation. Am J Gastroenterol. 2019;114(3):500–10. https://doi.org/10.14309/ajg.0000000000000113.
15. Bassotti G, Battaglia E, Bellone G, et al. Interstitial cells of Cajal, enteric nerves, and glial cells in colonic diverticular disease. J Clin Pathol. 2005;58(9):973–7. https://doi.org/10.1136/jcp.2005.026112.
16. Bassotti G, Battaglia E, De Roberto G, Morelli A, Tonini M, Villanacci V. Alterations in colonic motility and relationship to pain in colonic diverticulosis. Clin Gastroenterol Hepatol. 2005;3(3):248–53. http://www.ncbi.nlm.nih.gov/pubmed/15765444. Accessed June 24, 2019.
17. Barbaro MR, Cremon C, Fuschi D, et al. Nerve fiber overgrowth in patients with symptomatic diverticular disease. Neurogastroenterol Motil. 2019;31:e13575. https://doi.org/10.1111/nmo.13575.
18. Violi A, Cambiè G, Miraglia C, et al. Epidemiology and risk factors for diverticular disease. Acta Biomed. 2018;89(9-S):107–12. https://doi.org/10.23750/abm.v89i9-S.7924.
19. Tursi A, Papa V, Lopetuso LR, Settanni CR, Gasbarrini A, Papa A. Microbiota composition in diverticular disease: implications for therapy. Int J Mol Sci. 2022;23(23):14799. https://doi.org/10.3390/ijms232314799.
20. Spiller R. Is it diverticular disease or is it irritable bowel syndrome? Dig Dis. 2012;30(1):64–9. https://doi.org/10.1159/000335721.
21. Tursi A, Elisei W, Franceschi M, Picchio M, Di Mario F, Brandimarte G. The prevalence of symptomatic uncomplicated diverticular disease could be lower than expected: a single-center colonoscopy-based cohort study. Eur J Gastroenterol Hepatol. 2021;33(1S Suppl 1):e478–83. https://doi.org/10.1097/MEG.0000000000002142.
22. Tursi A. Diverticulosis today: unfashionable and still under-researched. Ther Adv Gastroenterol. 2016;9(2):213–28. https://doi.org/10.1177/1756283X15621228 21.
23. Chan CC, Lo KK, Chung EC, Lo SS, Hon TY. Colonic diverticulosis in Hong Kong: distribution pattern and clinical significance. Clin Radiol. 1998;53(11):842–4. http://www.ncbi.nlm.nih.gov/pubmed/9833789. Accessed June 24, 2019.

24. Peery AF, Keku TO, Martin CF, et al. Distribution and characteristics of colonic diverticula in a United States screening population. Clin Gastroenterol Hepatol. 2016;14(7):980–985.e1. https://doi.org/10.1016/j.cgh.2016.01.020.
25. Lacy BE, Patel NK. Rome criteria and a diagnostic approach to irritable bowel syndrome. J Clin Med. 2017;6(11):99. https://doi.org/10.3390/jcm6110099.
26. Chey WY, Jin HO, Lee MH, Sun SW, Lee KY. Colonic motility abnormality in patients with irritable bowel syndrome exhibiting abdominal pain and diarrhea. Am J Gastroenterol. 2001;96(5):1499–506. https://doi.org/10.1111/j.1572-0241.2001.03804.x.
27. Agrawal A, Houghton LA, Reilly B, Morris J, Whorwell PJ. Bloating and distension in irritable bowel syndrome: the role of gastrointestinal transit. Am J Gastroenterol. 2009;104(8):1998–2004. https://doi.org/10.1038/ajg.2009.251.
28. Simrén M, Castedal M, Svedlund J, Abrahamsson H, Björnsson E. Abnormal propagation pattern of duodenal pressure waves in the irritable bowel syndrome (IBS) [correction of (IBD)]. Dig Dis Sci. 2000;45(11):2151–61. http://www.ncbi.nlm.nih.gov/pubmed/11215731. Accessed June 24, 2019.
29. Bouin M, Plourde V, Boivin M, et al. Rectal distention testing in patients with irritable bowel syndrome: sensitivity, specificity, and predictive values of pain sensory thresholds. Gastroenterology. 2002;122(7):1771–7. http://www.ncbi.nlm.nih.gov/pubmed/12055583. Accessed June 24, 2019.
30. Whitehead WE, Holtkotter B, Enck P, et al. Tolerance for rectosigmoid distention in irritable bowel syndrome. Gastroenterology. 1990;98(5 Pt 1):1187–92. http://www.ncbi.nlm.nih.gov/pubmed/2323511. Accessed June 24, 2019.
31. Chadwick VS, Chen W, Shu D, et al. Activation of the mucosal immune system in irritable bowel syndrome. Gastroenterology. 2002;122(7):1778–83. http://www.ncbi.nlm.nih.gov/pubmed/12055584. Accessed June 24, 2019.
32. Guilarte M, Santos J, de Torres I, et al. Diarrhoea-predominant IBS patients show mast cell activation and hyperplasia in the jejunum. Gut. 2007;56(2):203–9. https://doi.org/10.1136/gut.2006.100594.
33. Liebregts T, Adam B, Bredack C, et al. Immune activation in patients with irritable bowel syndrome. Gastroenterology. 2007;132(3):913–20. https://doi.org/10.1053/j.gastro.2007.01.046.
34. Nam SY, Kim BC, Ryu KH, Park BJ. Prevalence and risk factors of irritable bowel syndrome in healthy screenee undergoing colonoscopy and laboratory tests. J Neurogastroenterol Motil. 2010;16(1):47–51. https://doi.org/10.5056/jnm.2010.16.1.47.
35. Choung RS, Talley NJ. Food allergy and intolerance in IBS. Gastroenterol Hepatol (N Y). 2006;2(10):756. https://www.ncbi.nlm.nih.gov/pmc/articles/PMC5358086/. Accessed June 24, 2019.
36. Thabane M, Kottachchi DT, Marshall JK. Systematic review and meta-analysis: the incidence and prognosis of post-infectious irritable bowel syndrome. Aliment Pharmacol Ther. 2007;26(4):535–44. https://doi.org/10.1111/j.1365-2036.2007.03399.x.
37. Chang L. The role of stress on physiologic responses and clinical symptoms in irritable bowel syndrome. Gastroenterology. 2011;140(3):761–5. https://doi.org/10.1053/j.gastro.2011.01.032.
38. Nicholl BI, Halder SL, Macfarlane GJ, et al. Psychosocial risk markers for new onset irritable bowel syndrome--results of a large prospective population-based study. Pain. 2008;137(1):147–55. https://doi.org/10.1016/j.pain.2007.08.029.
39. Endo Y, Shoji T, Fukudo S. Epidemiology of irritable bowel syndrome. Ann Gastroenterol. 2015;28(2):158–9. http://www.ncbi.nlm.nih.gov/pubmed/25830818. Accessed June 24, 2019.
40. Canavan C, West J, Card T. The epidemiology of irritable bowel syndrome. Clin Epidemiol. 2014;6:71–80. https://doi.org/10.2147/CLEP.S40245.
41. Lahner E, Bellisario C, Hassan C, Zullo A, Esposito G, Annibale B. Probiotics in the treatment of diverticular disease. A systematic review. J Gastrointestin Liver Dis. 2016;25(1):79–86. https://doi.org/10.15403/jgld.2014.1121.251.srw.
42. Carabotti M, Annibale B, Severi C, Lahner E. Role of fiber in symptomatic uncomplicated diverticular disease: a systematic review. Nutrients. 2017;9(2):161. https://doi.org/10.3390/nu9020161.
43. Iannone A, Ruospo M, Wong G, et al. Mesalazine for people with diverticular disease: a systematic review of randomized controlled trials. Can J Gastroenterol Hepatol. 2018;2018:1–12. https://doi.org/10.1155/2018/5437135.
44. Hall J, Hardiman K, Lee S, Lightner A, Stocchi L, Paquette IM, Steele SR, Feingold DL, Prepared on behalf of the Clinical Practice Guidelines Committee of the American Society of Colon and Rectal Surgeons. The American Society of Colon and Rectal Surgeons clinical practice guidelines for the treatment of left-sided colonic diverticulitis. Dis Colon Rectum. 2020;63(6):728–47. https://doi.org/10.1097/DCR.0000000000001679.
45. Carabotti M, Annibale B. Treatment of diverticular disease: an update on latest evidence and clinical implications. Drugs Context. 2018;7:212526. https://doi.org/10.7573/dic.212526.
46. Gerson LB. Antidepressants for irritable bowel syndrome: reappraisal for the nondepressed. Gastroenterology. 2010;138(2):775–7. https://doi.org/10.1053/j.gastro.2009.12.015.
47. Ford AC, Quigley EMM, Lacy BE, et al. Effect of antidepressants and psychological therapies, including hypnotherapy, in irritable bowel syndrome: systematic review and meta-analysis. Am J Gastroenterol. 2014;109(9):1350–65. https://doi.org/10.1038/ajg.2014.148.

17 Elective Surgery for Recurrent Diverticulitis: When and Why?

Sook C. Hoang and Traci L. Hedrick

Introduction

Diverticular disease represents a significant public health burden, accounting for 312,000 admissions and 1.5 million inpatient bed days resulting in a total cost of $2.6 billion dollars annually [1]. Sixty percent of people in Western and industrialized nations have evidence of diverticulosis by the age of 60 [2]. The actual number of patients with diverticulosis who progress to diverticulitis is difficult to accurately discern but ranges between 4 and 15% throughout the literature [3]. Notably, the incidence of diverticulitis is increasing, with the largest gains in patients aged 18–44 [4]. Diverticulitis is associated with negative impacts on quality of life and lost wages, which can be debilitating for patients and their families [5].

Acute diverticulitis can result in complicated or uncomplicated disease. The majority of cases (>75%) are uncomplicated with recurrence rates ranging between 20% and 30% after successful nonoperative management [6]. Complicated diverticulitis, defined by abscess, fistula, or stricture formation, affects up to 25% of patients with symptomatic diverticulitis and is associated with recurrence rates ranging from 20% to 40% following initial nonoperative management [7–9]. Traditionally, surgery was recommended for all patients following a single episode of complicated diverticulitis and two episodes of uncomplicated diverticulitis. However, this paradigm resulted in overtreatment for many patients, and more recently there has been a philosophical shift toward more nonoperative management [10]. There is a growing national trend toward nonoperative management of acute diverticulitis, with a declining number of patients undergoing colectomy for diverticulitis. Despite this, there is no increase in the proportion of patients with free perforation as a complication of diverticulitis [11]. As such, the decision to proceed with surgery in the setting of recurrent diverticulitis has become highly nuanced, requiring careful consideration of patient preference and the risk of recurrent or progressive disease.

Risk Factors for Recurrent Diverticulitis

Knowledge of associated risk factors for recurrent diverticulitis is helpful in successfully managing patients and informing them about their individual risk. In a 2018 large population-based study conducted through the National Health Service, El-Sayed et al. [12] identified 65,162 patients presenting with a first episode of acute diverticulitis and followed them for a minimum of 4 years. These authors found that the rate of

S. C. Hoang (✉) · T. L. Hedrick
Department of Surgery, University of Virginia Health System, Charlottesville, VA, USA
e-mail: sh7je@uvahealth.org; th8q@hscmail.mcc.virginia.edu

M. Boutros et al. (eds.), *Diverticulitis*, https://doi.org/10.1007/978-3-032-21720-2_17

hospital admission for recurrent acute diverticulitis was 11.2%. Risk factors for recurrent attacks and the need for surgery included younger patient age, female sex, smoking, obesity, increased comorbidities, dyslipidemia, and complicated disease at first attack. Age was inversely related to recurrence with an increased risk of emergency surgery in younger patients. There are a multitude of other studies demonstrating an increased risk of recurrence in patients younger than 50, although the association with increased risk of emergency surgery has not been consistently demonstrated [6, 13, 14]. It is well documented that recurrence rates increase with each subsequent attack of diverticulitis. Broderick-Villa et al. [15] found that the risk of a second recurrence increases threefold following an initial recurrence in 3165 patients with acute diverticulitis within the Southern Kaiser Permanente system. A first recurrent episode was the only factor predictive of subsequent recurrences.

Other risk factors for recurrent diverticulitis include the severity of initial attack, family history of diverticulitis, smoking, length of involved colon >5 cm, and presence of retroperitoneal abscess [8, 16, 17]. Certain other patient factors may play a role in predicting a more virulent course of acute diverticulitis and thereby increase the patient's risk of recurrence.

Based mainly on small retrospective case series, it does seem that immunocompromised patients tend to present with more severe disease. Biondo et al. [18] performed one of the largest cohort studies to date where 931 consecutive patients admitted with a diagnosis of diverticulitis to a Spanish hospital were tracked prospectively over 14 years. The following patient groups were classified as immunocompromised: transplant recipients, those with chronic renal failure on dialysis, patients with active extracolonic malignancy, and patients on chronic immunosuppressant medication, making up a fairly heterogeneous population of 166 immunocompromised patients. There were no differences in the recurrence rates following a single episode of uncomplicated diverticulitis between immunocompromised and immunocompetent patients (13.6% vs. 22.1%, $p = 0.092$) and only 1.2% of immunocompromised patients initially managed nonoperatively required subsequent emergency surgery. However, the recurrence rate following a bout of complicated diverticulitis (abscess) was 46.2% in the immunocompromised patient versus 15.2% in the immunocompetent patient ($p < 0.001$). Klarenbeek et al. [19] also found that a history of chronic renal failure, collagen vascular disease or immunosuppressive medications significantly increased rates of recurrence and perforation in a group of patients with both complicated and uncomplicated diverticulitis managed nonoperatively. Additionally, glucocorticoid use, chronic obstructive pulmonary disease, and hypoalbuminemia may also predispose patients to recurrence and perforation [20, 21].

It has been theorized that 5-ASA agents may prevent recurrent diverticulitis in patients with uncomplicated disease. However, this has been studied in several prospective double-blind randomized controlled trials (DIVA trial, PREVENT-1 and PREVENT-2 trials) and a 2017 Cochrane Review, which have all failed to demonstrate efficacy in preventing recurrences within 1 to 2 years with mesalamine [22–24]. Similarly, although inadequate fiber intake has been implicated in the development of diverticular disease, the use of fiber has not consistently been shown to prevent of recurrent episodes of diverticulitis [25, 26].

'Ticking Time Bomb' Theory

It is a common misperception perpetuated among patients and many referring providers that recurrent uncomplicated diverticulitis will progress over time to perforation requiring emergent surgery and colostomy. Historical understanding of diverticular disease arose from studies conducted initially by T.G. Parks in the 1970s who reported recurrence rates of 25% following an initial attack of acute diverticulitis [27]. Additionally, mortality rates increased from 4.7% following the first episode to 7.8% in subsequent episodes, with high rates of stoma formation [27]. Based on these data, it became surgical dogma to recommend elective resection following two episodes of uncomplicated diverticulitis. It is important to note that these initial studies were performed prior to the use of CT scans. Therefore, the ability to accurately diagnose diverticular disease can be questioned. Additionally, many of the initial studies associating recurrent diverticulitis with higher mortality rates were limited by small cohort size and a retrospective study design [28].

It is now generally accepted that recurrent diverticulitis is not a progressive disease and in the majority of cases, patients will develop a recurrent attack similar in severity to their prior episodes [20]. Less than 5% of patients progress to complicated disease in the form of an abscess, free perforation or fistula in the 5 years following an episode of uncomplicated diverticulitis [8, 16, 29]. More importantly, the risk for free perforation is believed to be greatest at the first attack and decreases with each subsequent attack [30]. This was demonstrated by Ritz et al. [31] who found that the risk of free perforation was 25% in patients presenting with their first attack, 12% in their second attack, 6% with their third attack, and 1% thereafter. In fact, multiple studies have found that the majority of patients (~90%) who require emergency surgery for acute diverticulitis had no previous history of acute diverticulitis [32, 33], again suggesting that the initial severity of a patient's diverticulitis attack, rather than the number of episodes, predicts the severity of the disease course.

The fear of eventually needing a colostomy has been a historical motivator in advocating for elective resection in patients with recurrent uncomplicated diverticulitis. However, based on the low rates of disease progression, the likelihood of eventually needing a colostomy in the setting of recurrent disease is less than 5% [8, 16, 20, 29, 34]. Given that the risk of colostomy secondary to anastomotic leak following an elective sigmoid resection is somewhat similar, it is unfounded to use the fear of a colostomy as a justification for prophylactic resection in the setting of recurrent uncomplicated diverticulitis. This was demonstrated by Salem et al. [35] who found that there was no increased risk for colostomy or mortality if surgery was performed after the first attack versus the fourth attack of acute diverticulitis.

Based on these data, patients can be reassured that recurrent diverticulitis does not represent a "ticking time bomb." The index episode usually predicts the severity of a patient's disease course and the risk of requiring an emergent operation in the setting of recurrent disease managed conservatively is low.

Recurrent Versus Persistent Diverticulitis

The distinction between recurrent and persistent (i.e., smoldering) disease in the setting of diverticulitis is not well defined [36, 37]. Varying time points ranging from 30-, 60-, and 90-day cut-offs are used throughout the literature in an attempt to separate recurrent and persistent diverticulitis into two clinical entities [38]. However, some studies neglect to include any type of time frame at all in the definition of recurrent diverticulitis. This lack of distinction makes it difficult to identify risk factors and treatment strategies specific for each disease type and is an area where further research efforts are required for clarification. For the purposes of this chapter, we will discuss both scenarios when considering the role of elective surgery in the setting of diverticulitis.

Elective Surgery for Uncomplicated Diverticulitis

A history of two episodes of diverticulitis is no longer considered an indication for surgery in the setting of uncomplicated diverticulitis. Rather than an absolute number of recurrent episodes, the decision to proceed with surgery should be individualized, taking into account the impact of each recurrence on the patient's quality of life [10]. Surgery is generally indicated when recurrence, or the fear of recurrence, interferes with the patients' personal and professional well-being. This will also depend on the patient's operative risk in weighing the risks and benefits of elective surgery.

It is increasingly recognized that patients with a history of diverticulitis may experience chronic gastrointestinal symptoms even in the absence of inflammation [39]. In addition to the chronic gastrointestinal manifestations, diverticulitis has also been associated with an increased incidence of anxiety and depression among patients. Patients with diverticulitis experience higher emotional distress and impaired social functioning compared to patients without the disease [40]. As such, quality of life is one of the most important considerations in determining when to recommend elective resection for recurrent diverticulitis. The DIRECT trial was a randomized controlled trial (RCT) focused specifically on patient-reported outcomes with a health-related quality of life primary endpoint (Gastrointestinal Quality of Life Index (GIQLI)) [41]. One-hundred and nine patients with either persistent abdominal complaints after a single attack of diverticulitis or recurrent diverticulitis (defined as three or more attacks in 2 years) were randomized to conservative management or elective laparoscopic sigmoidectomy. Surgery was associated with improved short-term (6-month) and long-term (5-year) quality of life compared to non-surgical management [41]. In addition to improved Gastrointestinal Quality of Life Index (GIQLI) scores, patients in the surgery group also reported higher generic quality of life scores, as measured by the Short Form-36 (SF-36), and lower pain scores at 5 years compared with conservative management. Importantly, 46% of patients in the conservative group ultimately required surgery over the study period due to ongoing symptoms. The Sigma-trial also reported greater quality of life scores at short-term follow-up (6 weeks) in patients undergoing laparoscopic surgery, but not open surgery, for the treatment of diverticular disease [42]. Follow-up of the LASER trial showed that elective sigmoid resection was effective in preventing recurrent diverticulitis and improved quality of life over conservative treatment within 2 years [43]. Several other cohort studies have similarly demonstrated improvements in quality-of-life outcomes with high patient satisfaction following laparoscopic sigmoidectomy for diverticular disease [44, 45].

Alternatively, a few small cohort studies have found that up to 25% of patients may experience ongoing abdominal discomfort even after surgical resection for diverticulitis [46–48]. The presence of preoperative irritable bowel syndrome (IBS) was associated with persistent abdominal discomfort and lower patient satisfaction following laparoscopic sigmoid colectomy for diverticular disease [46]. This highlights the importance of careful patient selection in the surgical management of recurrent diverticulitis as ongoing abdominal symptoms may be secondary to a functional bowel disorder such as IBS, which may not be alleviated with surgical resection. On the other hand, many patients who have been previously diagnosed with IBS may actually have been suffering from symptoms of chronic diverticular disease and will experience significant improvement in these "IBS-type symptoms" following surgery. These data emphasize the importance of communication in setting expectations before surgery. It is imperative that patients be properly informed so that they can actively participate in the decision to proceed with surgery after weighing the risks and benefits of surgery.

Although not necessarily unique to diverticular disease, patients may also experience changes in bowel function following sigmoid colectomy (i.e., "sigmoidectomy syndrome") [49]. Levack et al. [49] surveyed 325 patients after laparoscopic or open sigmoidectomy for diverticulitis assessing specifically patients' functional outcomes. Of the patients surveyed, 25% of patients reported fecal incontinence, 19.6% reported fecal urgency and 20.8% of patients reported incomplete emptying following surgery. Female patients were most susceptible to fecal incontinence (OR 2.3, $p = 0.008$), fecal urgency (OR 1.3, $p < 0.05$), and incomplete emptying (OR 1.4, $p < 0.05$) [49]. Although this study was limited by the lack of preoperative baseline functional data, the incidence of bowel dysfunction after elective sigmoid resection warrants attention and discussion with patients prior to surgery. Urinary and sexual dysfunction are also known risks of sigmoid resection with incidence rates less than 10%. However, Forgione et al.

Table 17.1 Societal guidelines indications for elective surgery in the setting uncomplicated and complicated diverticulitis

Society	Recommendations for elective resection
American Society of Colon and Rectal Surgeons (ASCRS) [10, 75]	The decision to recommend elective sigmoid colectomy after recovery from uncomplicated acute diverticulitis should be individualized. Elective colectomy should typically be considered after the patient recovers from an episode of complicated diverticulitis. (Grade of recommendation: Strong recommendation based on moderate-quality evidence, 1B)
American Gastroenterology Association (AGA) [73]	Suggest against elective colonic resection in patients with an initial episode of acute uncomplicated diverticulitis. The decision to perform elective prophylactic colonic resection in this setting should be individualized. (Conditional recommendation, very-low quality of evidence)
European Association for Endoscopic Surgery (EAES) and Society of American Gastrointestinal and Endoscopic Surgeons (SAGES) consensus statement [38]	Following a single episode of successfully treated Hinchey I/II acute diverticulitis, surgery should not be routinely offered solely to avoid further episodes (LoE: Low. Strength of recommendation: Weak). Recommend elective resection in patients with symptomatic diverticular disease that is negatively impacting quality of life. (LoE: Moderate. Strength of recommendation: Strong)
Association of Coloproctology of Great Britain and Ireland (ACPGBI) [74]	The decision on elective resection should be made on an individual basis after the assessment of the particular circumstances of the patient. (Grade C: Evidence of type IIa, IIb or III but inconsistent findings)

[45] did not identify any alterations to sexual and urinary function postoperatively in the setting of diverticular disease.

Indications for surgery in the setting of recurrent uncomplicated diverticulitis continue to evolve as the importance of patient-reported outcomes becomes increasingly recognized. In keeping with most societal guidelines (Table 17.1), the recommendation requires an individualized approach taking the impact of recurrences, the presence of ongoing symptoms, and the patient's operative risk into account [50–52].

Elective Surgery for Complicated Diverticulitis

Complicated diverticulitis is a broad term that describes a heterogenous group of patients with associated abscess, fistula, obstruction, stricture, and free perforation. The decision to operate on patients with fistula, stricture, obstruction, and free perforation is straightforward, as these patients clearly need operative management to achieve symptomatic relief or sepsis control. Traditionally, elective surgery has been recommended following nonoperative management of complicated diverticulitis with abscess to prevent progression or recurrence. However, given that the vast majority of patients can safely be managed with a combination of percutaneous drainage and antibiotics, more surgeons are opting for a watch-and-wait approach [53, 54].

Recurrence rates vary widely throughout the literature in the setting of diverticulitis with abscess. In a population-based study of 14,124 patients, Li et al. [16] demonstrated an 11% risk of recurrence in the subsequent 4 years following successful resolution of a complicated acute diverticulitis episode. Dharmarajan et al. [55] retrospectively identified 136 patients with complicated diverticulitis (perforation or abscess) managed at their institution. Ninety-five percent of patients were successfully treated nonoperatively with only 5% of patients requiring surgery for failed nonoperative management. Broderick-Villa et al. [15] did not find patients who underwent percutaneous abscess drainage to have an increased risk for recurrent disease. Other studies have described similar findings of patients managed successfully without surgical resection after an episode of complicated disease [56].

Despite these encouraging findings, other studies have reported higher rates of recurrence following nonoperative management in complicated disease. In particular, several retrospective cohort studies have demonstrated recurrence rates up to 40% in the setting of pelvic abscesses [57, 58]. In a systemic review and meta-analysis of 22 studies representing 1051 patients, Lamb and Kaiser [9] sought to determine the role of elective resection after successful nonoperative management of complicated diverticulitis with abscess. The authors found that 70% of patients were successfully managed nonoperatively during their index presentation. However, the recurrence rate following successful nonoperative management varied widely between 3 and 68%, with an overall recurrence rate of 28%. Interestingly, the recurrence rate was much higher in patients awaiting elective resection (39%) versus those in which no surgery was planned (18%), suggesting that surgeons used accurate clinical judgment in deciding who would benefit from elective resection. Of the 1051 patients included in the study, 65% ultimately underwent resection and only 28% of patients did not require an operation nor had a recurrence at follow-up. Importantly, recurrences were generally mild and less than 1% of patients progressed to perforation requiring emergent surgery.

Similar to uncomplicated disease, it is unlikely that patients successfully treated nonoperatively for diverticular abscess will progress over time to a more virulent presentation. Therefore, it is reasonable to consider a watch-and-wait approach in patients whose symptoms completely resolve following an episode of complicated diverticulitis with abscess. Society of American Gastrointestinal and Endoscopic Surgeons (SAGES)/European Association for Endoscopic Surgery (EAES) recommends a wait-and-watch approach following a single episode of successfully treated Hinchey I/II diverticulitis unless the patient has ongoing symptoms [38]. The American Society of Colon and Rectal Surgeons (ASCRS) clinical practice guidelines from 2014 recommend elective colectomy for patients who recover from an episode of complicated diverticulitis with abscess ≥5 cm or pelvic abscesses (Hinchey II) as there is a risk of disease recurrence up to 40% [10, 50]. Notably, the updated ASCRS clinical practice guidelines from 2020 now recommends a consideration for elective colectomy after nonoperative management of diverticulitis with abscess which is a change from the 2014 guidelines further supporting an individualized approach to the surgical management of acute diverticulitis with abscess [75].

Timing of Operative Intervention

The optimal timing of operative intervention in the setting of recurrent diverticulitis is dictated by the degree of inflammation and the persistence of symptoms. Theoretically, operative morbidity is reduced by delaying surgery to allow for resolution of the acute inflammation [59, 60]. A meta-analysis of small cohort studies comparing differences in morbidity between early (< 6 weeks) versus late (> 6 weeks) elective resection for diverticular disease found no difference in morbidity or mortality [61]. However, earlier surgery was associated with longer length of stay, longer operative time, and greater conversion to open surgery compared to the later surgery [61]. Other studies have similarly found a greater conversion rate to laparotomy when elective surgery is performed during the same admission [62]. Based on these data, SAGES/EAES recommended that consideration be given to delaying elective sigmoid resection for a minimum of 6 weeks from the most recent episode of acute diverticulitis [38]. This also allows for recovery of the patient's nutritional and functional status, and for medical conditions to be optimized. Conversely, this must be weighed against the risk of recurrence in the intervening time period and the trajectory of the patients' clinical course. The presence of smoldering disease with severe ongoing abdominal pain and weight loss will certainly dictate early intervention in a subset of patients [63].

Technical Considerations

When feasible, minimally invasive laparoscopic or robotic surgery is the preferred surgical approach for elective sigmoid resection [10, 38]. Multiple studies have demonstrated the benefit of laparoscopic resection compared to open resection for diverticular disease [42, 64]. In the Sigma trial, a randomized controlled trial comparing laparoscopic versus open elective sigmoidectomy for diverticular disease, patients in the laparoscopy group experienced a reduction in major complication rate, shorter length of hospital stay, and reduced pain scores compared to the open surgery group. Patients in the laparoscopy group also demonstrated better quality of life at 6 weeks postoperatively [42]. At long-term follow-up (6 months), there were no differences in late complications (incisional hernias, adhesive bowel obstruction, recurrence of diverticular disease) in the laparoscopic compared to the open surgery group. Other randomized controlled trials have demonstrated similar findings with less postoperative morbidity, pain, and length of hospital stay when comparing laparoscopy to open surgery [65, 66]. Other outcomes, including anastomotic leak, recurrence of diverticular disease, anastomotic stricture, and postoperative bowel obstruction, have been shown to be similar in open and laparoscopic surgery for diverticular disease [64]. Overall, the risk of anastomotic leak ranges from 1% to 6% and the risk of hernia ranges from 7–11%. Furthermore, there is a protective stoma rate of 1–4% [42, 67]. Therefore, when assessing a patient with recurrent diverticulitis for surgical candidacy, the risk of complications against the potential benefits should be closely weighed.

Select Populations

Young Patients

Management of acute diverticulitis in the young has been a fiercely debated topic, particularly given that this is the fastest growing demographic with diverticulitis [38, 68]. Traditionally, elective resection was recommended following a single episode of uncomplicated diverticulitis based on the premise that young age was associated with worse clinical outcomes [35, 69]. It has been consistently documented that young patients (<50 years of age) have a greater risk for recurrent disease [15, 38]. However, the association of young age with increased risk for morbidity and complicated disease requiring emergency surgery has been inconsistently demonstrated [18, 57, 70]. Many of the studies demonstrating a more virulent course in the young were plagued by misdiagnosis prior to the routine use of CT scan, as well as significant selection bias. While the rates of colectomy are demonstrably higher in young patients, it remains unclear if this association is due to more virulent disease or patient and surgeon preference [71]. As such, routine resection following a single episode of diverticulitis is no longer recommended. Rather, recommendations for surgery are based on the functional impact of recurrence with a focus on quality of life, regardless of age [10].

Immunosuppression

As previously mentioned, immunosuppressed patients are at increased risk of recurrence and typically present with more advanced diverticular disease than immunocompetent individuals. Additionally, clinical outcomes following emergency surgery for diverticulitis in immunocompromised patients are dismal, with mortality and morbidity rates up to 30% and 50%, respectively [18, 72–74]. Because postoperative outcomes are far better in the elective setting, ASCRS clinical practice guidelines recommended a lower threshold for elective resection in immunosuppressed patients following an attack of acute diverticulitis [3]. The 2020 ASCRS guideline states that the decision to offer sigmoid colectomy after recovery from uncomplicated acute diverticulitis in immunosuppressed patients should be individualized. Grade of Recommendation: Strong recommendation based on low-quality evidence, 1C [50]. The American Gastroenterological Association (AGA) clinical practice update in 2021 stated that after recovery from an episode of diverticulitis successfully managed without surgery, a patient who is chronically immunosuppressed should consult with a colorectal surgeon to discuss elective resection [51]. When elective resection is undertaken, expert consensus also recommends consideration of a protective stoma, particularly in transplant patients or patients on high doses of immunosuppressive medications [38]. A more detailed review of diverticulitis in the immunosuppressed patient can be found in Chap. 23.

Recurrence After Elective Surgery

The recurrence rate following resection for diverticulitis ranges between 5% and 8%, with a median time to recurrence of 29 months [67]. Risk factors associated with recurrence after surgery include younger age and persistence of postoperative abdominal pain. Persistence of abdominal pain after surgery was present in 22% of patients with recurrent diverticulitis following elective resection, suggesting an inadequate resection at the index operation [47]. Thaler et al. [67] compared patients who underwent laparoscopic sigmoid resection compared to patients who had an open resection and found no difference in recurrence rates. Additionally, they evaluated the association between recurrence following surgery and other technical aspects, including splenic flexure mobilization, specimen length, presence of inflammation at the proximal resection margin, and presence of tinea coli at the distal resection margin. The only variable associated with recurrence following surgery was the presence of tinea coli at the distal resection margin indicating residual sigmoid colon, demonstrating the importance of resecting down to the rectosigmoid junction [67]. The rectosigmoid junction can occasionally be difficult to recognize, particularly in the setting of significant inflammation or visceral obesity. The inability to advance the EEA stapler all the way up to the transected staple line is often a clear indication of residual sigmoid colon. This is due to the reduced caliber of the sigmoid colon lumen as compared to the rectal lumen, which should easily accommodate a 29 mm stapler. One should avoid the temptation to downsize to a smaller stapler or bring the anvil through the anterior rectal wall leaving a blind end of defunctionalized colon, which is at risk for ongoing inflammation. Instead, further dissection with transection of the residual sigmoid colon should be undertaken.

Conclusion

As the population ages and the incidence of diverticular disease continues to increase, it is imperative that surgeons have an in-depth knowledge of the relevant literature. Indications for surgery in the setting of recurrent diverticulitis have evolved over time to a more patient-centered approach. In general, elective resection is warranted when the impact of recurrences and/or the presence of ongoing symptoms interferes with quality of life, taking the patient's operative risk into account. This approach requires careful patient selection and expectation management in the preoperative setting to assure a successful long-term outcome.

References

1. Sandler RS, Everhart JE, Donowitz M, Adams E, Cronin K, Goodman C, et al. The burden of selected digestive diseases in the United States. Gastroenterology. 2002;122(5):1500–11.
2. Peery AF, Barrett PR, Park D, Rogers AJ, Galanko JA, Martin CF, et al. A high-fiber diet does not protect against asymptomatic diverticulosis. Gastroenterology. 2012;142(2):266–72.e1.
3. Shahedi K, Fuller G, Bolus R, Cohen E, Vu M, Shah R, et al. Long-term risk of acute diverticulitis among patients with incidental diverticulosis found during colonoscopy. Clin Gastroenterol Hepatol. 2013;11(12):1609–13.
4. Etzioni DA, Mack TM, Beart RW Jr, Kaiser AM. Diverticulitis in the United States: 1998–2005: changing patterns of disease and treatment. Ann Surg. 2009;249(2):210–7.
5. Iyer R, Longstreth GF, Chu LH, Chen W, Yen L, Hodgkins P, et al. Acute colonic diverticulitis: diagnostic evidence, demographic and clinical features in three practice settings. J Gastrointestin Liver Dis. 2014;23(4):379–86.

6. Regenbogen SE, Hardiman KM, Hendren S, Morris AM. Surgery for diverticulitis in the 21st century: a systematic review. JAMA Surg. 2014;149(3):292–303.
7. Schaffzin DM, Wong WD. Nonoperative management of complicated diverticular disease. Clin Colon Rectal Surg. 2004;17(3):169–76.
8. Hall JF, Roberts PL, Ricciardi R, Read T, Scheirey C, Wald C, et al. Long-term follow-up after an initial episode of diverticulitis: what are the predictors of recurrence? Dis Colon Rectum. 2011;54(3):283–8.
9. Lamb MN, Kaiser AM. Elective resection versus observation after nonoperative management of complicated diverticulitis with abscess: a systematic review and meta-analysis. Dis Colon Rectum. 2014;57(12):1430–40.
10. Feingold D, Steele SR, Lee S, Kaiser A, Boushey R, Buie WD, et al. Practice parameters for the treatment of sigmoid diverticulitis. Dis Colon Rectum. 2014;57(3):284–94.
11. Ricciardi R, Baxter NN, Read TE, Marcello PW, Hall J, Roberts PL. Is the decline in the surgical treatment for diverticulitis associated with an increase in complicated diverticulitis? Dis Colon Rectum. 2009;52(9):1558–63.
12. El-Sayed C, Radley S, Mytton J, Evison F, Ward ST. Risk of recurrent disease and surgery following an admission for acute diverticulitis. Dis Colon Rectum. 2018;61(3):382–9.
13. Guzzo J, Hyman N. Diverticulitis in young patients: is resection after a single attack always warranted? Dis Colon Rectum. 2004;47(7):1187–90. discussion 90-1
14. Hjern F, Josephson T, Altman D, Holmstrom B, Johansson C. Outcome of younger patients with acute diverticulitis. Br J Surg. 2008;95(6):758–64.
15. Broderick-Villa G, Burchette RJ, Collins JC, Abbas MA, Haigh PI. Hospitalization for acute diverticulitis does not mandate routine elective colectomy. Arch Surg. 2005;140(6):576–81. discussion 81-3
16. Li D, de Mestral C, Baxter NN, McLeod RS, Moineddin R, Wilton AS, et al. Risk of readmission and emergency surgery following nonoperative management of colonic diverticulitis: a population-based analysis. Ann Surg. 2014;260(3):423–30. discussion 30-1
17. Humes DJ, Ludvigsson JF, Jarvholm B. Smoking and the risk of hospitalization for symptomatic diverticular disease: a population-based cohort study from Sweden. Dis Colon Rectum. 2016;59(2):110–4.
18. Biondo S, Pares D, Marti Rague J, Kreisler E, Fraccalvieri D, Jaurrieta E. Acute colonic diverticulitis in patients under 50 years of age. Br J Surg. 2002;89(9):1137–41.
19. Klarenbeek BR, Samuels M, van der Wal MA, van der Peet DL, Meijerink WJ, Cuesta MA. Indications for elective sigmoid resection in diverticular disease. Ann Surg. 2010;251(4):670–4.
20. Chapman JR, Dozois EJ, Wolff BG, Gullerud RE, Larson DR. Diverticulitis: a progressive disease? Do multiple recurrences predict less favorable outcomes? Ann Surg. 2006;243(6):876–30. discussion 80-3
21. Yoo PS, Garg R, Salamone LF, Floch MH, Rosenthal R, Longo WE. Medical comorbidities predict the need for colectomy for complicated and recurrent diverticulitis. Am J Surg. 2008;196(5):710–4.
22. Stollman N, Magowan S, Shanahan F, Quigley EM. A randomized controlled study of mesalamine after acute diverticulitis: results of the DIVA trial. J Clin Gastroenterol. 2013;47(7):621–9.
23. Raskin JB, Kamm MA, Jamal MM, Marquez J, Melzer E, Schoen RE, et al. Mesalamine did not prevent recurrent diverticulitis in phase 3 controlled trials. Gastroenterology. 2014;147(4):793–802.
24. Carter F, Alsayb M, Marshall JK, Yuan Y. Mesalamine (5-ASA) for the prevention of recurrent diverticulitis. Cochrane Database Syst Rev. 2017;10:Cd009839.
25. Maconi G, Barbara G, Bosetti C, Cuomo R, Annibale B. Treatment of diverticular disease of the colon and prevention of acute diverticulitis: a systematic review. Dis Colon Rectum. 2011;54(10):1326–38.
26. Unlu C, Daniels L, Vrouenraets BC, Boermeester MA. A systematic review of high-fibre dietary therapy in diverticular disease. Int J Color Dis. 2012;27(4):419–27.
27. Parks TG. Natural history of diverticular disease of the colon. A review of 521 cases. Br Med J. 1969;4(5684):639–42.
28. Hackford AW, Schoetz DJ Jr, Coller JA, Veidenheimer MC. Surgical management of complicated diverticulitis. The Lahey clinic experience, 1967 to 1982. Dis Colon Rectum. 1985;28(5):317–21.
29. Shaikh S, Krukowski ZH. Outcome of a conservative policy for managing acute sigmoid diverticulitis. Br J Surg. 2007;94(7):876–9.
30. Pittet O, Kotzampassakis N, Schmidt S, Denys A, Demartines N, Calmes JM. Recurrent left colonic diverticulitis episodes: more severe than the initial diverticulitis? World J Surg. 2009;33(3):547–52.
31. Ritz JP, Lehmann KS, Frericks B, Stroux A, Buhr HJ, Holmer C. Outcome of patients with acute sigmoid diverticulitis: multivariate analysis of risk factors for free perforation. Surgery. 2011;149(5):606–13.
32. Lorimer JW. Is prophylactic resection valid as an indication for elective surgery in diverticular disease? Can J Surg. 1997;40(6):445–8.
33. Nylamo E. Diverticulitis of the colon: role of surgery in preventing complications. Ann Chir Gynaecol. 1990;79(3):139–42.
34. Chautems RC, Ambrosetti P, Ludwig A, Mermillod B, Morel P, Soravia C. Long-term follow-up after first acute episode of sigmoid diverticulitis: is surgery mandatory?: a prospective study of 118 patients. Dis Colon Rectum. 2002;45(7):962–6.
35. Salem L, Veenstra DL, Sullivan SD, Flum DR. The timing of elective colectomy in diverticulitis: a decision analysis. J Am Coll Surg. 2004;199(6):904–12.
36. Gervaz P, Ambrosetti P. Time for a (re) definition of (recurrent) sigmoid diverticulitis? Ann Surg. 2011;254(6):1076–7.
37. Garfinkle R, Kugler A, Pelsser V, Vasilevsky CA, Morin N, Gordon P, et al. Diverticular abscess

managed with long-term definitive nonoperative intent is safe. Dis Colon Rectum. 2016;59(7):648–55.
38. Francis NK, Sylla P, Abou-Khalil M, Arolfo S, Berler D, Curtis NJ, et al. EAES and SAGES 2018 consensus conference on acute diverticulitis management: evidence-based recommendations for clinical practice. Surg Endosc. 2019;33(9):2726–41.
39. Jung HK, Choung RS, Locke GR 3rd, Schleck CD, Zinsmeister AR, Talley NJ. Diarrhea-predominant irritable bowel syndrome is associated with diverticular disease: a population-based study. Am J Gastroenterol. 2010;105(3):652–61.
40. Bolster LT, Papagrigoriadis S. Diverticular disease has an impact on quality of life—results of a preliminary study. Color Dis. 2003;5(4):320–3.
41. van de Wall BJM, Stam MAW, Draaisma WA, Stellato R, Bemelman WA, Boermeester MA, et al. Surgery versus conservative management for recurrent and ongoing left-sided diverticulitis (DIRECT trial): an open-label, multicentre, randomised controlled trial. Lancet Gastroenterol Hepatol. 2017;2(1):13–22.
42. Klarenbeek BR, Bergamaschi R, Veenhof AA, van der Peet DL, van den Broek WT, de Lange ES, et al. Laparoscopic versus open sigmoid resection for diverticular disease: follow-up assessment of the randomized control sigma trial. Surg Endosc. 2011;25(4):1121–6.
43. Ibrahim AM, Lillemoe KD, Klingensmith ME, Dimick JB. Visual abstracts to disseminate research on social media: a prospective, Case-control Crossover Study. Ann Surg. 2017 Dec;266(6):e46–8. https://doi.org/10.1097/SLA.0000000000002277.
44. Pasternak I, Wiedemann N, Basilicata G, Melcher GA. Gastrointestinal quality of life after laparoscopic-assisted sigmoidectomy for diverticular disease. Int J Color Dis. 2012;27(6):781–7.
45. Forgione A, Leroy J, Cahill RA, Bailey C, Simone M, Mutter D, et al. Prospective evaluation of functional outcome after laparoscopic sigmoid colectomy. Ann Surg. 2009;249(2):218–24.
46. Ambrosetti P, Francis K, Weintraub D, Weintraub J. Functional results following elective laparoscopic sigmoidectomy after CT-proven diagnosis of acute diverticulitis evaluation of 43 patients and review of the literature. J Gastrointest Surg. 2007;11(6):767–72.
47. Andeweg C, Peters J, Bleichrodt R, van Goor H. Incidence and risk factors of recurrence after surgery for pathology-proven diverticular disease. World J Surg. 2008;32(7):1501–6.
48. Egger B, Peter MK, Candinas D. Persistent symptoms after elective sigmoid resection for diverticulitis. Dis Colon Rectum. 2008;51(7):1044–8.
49. Levack MM, Savitt LR, Berger DL, Shellito PC, Hodin RA, Rattner DW, et al. Sigmoidectomy syndrome? Patients' perspectives on the functional outcomes following surgery for diverticulitis. Dis Colon Rectum. 2012;55(1):10–7.
50. Hall J, Hardiman K, Lee S, et al. Prepared on behalf of the clinical practice guidelines Committee of the American Society of colon and Rectal surgeons. The American Society of Colon and Rectal Surgeons clinical practice guidelines for the treatment of left-sided colonic diverticulitis. Dis Colon Rectum. 2020;63(6):728–47. https://doi.org/10.1097/DCR.0000000000001679.
51. Sartelli M, Weber DG, Kluger Y, et al. 2020 update of the WSES guidelines for the management of acute colonic diverticulitis in the emergency setting. World J Emerg Surg. 2020;15(1):32. https://doi.org/10.1186/s13017-020-00313-4. PMID: 32381121; PMCID: PMC7206757
52. Peery AF, Shaukat A, Strate LL. AGA clinical practice update on medical management of colonic diverticulitis: expert review. Gastroenterology. 2021;160(3):906–911.e1. https://doi.org/10.1053/j.gastro.2020.09.059. Epub 2020 Dec 3. PMID: 33279517; PMCID: PMC7878331
53. Kumar RR, Kim JT, Haukoos JS, Macias LH, Dixon MR, Stamos MJ, et al. Factors affecting the successful management of intra-abdominal abscesses with antibiotics and the need for percutaneous drainage. Dis Colon Rectum. 2006;49(2):183–9.
54. Brandt D, Gervaz P, Durmishi Y, Platon A, Morel P, Poletti PA. Percutaneous CT scan-guided drainage vs. antibiotherapy alone for Hinchey II diverticulitis: a case-control study. Dis Colon Rectum. 2006;49(10):1533–8.
55. Dharmarajan S, Hunt SR, Birnbaum EH, Fleshman JW, Mutch MG. The efficacy of nonoperative management of acute complicated diverticulitis. Dis Colon Rectum. 2011;54(6):663–71.
56. Gaertner WB, Willis DJ, Madoff RD, Rothenberger DA, Kwaan MR, Belzer GE, et al. Percutaneous drainage of colonic diverticular abscess: is colon resection necessary? Dis Colon Rectum. 2013;56(5):622–6.
57. Kaiser AM, Jiang JK, Lake JP, Ault G, Artinyan A, Gonzalez-Ruiz C, et al. The management of complicated diverticulitis and the role of computed tomography. Am J Gastroenterol. 2005;100(4):910–7.
58. Ambrosetti P. Value of CT for acute left-colonic diverticulitis: the surgeon's view. Dig Dis. 2012;30(1):51–5.
59. Siewert JR, Huber FT, Brune IB. Early elective surgery of acute diverticulitis of the colon. Chirurg. 1995;66(12):1182–9.
60. Reissfelder C, Buhr HJ, Ritz JP. What is the optimal time of surgical intervention after an acute attack of sigmoid diverticulitis: early or late elective laparoscopic resection? Dis Colon Rectum. 2006;49(12):1842–8.
61. Khan RMA, Hajibandeh S. Early elective versus delayed elective surgery in acute recurrent diverticulitis: a systematic review and meta-analysis. Int J Surg. 2017;46:92–101.
62. Hoffmann H, Dell-Kuster S, Genstorfer J, Kettelhack C, Langer I, Rosenthal R, et al. Surgical treatment of acute recurrent diverticulitis: early elective or late elective surgery. An analysis of 237 patients. World J Surg. 2012;36(4):898–907.
63. Vaghiri S, Prassas D, Knoefel WT, Krieg A. The optimal timing of elective surgery in sigmoid diverticular

disease: a meta-analysis. Langenbeck's Arch Surg. 2022;407(8):3259–74. https://doi.org/10.1007/s00423-022-02698-z. Epub 2022 Oct 10. PMID: 36214867; PMCID: PMC9722804
64. Siddiqui MR, Sajid MS, Qureshi S, Cheek E, Baig MK. Elective laparoscopic sigmoid resection for diverticular disease has fewer complications than conventional surgery: a meta-analysis. Am J Surg. 2010;200(1):144–61.
65. Gervaz P, Inan I, Perneger T, Schiffer E, Morel P. A prospective, randomized, single-blind comparison of laparoscopic versus open sigmoid colectomy for diverticulitis. Ann Surg. 2010;252(1):3–8.
66. Rink AD, John-Enzenauer K, Haaf F, Straub E, Nagelschmidt M, Vestweber KH. Laparoscopic-assisted or laparoscopic-facilitated sigmoidectomy for diverticular disease? A prospective randomized trial on postoperative pain and analgesic consumption. Dis Colon Rectum. 2009;52(10):1738–45.
67. Thaler K, Weiss EG, Nogueras JJ, Arnaud JP, Wexner SD, Bergamaschi R. Recurrence rates at minimum 5-year follow-up: laparoscopic versus open sigmoid resection for uncomplicated diverticulitis. Surg Laparosc Endosc Percutan Tech. 2003;13(5):325–7.
68. Etzioni DA, Cannom RR, Ault GT, Beart RW Jr, Kaiser AM. Diverticulitis in California from 1995 to 2006: increased rates of treatment for younger patients. Am Surg. 2009;75(10):981–5.
69. Konvolinka CW. Acute diverticulitis under age forty. Am J Surg. 1994;167(6):562–5.
70. Faria GR, Almeida AB, Moreira H, Pinto-de-Sousa J, Correia-da-Silva P, Pimenta AP. Acute diverticulitis in younger patients: any rationale for a different approach? World J Gastroenterol. 2011;17(2):207–12.
71. Razik R, Chong CA, Nguyen GC. Younger age and prognosis in diverticulitis: a nationwide retrospective cohort study. Can J Gastroenterol. 2013;27(2):95–8.
72. Reshef A, Gurland B, Zutshi M, Kiran RP, Hull T. Colectomy with ileorectal anastomosis has a worse 30-day outcome when performed for colonic inertia than for a neoplastic indication. Color Dis. 2013;15(4):481–6.
73. Stollman N, Smalley W, Hirano I. American Gastroenterological Association Institute guideline on the management of acute diverticulitis. Gastroenterology. 2015;149(7):1944–9.
74. Fozard JB, Armitage NC, Schofield JB, Jones OM. ACPGBI position statement on elective resection for diverticulitis. Color Dis. 2011;13(Suppl 3):1–11.
75. Hall J, Hardiman K, Lee S, Lightner A, Stocchi L, Paquette IM, Steele SR, Feingold DL; Prepared on behalf of the Clinical Practice Guidelines Committee of the American Society of Colon and Rectal Surgeons. The American Society of Colon and Rectal Surgeons Clinical Practice Guidelines for the Treatment of Left-Sided Colonic Diverticulitis. Dis Colon Rectum. 2020 Jun;63(6):728–747. https://doi.org/10.1097/DCR.0000000000001679. PMID: 32384404.

18 Elective Surgery for Complicated Diverticulitis

Steven D. Wexner, Paul A. Kolarsick, and Paul Strombom

Introduction

The prevalence of diverticular disease has increased in industrialized countries during the past century. Approximately one in five patients with diverticulosis will develop diverticulitis, a disease process that accounts for approximately 300,000 annual hospitalizations in the United States [1]. Complicated or complex diverticulitis, classically defined as diverticulitis associated with free perforation, abscess, fistula, stricture, or obstruction, accounts for 15–20% of patients with diverticulitis [2, 3].

In the acute setting, surgical management is indicated for those patients with purulent or feculent generalized peritonitis, hemodynamic instability as well as those who fail to improve with medical management including bowel rest and antibiotics with or without percutaneous drainage (PD). In addition, those patients with larger abscesses that are not amenable to percutaneous drainage may be considered for early intervention in the acute setting since antibiotics alone are often insufficient.

Elective resection was previously recommended after two episodes of acute, uncomplicated diverticulitis; young, male patients were thought to benefit from resection after a single episode. The rationale for these recommendations was based largely on the work of Parks who reported that 70% of patients will respond to medical therapy with the first episode of acute diverticulitis, while only 6% will respond during a third episode. Furthermore, mortality was reported to increase with subsequent attacks from 4.7% on the first admission to 7.8% each subsequent admission [4].

More recent data have not supported this practice as the risk of recurrence requiring urgent Hartmann's procedure after an initial bout of diverticulitis has been found to be low, on the order of one in 2000 patient-years of follow-up, making the chance of emergency surgery with colostomy within range of the risk profile associated with elective resection itself [5].

In the case of complicated diverticulitis, it is still generally recommended by society guidelines that management involve elective surgical resection, although there is no complete accord [6, 7]. The natural history and management of the various manifestations of complicated diverticulitis are distinct and deserve individual consider-

S. D. Wexner (✉)
Ellen Leifer Shulman and Steven Shulman Digestive Disease Center, Cleveland Clinic Florida, Weston, FL, USA
e-mail: wexners@ccf.org; Steven.d.wexner@medstar.net; steven.d.wexner@medstar.edu

P. A. Kolarsick
Monmouth Medical Center, Department of Surgery, Long Branch, NJ, USA

P. Strombom
Northwell Health Physician Partners Surgical Specialties at Phelps, Sleepy Hollow, NY, USA

M. Boutros et al. (eds.), *Diverticulitis*, https://doi.org/10.1007/978-3-032-21720-2_18

ation. Technical considerations for elective surgical management of complicated diverticulitis will also be discussed.

Abscess

Acute diverticulitis complicated by abscess formation has been reported to affect between 10% and 25% of patients with acute diverticulitis (Fig. 18.1) [8–13]. Historically treated as a surgical emergency, the development of axial imaging with computed tomography (CT) and advances in interventional radiology techniques, as well as improvements in antimicrobial therapy, parenteral nutrition and critical care delivery, have driven the evolution of disease management. The majority of patients are now initially treated nonoperatively with antibiotics and percutaneous drainage if amenable.

Up to 25% of acute diverticulitis episodes are associated with complications requiring urgent surgery [14]. Kaiser et al. [11] reported that 22.2% of patients with diverticular abscesses underwent urgent resection with nearly one-third of these requiring a two-stage procedure. More recently, Devaraj et al. [15] reported that 11.9% of patients with diverticular abscess failed medical management during the index hospitalization; 80% of them underwent colostomy creation and required a significantly longer length of hospital stay. A recent systematic review found that urgent surgery was performed at index hospitalization in 30% of patients with diverticular abscess [16]. Following urgent surgery for diverticulitis, over a third of patients will remain with definitive stoma [17, 18].

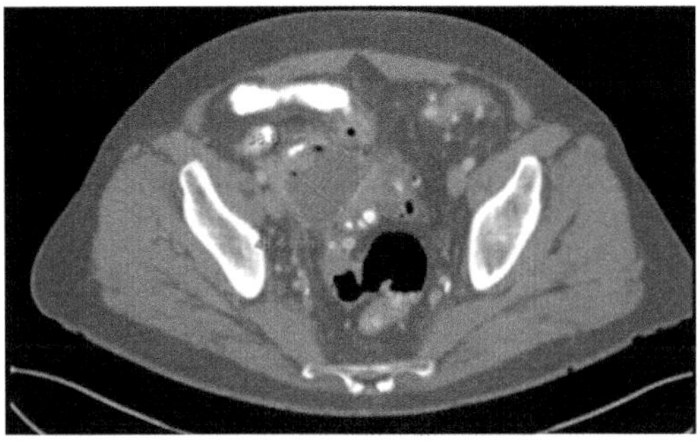

Fig. 18.1 Diverticulitis complicated by abscess formation on CT

Abscesses up to 3–4 cm will often resolve with antibiotics alone and drainage may be unnecessary [7, 19–21]. Different guidelines propose different abscess diameter cutoffs, such as 3, 4–5, or 4 cm, for distinguishing between small and large abscesses [22]. A retrospective study of 114 patients with abdominal abscesses of various etiologies demonstrated that up to 54% responded to treatment without percutaneous drainage. Failure of medical treatment was associated with abscesses >6.5 cm as well as presentation with fever of greater than 101.2° [23].

CT-guided percutaneous drainage (PD) has been increasingly used since the 1980s to treat larger abscesses [6]. A recent meta-analysis found PD to be successful in 49% of patients with diverticular abscesses greater than 3 cm in size [16]. Devaraj reported PD was successful in resolving acute symptomatology in 93.8%, which is consistent with other reports [11, 15]. It has been suggested that PD be limited to two attempts prior to consideration for surgical treatment [24].

Percutaneous drainage makes it possible for the majority of patients with diverticular abscesses to avoid an urgent operation in the acute setting when there is a higher risk of morbidity and colostomy creation. Instead, many patients are able to undergo elective, one-stage procedures, often benefiting from a laparoscopic approach [11, 21, 25, 26].

Elective surgery is indicated if the risk of recurrence or future complications outweighs the risks associated with elective resection. Free perforation is often the first manifestation of complicated diverticulitis and is less common during subsequent episodes [27, 28]. It has even been hypothesized that the healed diverticulum may produce a buttressing effect, protecting against more severe presentations in the future [29].

Immunocompromised patients are generally recommended to undergo resection though some studies even question this paradigm following successful medical treatment [30–32]. Due to the high risk of early, severe, and frequent relapses after nonoperative management of complicated diverticulitis in the immunosuppressed, a recent consensus statement from the European Association of Endoscopic Surgeons (EAES) and the Society of American Gastrointestinal and Endoscopic Surgeons (SAGES) recommended early resectional surgical management [7, 33].

There is a body of literature which advocates for continued expectant management after recovery from acute diverticulitis complicated by abscess [26, 34–37]. These studies generally report low recurrence rates, successful treatment of recurrence with conservative measures, and low rates of urgent surgery during the follow-up period.

Kaiser et al. [11] reported that only 23% of patients who responded to medical treatment developed recurrent diverticulitis in the follow-up period. Buchwald et al. [38] reported a 28% recurrence rate at a median of 110 months of follow-up for those treated conservatively with or without PD. Jalouta et al. [3] reported a 5-year recurrence-free survival rate of 77% for those treated expectantly after PD of diverticular abscesses. Gaertner et al. [35] found a recurrence-free survival rate of 58% at greater than 7 years of follow-up among those treated with PD.

In a retrospective cohort of 3165 patients hospitalized for acute diverticulitis, Broderick-Villa et al. reported that 19% required emergent operation. Of the remaining patients treated nonoperatively only 7.3% underwent elective resection. The authors noted an overall recurrence rate of 13.3%. They found no association between higher recurrence and those who required initial PD; however, only 44 patients in total underwent PD (9 of whom underwent elective resection). Disease severity or Hinchey classification was not reported [34].

Gaertner et al. [35] described 32 patients with diverticular abscess managed with PD and found that 58% did not recur at follow-up at greater than 7 years, and 42% of those who did recur were treated successfully again without surgical intervention. Buchwald et al. [38] reported that only four of the 21 patients who suffered recurrences after initial conservative treatment required surgery. The authors concluded that observation after percutaneous drainage of diverticular abscess was safe and select patients can be managed without elective resection. Of note, 218 patients in Gaertner's study were initially treated with PD and 159 of them did undergo resection (22 emergently); the indications for elective resection were not clearly defined.

A retrospective study by Bridoux et al. [39] that included 114 patients with complicated diverticulitis (defined as the presence of abscess or extraluminal air) included 62 patients with pelvic or mesocolic abscess. Of the remaining 105 patients who did not require urgent operation, 22.9% underwent elective resection for persistent or recurrent symptoms, complications, or surgeon decision for prevention. Among the 81 patients (71%) who did not undergo surgery, only 6 had recurrence at a median of 12 months follow-up, though 16 reported abdominal pain.

Elagili et al. [37] studied 18 patients with diverticular abscesses of at least 3 cm in size who refused surgery after PD or had comorbidities that prohibited surgical management. Of the 15 patients who did not die of pre-existing comorbidities, 7 developed recurrent diverticulitis and 3 underwent surgery (with 1 requiring an urgent Hartmann's procedure).

Many of these retrospective studies supporting nonoperative management of diverticulitis complicated by abscess formation suffer inherent selection bias. Large proportions of patients undergo elective resection and it is often not clear how patients were initially selected for surgical management. Presumably, those with the worst disease underwent early elective resections while those refusing elective surgery may be presumed to have had no further symptoms following initial treatment with or without drainage. This highly select group who recover completely may have an acceptably low risk of recurrence to consider avoiding resection.

For example, the majority of patients (73%) in Gaertner's study [35] underwent elective resection without clear selection criteria; when the total study population is analyzed, colectomy-free survival was only 17%. In Ambrosetti's study [25], 25% of the 73 patients with diverticular abscess required surgery at their initial hospitalization and an additional 34% underwent elective surgery. Lamb et al. [16] noted that one quarter of patients from their cumulative cohort underwent surgery during the index hospitalization and were therefore not a part of the analysis pool, making it unknown how those worst patients would have fared with continued conservative management.

Similarly, studies suggesting low risk of subsequent and more severe attacks may be underestimating the true recurrence risk since surgical intervention eliminated the worst disease. Studies arguing for conservative management of recurrences are often limited by small size and lack of long-term follow-up.

Recurrence rates in excess of 40% for pelvic abscesses treated medically with or without percutaneous drainage have been reported in other retrospective data [11]. In a trial of 107 patients with initial presentation of diverticulitis with extraluminal air and/or abscess (49 with abscesses) randomized to elective surgery or observation, the observation group overall had a rate of recurrent diverticulitis of 32%, at an average of 7 months. This finding did not account for the 12% who had failed initial non-operative management [40].

In their systematic review and metanalysis of 22 studies including 1051 patients with acute diverticulitis with abscess, Lamb and Kaiser [16] noted an overall recurrence rate of 39% in those awaiting elective resection and 18% in the non-operative group, though there was large variation amongst studies ranging to as high as a 68% recurrence rate, particularly with pelvic or distant abscesses. Only 28% of the entire cohort had neither surgery or recurrence during the follow-up period.

Devaraj et al. [15] retrospectively reviewed 210 patients with diverticular abscesses, of whom 185 were successfully managed nonoperatively at the index hospitalization. This hospital system and patient population lacked the resources to offer routine elective sigmoid resection to a majority of patients; of the 37 patients who underwent elective surgery, only 6 were asymptomatic patients with the intention of preventing future attacks. Recurrence occurred in 61% after an average of 5.3 month and 42% experienced more than 1 episode. Recurrences were more severe than the index presentation in 46% with nearly two-thirds having recurrent abscess, fistula, stricture, or peritonitis. In all, 59% would eventually undergo surgery.

Abscess characteristics have been found to be associated with outcomes in multiple studies (Table 18.1). Patients with pelvic abscesses have been shown to have higher rates of recurrence compared to those with pericolic abscesses and are less likely to recover with non-operative treatment [11, 15, 16, 26, 34, 40]. In a retrospective evaluation, Ambrosetti et al. [26] found that patients with pelvic abscesses were more likely to require surgery during initial hospitalization compared to those with mesocolic abscesses (39% vs. 15%, respectively) and were also more likely to require surgery overall (71% vs. 51%, respectively).

Mesocolic abscesses >5 cm have also been shown to have higher recurrence rates, up to 40% in some studies [11, 35, 41, 42]. After PD, Devaraj et al. [15] reported a 74% recurrence, associated with larger abscess size; PD did not reduce the rate of recurrence in this study and 29% of patients with recurrence after initially successful PD required an urgent operation. Kaiser et al. [11] reported a 42% recurrence rate after successful PD. Conversely, in a systematic review of 8766 patients with modified Hinchey IB and II diverticular abscesses, Gregersen et al. [42] found that patients treated initially with PD had a lower rate of recurrence compared to those treated with antibiotics alone (15.9% vs. 22.2%, respectively).

Elective surgery has an associated risk of morbidity and mortality; however, these issues must be weighed against the potential adverse effects of nonoperative management on patient quality of life as well as the costs associated with recurrent hospitalizations, imaging, and drainage procedures, long-term antibiotics and parenteral nutrition. Devaraj et al. [15] found that deferring resection was associated with higher colostomy

Table 18.1 Characteristics associated with adverse outcomes after diverticular disease

Pelvic abscess
Larger mesocolic abscess (especially >5 cm)
Abscess requiring percutaneous drainage
Immunocompromised status

rate than elective surgery (56% vs. 3%, respectively). Urgent operation was required in over a quarter of recurrences. Kaiser et al. [11] found that without elective resection, there was up to a 40% risk of ostomy creation compared to a 0% risk during elective procedures, leading the authors to conclude that successful drainage should be considered a temporary bridge to surgical resection rather than definitive treatment.

Current practice guidelines from the American Society of Colon and Rectal Surgeons recommend elective colectomy for patients who recover from an episode of diverticulitis complicated by abscess [6]. Medical management alone frequently results in chronic or recurrent diverticular symptoms, especially pelvic abscesses and those greater than five centimeters in size [6, 16]. A recent consensus statement from EAES and SAGES advises against routine surgical resection following a single episode of Hinchey I or II diverticulitis, though this is a weak recommendation with a low level of evidence [7]. While understanding of the natural history of diverticulitis complicated by abscess continues to evolve, the decision to offer operative treatment over conservative management should ultimately be decided on a case-by-case basis, taking into account patient and abscess characteristics.

Stricture

Bowel wall thickening, contraction, and fibrosis secondary to chronic inflammation can result in a stricture (Fig. 18.2). While the majority of large bowel obstructions are due to malignancy, up to 10% develop as a result of diverticular disease [43]. Stricture development has been reported to occur in only 0.09% of patients with diverticular disease [44]. Elective resection of diverticular stricture is commonly required to provide symptomatic relief. Klarenbeek et al. [31] found that symptoms of stenosis were an indication for elective resection in up to 40% of patients.

Evaluation of colonic stricture should include colonoscopy, water-soluble contrast enema, and CT to exclude any neoplastic process, although diverticulitis has not been shown to increase the risk of malignancy [45]. However, colonoscopic evaluation may be limited in the setting of stricture. Furthermore, strictures of malignant origin may also be difficult to access in the setting of chronic diverticulitis. One meta-analysis found a 10.8% proportional pooled rate of malignancy in patients with complicated diverticulitis while the risk in uncomplicated diverticulitis was only 0.7% [46]. In their study of 16 patients who underwent elective resection for diverticular stricture, Venara et al. [47] found adenocarcinoma in 2 patients (12.5%), one of which was a T3 tumor likely causing the stricture. If unable to adequately assess a strictured area endoscopically, an oncologic resection is advisable.

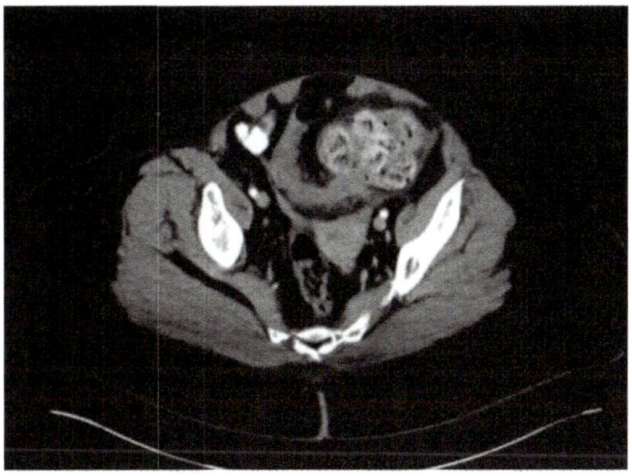

Fig. 18.2 Diverticular stricture on CT

The majority of the literature on colonic stenting has been related to malignant stenosis; benign disease has been reported as an indication for stenting in only 3% of cases [48]. A systematic review of colonic stenting in 122 patients with benign conditions (including 54% of diverticular etiology) found a high initial technical success rate but overall high rates of reobstruction (14%) and perforation (12%); less than half of patients ultimately avoided stoma creation [49]. These complication rates are significantly higher than for stenting in malignant obstruction, leading the authors to conclude that stenting cannot be recommended for colorectal obstruction of benign etiology. In contrast, other authors' experience with colonic stenting of diverticulitis-associated strictures has been largely very favorable; in >75% of patients [50].

Fistula

Fistulas can occur in approximately 2–4% of patients with diverticular disease [48, 49]. Various types of fistulas can develop including colovesicular, colovaginal, coloenteric, colouterine and colocutaneous fistulas. Colovesicular fistulas are the most common of these fistulas accounting for approximately 65% of all diverticular fistulas (Fig. 18.3) [51]. Furthermore, diverticulitis is responsible for most colovesicular fistulas, ranging from 40% to 90% in reported studies. Colovesicular fistulas are more common in men, and when they occur in women, the patient frequently has a prior history of hysterectomy although it is still possible to develop these fistulas with the uterus in situ [52–54]. Patients with colovesicular fistulas can present with a variety of symptoms including pneumaturia, fecaluria, and recurrent urinary tract infections that are generally polymicrobial when cultured. More rarely, patients will present with urine per rectum, diarrhea, or hematuria. Patients may have a prior history of diverticulitis, but more than half will present for the first time with these new-onset symptoms [55]. These patients presenting with new symptoms of a fistula may recall an episode of abdominal pain that resolved spontaneously before developing their symptoms.

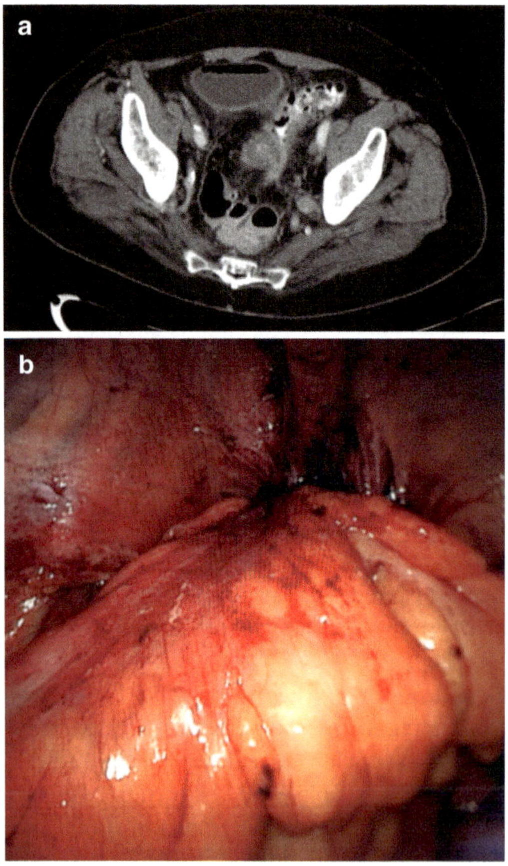

Fig. 18.3 Colovesicular fistula on CT (**a**) and laparoscopy (**b**)

Various diagnostic tests have been described in the literature to make the diagnosis of colovesicular fistula. Computed tomography demonstrating air in the bladder, absent prior instrumentation, is pathognomonic for a colovesicular fistula. A colovesicular fistula can arise in the setting of a perforating colon cancer or an advanced bladder tumor; therefore, a colonoscopy and potentially cystoscopy to rule out malignancy may be warranted. The fistula frequently will not be identified on colonoscopy but the entirety of the colon can be surveyed and any concurrent malignancy or polyps can be managed accordingly. Cystoscopy may reveal an area of granulation tissue or inflammation most frequently at the dome of the bladder although it is unclear if this adds anything to the findings of CT and colonoscopy beyond ruling out a bladder malignancy.

If the patient is not acutely ill from urosepsis, colovesicular fistulas can be managed and treated in a relatively elective fashion. If the patient is particularly symptomatic from recurrent urinary tract infections, suppressive antibiotics can be used until surgery. Patients with bladder outlet obstruction symptoms may need a large-diameter bladder catheter placed with bladder irrigation to remove debris and relieve the obstruction. Although surgery in these settings is still technically elective, it is prudent not to significantly delay surgery given the extent of symptoms and risk of recurrent urinary infection.

The surgical management of colovesicular fistula relies upon removing the diseased portion of the colon with or without repair of the fistula on the bladder side. The sigmoid colon is most frequently involved in colovesicular fistulas, and it is important to maintain standard principles of sigmoid colectomy for diverticulitis when treating a colovesicular fistula, including removing all sigmoid colon down to the top of the rectum where tenia coalesce. The exact site of the fistula is not always readily identified as the fistula can be relatively small with significant surrounding inflammation and adhesions to the dome of the bladder. In these cases, the colon and the bladder can be separated bluntly, either using finger fracture if operating in open fashion or with blunt laparoscopic instruments when using minimally invasive techniques. If the fistula is not easily identified after separating the colon from the bladder, the bladder can be filled with methylene blue mixed with saline to try and identify the fistula [56]. If a leak is identified, postoperative bladder decompression with the urinary catheter is generally sufficient. However, a suture repair can be undertaken. If a leak is not identified after filling the bladder, no further intervention is needed and the bladder should heal without issue. Alternatively, if a large fistula is identified, repair of the bladder is warranted although this scenario is rare in diverticular fistulas. Data are relatively sparse regarding the management of colovesicular fistula in the setting of diverticulitis. Filling the bladder with methylene blue was only reported in one study although anecdotally it seems to be performed in multiple institutions.

After the sigmoid colon has been removed and the fistula has been evaluated, a primary anastomosis is generally acceptable in the absence of an abscess cavity or phlegmon (Fig. 18.4). A diverting loop ileostomy may be considered if there is significant persistent surrounding pelvic inflammation. Rarely, the rectum will be involved with the inflamed sigmoid colon and an anastomosis in the mid or distal rectum may need to be performed. Lastly, an omental flap can be mobilized to place healthy tissue between the prior fistula and the newly created anastomosis in hopes of preventing any recurrent fistulization.

Postoperative bladder decompression with an indwelling catheter may be undertaken for a variable length of time. There is little consensus as reports range from 3 to 14 days in studies with relatively small numbers and diverse patient groups [53–57]. However, there is more consensus that a postoperative cystogram can confirm that there is no persistent leak and that the urinary catheter can be safely removed. One study reported zero cases of a positive cystogram in patients who did not have a complicated bladder repair [57]. Although data are still lacking, it seems reasonable to have a stepwise protocol depending on the complexity of the fistula and subsequent repair. For example, a negative methylene blue leak test would indicate standard postoperative removal of the catheter is safe, while a simple bladder repair may require 3–4 days of bladder decompression and a more complex bladder repair should be studied with a cystogram prior to removing the catheter on postoperative day 7. Further studies will be needed to clarify the safety of this protocol as described. Prolonged bladder catheterization may be required if the postoperative cystogram is positive for a persistent leak.

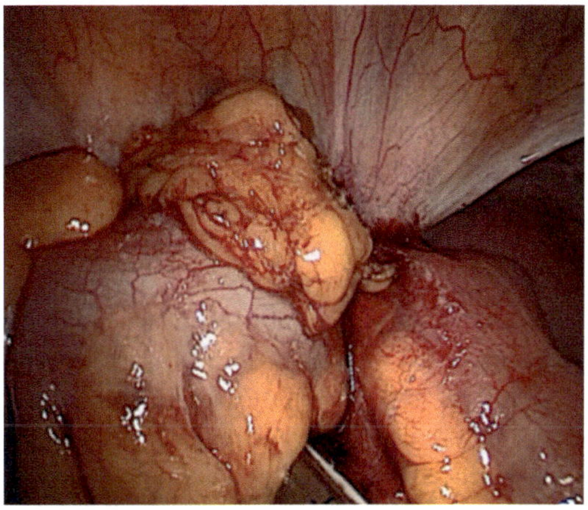

Fig. 18.4 Diverticulitis with phlegmon tethering small intestine

Nonoperative management of colovesicular fistulas is an option but should be reserved for those patients who are particularly high-risk and poor candidates for surgery. Prolonged antibiotics can be used to suppress symptoms of urinary tract infection, although these patients still may require frequent bladder catheterization due to obstructive symptoms [58]. If the patient is deemed a reasonable risk for surgery, it is recommended to proceed with surgery.

Colovaginal fistulas are the second most common diverticular fistula. Like women with colovesicular fistulas, the vast majority of women with colovaginal fistulas have had a prior hysterectomy. As with colovesicular fistulas, diverticulitis is the most common cause of colovaginal fistulas, representing 80–90% of cases [59, 60]. Most patients report discharge of gas or feces from the vagina. Various diagnostic imaging studies have been described including CT abdomen and pelvis with oral, rectal and IV contrast, which will demonstrate the presence of diverticulosis, perhaps thickening and inflammation of the sigmoid colon in proximity to the vagina, and occasionally contrast will identify the fistula passing into the vagina. One study showed that laparoscopic treatment of colovesical fistula is possible and has a shorter hospital stay than open surgery [61]. The CT also provides other clinical information such as phlegmon close to the ureters, and undrained abscesses that may need to be addressed prior to surgery. Other imaging tests include water-soluble contrast enemas, and vaginography, attempting to identify the fistula tract from either direction (Fig. 18.5). Lastly, colonoscopy is an important part of the clinical evaluation to rule out synchronous lesions and confirm that the fistula is not due to a colonic malignancy. At the time of colonoscopy, the exam can start by visually inspecting the vagina to try and identify the fistula tract and then continuing with the standard colonoscopy. This can be useful if the fistula has not already been identified on physical exam in the office or with prior imaging studies. Occasionally, the fistula cannot be definitively identified on exam or imaging but the patient remains symptomatic. In these rare cases, it is still reasonable to proceed to surgery, identify the sigmoid colon adhered to the top of the vagina and conclude that proceeding with sigmoidectomy as planned is acceptable.

Treatment of colovaginal fistulas generally consists of surgical resection of the diseased colonic segment. Like colovesicular fistula, these patients are usually stable and not at risk for impending sepsis; therefore, the evaluation can be completed in a timely fashion and surgery can be electively scheduled. The surgical approach is like that of colovesicular fistula, again requiring sigmoid colectomy to the top of the rectum. The fistula can be separated from the vagina bluntly with finger fracture or laparoscopic instruments. If the subsequent defect in the vagina is large, it can be repaired with interrupted simple sutures, but if small or not visible on inspection, no further repair is needed as the defect should heal once the inflammation has been removed. A primary anastomosis should be safe to perform in most patients and lastly an omental flap can be mobilized and brought into the pelvis to separate the fresh anastomosis from the vagina.

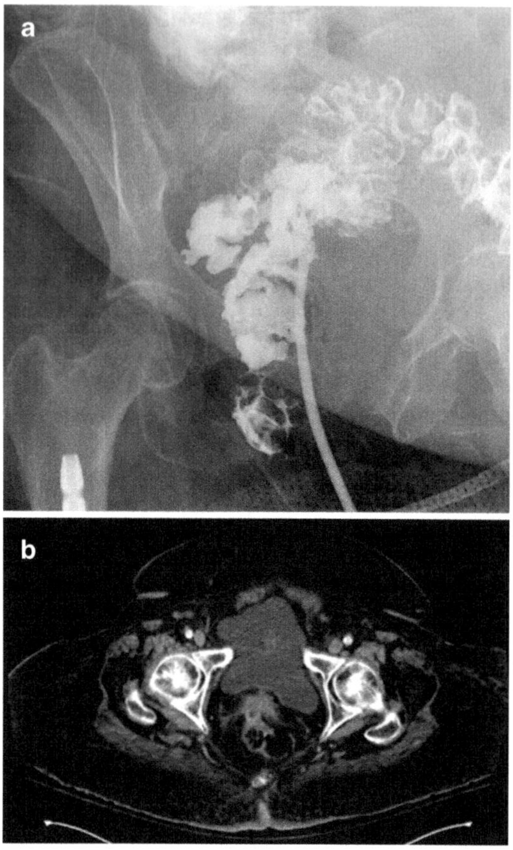

Fig. 18.5 Colovaginal fistula on vaginogram (**a**) and CT (**b**)

Operative Approaches to Complicated Diverticulitis

Sigmoid resection in the setting of complicated diverticulitis can be approached in many ways. First, preoperative and intraoperative considerations that can be applied to all surgical approaches will be discussed. Evidence regarding the timing of elective surgery is limited, retrospective, and with mixed results. Some studies have shown increased rates of conversion to open surgery when performed less than 6 weeks from the most recent attack, while others showed no difference. Although the data is limited, it seems reasonable to wait a minimum of 6 weeks to allow inflammation to resolve [62–64]. Preoperative mechanical oral cathartic bowel preparation combined with oral antibiotic preparation is recommended to decrease the risk of surgical site infection. This topic has been debated in the literature with most recent data suggesting a significant benefit to combined mechanical and oral antibiotic bowel [65–68]. In the specific setting of surgery for diverticulitis, there are no data currently to suggest improved outcomes with bowel preparation compared to no bowel preparation so this recommendation is inferred from the overarching data regarding colectomy in general. Intravenous antibiotic prophylaxis should be administered prior to incision. Ureteral stents can be used to assist in identifying the ureters during surgery and potentially decrease the risk of ureteral injury or at least easy recognition of any injury. Until recently, there were no data to support this claim and there are still no randomized controlled trials showing a significant difference. Many surgeons believe that stents only facilitate early identification and repair of injuries. Recently, however, Coakley et al. [69] published a study examining ureteral stents used in colectomy taking data from the National Surgical Quality Improvement Program. In total, 51,125 patients were included and there were 333 ureteral injuries reported (0.65%), consistent with previously reported data. Ureteral injuries most commonly occur in cases of diverticulitis, accounting for 36% of all injuries. The authors showed that only 4.9% of cases in the study used ureteral stents but on multivariable analysis there was a decreased risk of ureteral injury in patients with prophylactic stent placement (OR = 0.45, 95% CI, 0.25–0.81). It remains unclear if any randomized controlled trial will ever show a significant difference given the low rates of ureteral injury, but it seems reasonable to use ureteral stents in patients with complicated diverticulitis. Some potential complications noted in the literature include gross hematuria in 95% of cases, approximately a 6% risk of urinary tract infection and an increased risk of postoperative acute kidney injury, especially in the setting of bilateral stents (OR 3.82 95% CI 2.17–6.75) [70, 71].

Minimally invasive techniques are preferred, although the standard open approach is still acceptable. Hand-assisted laparoscopy offers a potential means of avoiding conversion to a standard open surgery.

Laparoscopy has become more widely accepted. Studies specifically assessing laparoscopy compared to open surgery solely in the setting of complicated diverticulitis are fewer but there are still some important points that can be gleaned from the literature. First, the rate of conversion from laparoscopy to laparotomy seems to be higher in the setting of complicated diverticulitis. Martel et al. [72] examined 183 consecutive cases of laparoscopic sigmoid colectomy for diverticulitis and compared the outcomes of uncomplicated versus complicated diverticulitis. Thirty-nine patients had a history of complicated diverticulitis and had a conversion rate of 23% compared to 4% in the uncomplicated cohort. Complication rates were also higher in the complicated diverticulitis group, but the anastomotic leak rates were not significantly different. Laparoscopy seems to be considered safe in each specific aspect of complicated diverticulitis including fistulas. A recent systematic review by Cirocchi et al. [73] covered 11 studies examining laparoscopy in the treatment of fistulas from diverticular disease. The authors concluded that laparoscopy is safe. Overall, the recurrence of fistula was low (0.8%), and the need for a Hartmann's procedure or proximal diversion was also low (1.4%) with no difference compared to open techniques. Furthermore, laparoscopy has been reported to result in less postoperative pain, faster gastrointestinal recovery, improved cosmesis and shorter hospital stay, although some of this data is quite limited. Of the four randomized controlled trials published so far, two of the studies showed decreased morbidity while the other two showed no difference. It should be noted that these trials did not specifically compare laparoscopic versus open approaches in complicated diverticulitis but also included uncomplicated symptomatic patients [74–77]. From the literature and our experience, it seems it is reasonable to recommend minimally invasive surgery in the management of complicated diverticular disease. Beyond our own personal recommendation to use minimally invasive surgery, the recent SAGES/EAES consensus statement similarly recommends the use of laparoscopy when feasible in the elective management of patients with diverticulitis; patients with 98 percent of members approve this recommendation [7]. Minimally invasive surgery will likely continue to increase its share of the surgeries performed as technology and experience continue to grow.

Data specifically comparing laparoscopic surgery to hand-assisted surgery in diverticulitis is limited. Lee et al. [78] examined results from a prospectively maintained database and found that hand-assisted surgery resulted in shorter operative times. In patients with complicated diverticulitis, the rate of conversion to laparotomy was less in the hand-assisted group but the data were limited with only 4 patients in the laparoscopic group and only 10 in the hand-assisted group. A randomized controlled trial comparing hand-assisted surgery to laparoscopy found decreased operating times for patients undergoing left colectomy and total abdominal colectomy but did not specifically compare patients with complicated diverticulitis [79]. Although the authors prefer a laparoscopic approach, proponents of hand-assisted surgery may claim that hand-assisted surgery potentially avoids a larger laparotomy incision and or facilitates resecting colovesicular fistulas.

Principles of Resection and Approaches to Dissection

Multiple studies have examined preserving the inferior mesenteric artery to decrease the risk of anastomotic leak with variable results. A recent systematic review by Cirocchi et al. [80] examined eight studies, two of which were randomized controlled studies. The analysis included 2190 patients undergoing sigmoid colectomy for diverticular disease and 1353 patients had IMA preservation while the remaining 837 patients underwent ligation of the IMA. There was no significant difference regarding anastomotic leak rate when comparing the two groups, while the IMA preservation group had a higher rate of conversion to open surgery (9% vs 5.1%).

Given the variability of presentation and complications from diverticulitis, there does not seem to be one specific surgical approach that is best suited for approaching the dissection. The surgical dissection for diverticulitis has been described in many ways, including a lateral-to-medial dissection, medial-to-lateral and a top-down approach starting at the descending colon away from the inflammation and approaching the pelvis after better delineating anatomy where the tissue is less inflamed and scarred. From our experience, it seems that it is best to be comfortable with performing the dissection in whichever manner suits the individual patient best. In some cases, the patient may have had a large mesenteric abscess making a medial-to-lateral approach difficult while a lateral-to-medial or top-down approach may be simpler and safer. In other cases, the sigmoid colon can be particularly scarred to the pelvic sidewall from prior inflammation and a medial to lateral approach can help start the dissection and facilitate identifying the ureter preventing injury. It is important to be flexible in one's approach and adjust one's plan based on the individual patient and anatomy encountered. Lastly, converting to laparotomy is the safest option if the case is not progressing or there is any question to the safety of proceeding in a minimally invasive fashion.

We recommend routine mobilization of the splenic flexure although data suggest that an individualized approach is safe. Routine mobilization of the flexure adds significant length and will decrease the risk of tension at the anastomosis. The proximal point of transection can be difficult to laparoscopically localize until the bowel is exteriorized and palpated by hand to detect areas of prior disease and wall thickening. If the splenic flexure has already been mobilized, the descending colon will likely reach the top of the rectum despite a larger than expected resection. Alternatively, splenic flexure mobilization does risk splenic injury as well as injury to the marginal artery in patients who may not need the additional length. Schlussel et al. [81] performed a retrospective review of sigmoid and left colectomy cases. Approximately half of the patients underwent splenic flexure mobilization and the authors showed no difference in major or minor complications, while patients undergoing splenic flexure mobilization required longer operative times. The authors concluded that selective splenic flexure mobilization was safe based on their findings.

Similar to the various approaches to the initial dissection of the sigmoid colon, there are multiple methods of splenic flexure mobilization. These techniques include an inframesocolic approach, a supramesocolic approach and a lateral to medial approach. The inframesocolic approach starts medially at the IMV and progresses toward the splenic flexure from beneath the mesocolon. The lesser sac can be entered by continuing the dissection superiorly and over the tail of the pancreas. The supramesocolic dissection approach starts by dividing the omentum to enter the lesser sac and continuing the dissection laterally along the transverse colon until the splenocolic ligament is divided. The lateral to medial approach continues the dissection of the white line of Toldt laterally until the spleen is separated from the colon and the colon is mobilized to the midline.

Some patients may have more inflammation than expected that involves the rectum. This scenario can occur in patients who previously had a large pelvic abscess and continue to have a smoldering infectious or inflammation while waiting for their elective surgery. Residual abscess may even be encountered at the time of surgery which may make the surgeon wary of creating a fresh anastomosis in the setting of active infection and inflammation. One option is to abandon the planned primary anastomosis and create a Hartmann's procedure. This maneuver will divert stool away from the pelvis allowing infection and inflammation to subside before creating a primary colorectal anastomosis at a later date. Alternatively, a primary anastomosis with diverting loop ileostomy can be performed. We are unaware of any data specifically comparing these options in the setting of elective surgery for complicated diverticulitis. However, randomized controlled trials have shown better outcomes for a primary anastomosis and diverting loop ileostomy in the setting of emergent surgery for perforated diverticulitis. Although outcomes and complications from the initial surgery in these studies are generally equivalent, all studies have shown a higher rate of stoma reversal in patients with a diverting loop ileostomy compared to patients with a Hartmann's stump and end colostomy. Furthermore, there is less morbidity at the time of stoma reversal for a diverting loop ileostomy compared to a Hartmann's closure [82–85]. Based on these data, we infer similar outcomes in the elective setting and prefer a primary anastomosis with diverting loop ileostomy over a Hartmann's procedure when encountering unexpected residual infection or inflammation in the pelvis. As always, the advisability of this approach must be undertaken in the context of the individual patient.

Conclusions

In conclusion, the prevalence of diverticulitis seems to have significantly increased. In addition, the age at which patients present with diverticulitis seems to have decreased. Despite this amalgamated increase in the potential number of patients who present with diverticulitis, evidence-based guidelines have decreased the need for surgical intervention based upon absolute criteria such as age, number of episodes, or severity of attack. The management of diverticulitis has become a very individualized personalized algorithm. When patients undergo surgery for perforation and/or abscess secondary to diverticulitis, primary anastomosis with loop ileostomy seems to have supplanted the Hartmann's procedure. Laparoscopic lavage seems to be less employed than it had transiently been. Elective management of individuals with chronic diverticulitis with strictures, colovesical or colovaginal fistulas, or chronic unrelenting symptoms is generally managed according to the individual patient. While in the emergent setting a bowel preparation would not be utilized, in the elective setting both a mechanical or oral cathartic, and oral antibiotic bowel preparation would be utilized. Ureteric catheters are employed in both the emergency and elective settings. We tend not to close either bladder or vaginal defects from fistulas unless they are quite large and tend to create proximal loop ileostomies only when significant residual pelvic inflammation remains after the resection and anastomosis. Laparoscopy has become the preferred access method of choice in both elective and emergency settings. We have found that the clear majority of operations in both scenarios can be successfully completed laparoscopically. We consider hand-assisted surgery in the realm of laparotomy and assiduously avoid its use, although it may prove useful to avoid full conversion to open surgery. Clearly, the management of diverticular disease is evolving toward a minimally invasive approach to both offering and performing surgery [86].

References

1. Neale JA. Surgical management of diverticular disease in the elective setting. Clin Colon Rectal Surg. 2018;31(4):236–42.
2. Hall J. Diverticular disease. In: Steele S, Hull T, Read T, Saclarides T, Senagore A, Whitlow C, editors. The ASCRS textbook of colon and rectal surgery. 3rd ed. Springer; 2016. p. 645–67.
3. Jalouta T, Jrebi N, Luchtefeld M, Ogilvie JW. Diverticulitis recurrence after percutaneous abscess drainage. Int J Color Dis. 2017;32(10):1367–73.
4. Parks TG. Papers and originals natural history of diverticular disease of the colon. A review of 52i cases. Br Med J. 1969;(December):639–42.
5. Janes S, Meagher A, Frizelle FA. Elective surgery after acute diverticulitis. Br J Surg. 2005;92(2):133–42.
6. Hall J, Hardiman K, Lee S, et al. The American Society of Colon and Rectal Surgeons clinical practice guidelines for the treatment of left-sided colonic diverticulitis. Dis Colon Rectum. 2020;6:728–47.
7. Francis NK, Sylla P, Abou-Khalil M, et al. EAES and SAGES 2018 consensus conference on acute diverticulitis management: evidence-based recommendations for clinical practice. Surg Endosc [Internet]. 2019. Available from: https://doi.org/10.1007/s00464-019-06882-z.
8. Beckham H, Whitlow CB. The medical and nonoperative treatment of diverticulitis. Clin Colon Rectal Surg. 2009;22(3):156–60.
9. Symeonidis N, Psarras K, Lalountas M, et al. Clinical features of colonic diverticular disease. Tech Coloproctol. 2011;15(S1):5–8.
10. Ambrosetti P, Robert J, Witzig J, et al. Incidence, outcome, and proposed management of isolated abscesses complicating acute left-sided colonic diverticulitis – a prospective study of 140 patients. Dis Colon Rectum. 1992;35(11):1072–6.
11. Kaiser AM, Jiang JK, Lake JP, et al. The management of complicated diverticulitis and the role of computed tomography. Am J Gastroenterol. 2005;100(4):910–7.
12. Hall JF, Roberts PL, Ricciardi R, et al. Long-term follow-up after an initial episode of diverticulitis: what are the predictors of recurrence? Dis Colon Rectum. 2011;54(3):283–8.
13. Schoetz DJ. Diverticular disease of the colon a century-old problem. Dis Colon Rectum. 1999;42(6):703–9.
14. Abbas S. Resection and primary anastomosis in acute complicated diverticulitis, a systematic review of the literature. Int J Color Dis. 2007;22(4):351–7.
15. Devaraj B, Liu W, Tatum J, Cologne K, Kaiser AM. Medically treated diverticular abscess associated with high risk of recurrence and disease complications. Dis Colon Rectum. 2016;59(3):208–15.
16. Lamb MN, Kaiser AM. Elective resection versus observation after nonoperative management of complicated diverticulitis with abscess: a systematic review and meta-analysis. Dis Colon Rectum. 2014;57(12):1430–40.
17. Bridoux V, Regimbeau JM, Ouaissi M, et al. Hartmann's procedure or primary anastomosis for generalized peritonitis due to perforated diverticulitis: a prospective multicenter randomized trial (DIVERTI). J Am Coll Surg [Internet]. 2017;225(6):798–805. Available from: https://doi.org/10.1016/j.jamcollsurg.2017.09.004.
18. Oberkofler CE, Rickenbacher A, Raptis DA, et al. A multicenter randomized clinical trial of primary anastomosis or Hartmann's procedure for perforated left colonic diverticulitis with purulent or fecal peritonitis. Ann Surg. 2012;256(5):819–27.

19. Siewert B, Tye G, Kruskal J, et al. CT-guided drainage in the treatment of diverticular abscesses: size matters. AJR Am J Roentgenol. 2006;186:680–6.
20. Dharmarajan S, Hunt SR, Birnbaum EH, Fleshman JW, Mutch MG. The efficacy of nonoperative management of acute complicated diverticulitis. Dis Colon Rectum. 2011;54(6):663–71.
21. Brandt D, Gervaz P, Durmishi Y, Platon A, Morel P, Poletti PA. Percutaneous CT scan-guided drainage vs. antibiotherapy alone for Hinchey II diverticulitis: a case-control study. Dis Colon Rectum. 2006;49(10):1533–8.
22. Cirocchi R, Duro F, Avenia S, et al. Guidelines for the treatment of abdominal abscesses in acute diverticulitis: an umbrella review. J Clin Med. 2023;12(17):5522. https://doi.org/10.3390/jcm12175522. PMID: 37685590; PMCID: PMC10488020.
23. Kumar RR, Kim JT, Haukoos JS, et al. Factors affecting the successful management of intra-abdominal abscesses with antibiotics and the need for percutaneous drainage. Dis Colon Rectum. 2006;49(2):183–9.
24. Shaikh S, Krukowski ZH. Outcome of a conservative policy for managing acute sigmoid diverticulitis. Br J Surg. 2007;94(7):876–9.
25. Durmishi Y, Gervaz P, Brandt D, et al. Results from percutaneous drainage of Hinchey stage II diverticulitis guided by computed tomography scan. Surg Endosc Other Interv Tech. 2006;20(7):1129–33.
26. Ambrosetti P, Chautems R, Soravia C, Peiris-Waser N, Terrier F. Long-term outcome of mesocolic and pelvic diverticular abscesses of the left colon: a prospective study of 73 cases. Dis Colon Rectum. 2005;48(4):787–91.
27. Collins D, Winter DC. Elective resection for diverticular disease: an evidence-based review. World J Surg. 2008;32(11):2429–33.
28. Jacobs DO. Diverticulitis. N Engl J Med. 2007;357(20):57–66.
29. Chapman JR, Dozois EJ, Wolff BG, Gullerud RE, Larson DR. Diverticulitis: a progressive disease? Do multiple recurrences predict less favorable outcomes? Ann Surg. 2006;243(6):876–80.
30. Perkins JD, Shield CF, Chang FC, Farha GJ. Acute diverticulitis. Comparison of treatment in immunocompromised and nonimmunocompromised patients. Am J Surg. 1984;148(6):745–8.
31. Klarenbeek BR, Samuels M, Van Der Wal MA, Van Der Peet DL, Meijerink WJ, Cuesta MA. Indications for elective sigmoid resection in diverticular disease. Ann Surg. 2010;251(4):670–4.
32. Biondo S, Borao JL, Kreisler E, et al. Recurrence and virulence of colonic diverticulitis in immunocompromised patients. Am J Surg. 2012;204(2):172–9.
33. Sartelli M, Weber DG, Kluger Y, et al. 2020 update of the WSES guidelines for the management of acute colonic diverticulitis in the emergency setting. World J Emerg Surg. 2020;15(1):32. https://doi.org/10.1186/s13017-020-00313-4. PMID: 32381121; PMCID: PMC7206757.
34. Broderick-Villa G, Burchette RJ, Collins JC, et al. Hospitalization for acute diverticulitis does not mandate routine elective colectomy. Arch Surg. 2005;140(6):576–83.
35. Gaertner WB, Willis DJ, Madoff RD, et al. Percutaneous drainage of colonic diverticular abscess: is colon resection necessary? Dis Colon Rectum. 2013;56(5):622–6.
36. Nelson RS, Ewing BM, Wengert TJ, Thorson AG. Clinical outcomes of complicated diverticulitis managed nonoperatively. Am J Surg. 2008;196(6):969–74.
37. Elagili F, Stocchi L, Ozuner G, Dietz DW, Kiran RP. Outcomes of percutaneous drainage without surgery for patients with diverticular abscess. Dis Colon Rectum. 2014;57(3):331–6.
38. Buchwald P, Dixon L, Wakeman CJ, Eglinton TW, Frizelle FA. Hinchey I and II diverticular abscesses: long-term outcome of conservative treatment. ANZ J Surg. 2017;87(12):1011–4.
39. Bridoux V, Antor M, Schwarz L, et al. Elective operation after acute complicated diverticulitis: is it still mandatory? World J Gastroenterol. 2014;20(25):8166–72.
40. You K, Bendl R, Taut C, et al. Randomized clinical trial of elective resection versus observation in diverticulitis with extraluminal air or abscess initially managed conservatively. Br J Surg. 2018;105(8):971–9.
41. Ambrosetti P, Becker C, Terrier F. Colonic diverticulitis: impact of imaging on surgical management – a prospective study of 542 patients. Eur Radiol. 2002;12(5):1145–9.
42. Gregersen R, Mortensen LQ, Burcharth J, Pommergaard HC, Rosenberg J. Treatment of patients with acute colonic diverticulitis complicated by abscess formation: a systematic review. Int J Surg [Internet]. 2016;2016(35):201–8. Available from: https://doi.org/10.1016/j.ijsu.2016.10.006.
43. Greenlee HB, Pienkos EJ, Vanderbilt PC, et al. Large bowel obstruction. Arch Surg. 1974;108:470–6.
44. Sugihara K, Muto T, Morioka Y, Asano A, Yamamoto T. Diverticular disease of the colon in Japan a review of 615 cases. Dis Colon Rectum. 1984;27(8):531–7.
45. Krones CJ, Klinge U, Butz N, et al. The rare epidemiologic coincidence of diverticular disease and advanced colonic neoplasia. Int J Color Dis. 2006;21(1):18–24.
46. Sharma PV, Eglinton T, Hider P, Frizelle F. Systematic review and meta-analysis of the role of routine colonic evaluation after radiologically confirmed acute diverticulitis. Ann Surg. 2014;259(2):263–72.
47. Venara A, Toque L, Barbieux J, Cesbron E, Ridereau-Zins C, Lermite E. Sigmoid stricture associated with diverticular disease should be an indication for elective surgery with lymph node clearance. J Visc Surg [Internet]. 2015;152(4):211–5.
48. Khot U, Wenk Lang A, Murali K, Parker M. Systematic review of the efficacy and safety of colorectal stents. Br J Surg. 2002;89(9):1096–102.

49. Currie A, Christmas C, Aldean H, Mobasheri M, Bloom ITM. Systematic review of self-expanding stents in the management of benign colorectal obstruction. Color Dis. 2014;16(4):239–45.
50. Fejleh MP, Tabibian JH. Colonoscopic management of diverticular disease. World J Gastrointest Endosc. 2020;12(2):53–9. https://doi.org/10.4253/wjge.v12.i2.53. PMID: 32064030; PMCID: PMC6965002.
51. Young-Fadok TM, Roberts PL, Spencer MP, Wolff BG. Colonic diverticular disease. Curr Probl Surg. 2000;37(7):457–514.
52. Woods RJ, Lavery IC, Fazio VW, Jagelman DG, Weakley FL. Internal fistulas in diverticular disease. Dis Colon Rectum. 1988;31(8):591–6. https://doi.org/10.1007/bf02556792.
53. Mileski WJ, Joehl RJ, Rege RV, Nahrwold DL. One-stage resection and anastomosis in the management of colovesical fistula. Am J Surg. 1987;153(1):75–9.
54. Najjar SF, Jamal MK, Savas JF, Miller TA. The spectrum of colovesical fistula and diagnostic paradigm. Am J Surg. 2004;188(5):617–21.
55. Melchior S, Cudovic D, Jones J, Thomas C, Gillitzer R, Thuroff J. Diagnosis and surgical management of colovesical fistulas due to sigmoid diverticulitis. J Urol. 2009;182(3):978–82.
56. Bertelson NL, Abcarian H, Kalkbrenner KA, et al. Diverticular colovesical fistula: what should we really be doing? Tech Coloproctol. 2018;22(1):31–6.
57. de Moya MA, Zacharias N, Osbourne A, et al. Colovesical fistula repair: is early Foley catheter removal safe? J Surg Res. 2009;156(2):274–7.
58. Amin M, Nallinger R, Polk HC Jr. Conservative treatment of selected patients with colovesical fistula due to diverticulitis. Surg Gynecol Obstet. 1984;159(5):442–4.
59. Bahadursingh AM, Longo WE. Colovaginal fistulas. Etiology and management. J Reprod Med. 2003;48(7):489–95.
60. Berger MB, Khandwala N, Fenner DE, Burney RE. Colovaginal fistulas: presentation, evaluation, and management. Female Pelvic Med Reconstr Surg. 2016;22(5):355–8.
61. Trejo-Avila M, Vergara-Fernández O. Open versus laparoscopic surgery for the treatment of diverticular colovesical fistulas: a systematic review and meta-analysis. ANZ J Surg. 2021;91(9):E570–7. https://doi.org/10.1111/ans.16985. Epub 2021 May 31. PMID: 34056819.
62. Warwas FB, Schneider B. Elective vs. early elective surgery in diverticular disease: a retrospective study on the optimal timing of non-emergency treatment. Int J Color Dis. 2018;33:531–9.
63. Natarajan S, Ewings EL, Vega RJ. Laparoscopic sigmoid colectomy after acute diverticulitis: when to operate? Surgery. 2004;136(4):725–30.
64. Zingg U, Pasternak I, Guertler L, et al. Early vs. delayed elective laparoscopic-assisted colectomy in sigmoid diverticulitis: timing of surgery in relation to the acute attack. Dis Colon Rectum. 2007;50(11):1911–7.
65. Van Sant HP, Slieker JC, Hop WC, et al. The influence of mechanical bowel preparation in elective colorectal surgery for diverticulitis. Tech Coloproctol. 2012;16(4):309–14.
66. Koller SE, Bauer KW, Egleston BL, et al. Comparative effectiveness and risks of bowel preparation before elective colorectal surgery. Ann Surg. 2018;267(4):734–42.
67. Kiran RP, Murray AC, Chiuzan C, Estrada D, Forde K. Combined preoperative mechanical bowel preparation with oral antibiotics significantly reduces surgical site infection, anastomotic leak, and ileus after colorectal surgery. Ann Surg. 2015;262(3):416–25; discussion 423–415.
68. Klinger AL, Green H, Monlezun DJ, et al. The role of bowel preparation in colorectal surgery: results of the 2012–2015 ACS-NSQIP data. Ann Surg. 2019;269(4):671–7.
69. Coakley KM, Kasten KR, Sims SM, Prasad T, Heniford BT, Davis BR. Prophylactic ureteral catheters for colectomy: a national surgical quality improvement program-based analysis. Dis Colon Rectum. 2018;61(1):84–8.
70. Blake MF, Dwivedi A, Tootla A, Tootla F, Silva YJ. Laparoscopic sigmoid colectomy for chronic diverticular disease. JSLS. 2005;9(4):382–5.
71. Hassinger TE, Mehaffey JH, Mullen MG, et al. Ureteral stents increase risk of postoperative acute kidney injury following colorectal surgery. Surg Endosc. 2018;32(7):3342–8. https://doi.org/10.1007/s00464-018-6054-y.
72. Martel G, Bouchard A, Soto CM, Poulin EC, Mamazza J, Boushey RP. Laparoscopic colectomy for complex diverticular disease: a justifiable choice? Surg Endosc. 2010;24:2273–80.
73. Cirocchi R, Farinella E, Trastulli S, Sciannameo F, Audisio R. Elective sigmoid colectomy for diverticular disease. Laparoscopic vs open surgery: a systematic review. Color Dis. 2012;14(6):671–83.
74. Klarenbeek BR, Veenhof AA, Bergamaschi R, et al. Laparoscopic sigmoid resection for diverticulitis decreases major morbidity rates: a randomized control trial: short-term results of the Sigma Trial. Ann Surg. 2009;249(1):39–44. https://doi.org/10.1097/SLA.0b013e31818e416a.
75. Gervaz P, Inan I, Perneger T, Schiffer E, Morel P. A prospective, randomized, single-blind comparison of laparoscopic versus open sigmoid colectomy for diverticulitis. Ann Surg. 2010;252(1):3–8.
76. Raue W, Paolucci V, Asperger W, Albrecht R, Buchler MW, Schwenk W, Group L-CT. Laparoscopic sigmoid resection for diverticular disease has no advantages over open approach: midterm results of a randomized controlled trial. Langenbeck's Arch Surg. 2011;396(7):973–80. https://doi.org/10.1007/s00423-011-0825-4.
77. Rink AD, John-Enzenauer K, Haaf F, Straub E, Nagelschmidt M, Vestweber KH. Laparoscopic-assisted or laparoscopic-facilitated sigmoidectomy for diverticular disease? A prospective randomized trial

on postoperative pain and analgesic consumption. Dis Colon Rectum. 2009;52(10):1738–45.
78. Lee SW, Yoo J, Dujovny N, Sonoda T, Milsom JW. Laparoscopic vs. hand-assisted laparoscopic sigmoidectomy for diverticulitis. Dis Colon Rectum. 2006;49(4):464–9. https://doi.org/10.1007/s10350-006-0500-y. PMID: 16518715.
79. Marcello PW, Fleshman JW, Milsom JW, et al. Hand-assisted laparoscopic vs. laparoscopic colorectal surgery: a multicenter, prospective, randomized trial. Dis Colon Rectum. 2008;51(6):818–26; discussion 826–8. https://doi.org/10.1007/s10350-008-9269-5. Epub 2008 Apr 17. PMID: 18418653.
80. Cirocchi R, Trastulli S, Farinella E, et al. Is inferior mesenteric artery ligation during sigmoid colectomy for diverticular disease associated with increased anastomotic leakage? A meta-analysis of randomized and non-randomized clinical trials. Color Dis. 2012;14(9):e521–9.
81. Schlussel AT, Wiseman JT, Kelly JF, et al. Location is everything: the role of splenic flexure mobilization during colon resection for diverticulitis. Int J Surg. 2017;40:124–9.
82. Binda GA, Karas JR, Serventi A, et al., Study Group on D. Primary anastomosis vs nonrestorative resection for perforated diverticulitis with peritonitis: a prematurely terminated randomized controlled trial. Color Dis. 2012;14:1403–10.
83. Oberkofler CE, Rickenbacher A, Raptis DA, et al. A multicenter randomized clinical trial of primary anastomosis or Hartmann's procedure for perforated left colonic diverticulitis with purulent or fecal peritonitis. Ann Surg. 2012;256:819–27.
84. Bridoux V, Regimbeau JM, Ouaissi M, et al. Hartmann's procedure or primary anastomosis for generalized peritonitis due to perforated diverticulitis: a prospective multicenter randomized trial (DIVERTI). J Am Coll Surg. 2017;225:798–805.
85. Lambrichts DPV, Vennix S, Musters GD, et al. Hartmann's procedure versus sigmoidectomy with primary anastomosis for perforated diverticulitis with purulent or faecal peritonitis (LADIES): a multicentre, parallel-group, randomised, open-label, superiority trial. Lancet Gastroenterol Hepatol. 2019;4(8):599–610.
86. Wexner SD, Yellinek S. Commentary: is preoperative bowel preparation needed before elective colectomy? Lancet. 2019;394(10201):808–10. https://doi.org/10.1016/S0140-6736(19)31269-3.

19 Elective Surgery for Diverticulitis: Technical Considerations

W. Donald Buie and Mark E. Lipson

Introduction

Elective surgery for recurrent diverticulitis can be technically challenging. As surgical treatment has evolved to more selective resection, patients presenting for elective procedures have often experienced repeated episodes of diverticulitis, resulting in significant fibrosis and chronic inflammation. Occasionally, patients have smoldering diverticulitis with incomplete resolution of inflammation but without overt signs of clinical infection. As a result, traditional surgical dissection planes may be distorted, obscured, or absent. In addition, the mesentery may be inflamed, thickened, and friable, making it prone to bleeding or fracture. Finally, the diverticulitis itself can involve, or place at risk, other critical structures, including small bowel, ureters, bladder, and vagina, all of which can pose technical challenges to a safe resection.

This chapter will outline the technical aspects of elective surgery for recurrent diverticulitis. It is divided into three sections: preoperative considerations, surgical principles/operative techniques, and surgical management of complex disease.

Preoperative Considerations

Timing

Timing is critical for elective diverticular resection. When possible, all acute inflammation should be settled both biochemically and clinically. Abscesses should be resolved with drainage and/or antibiotics. The patient should be fully recovered with normal weight, functional status, and resolution of abdominal pain. Incomplete recovery may be related to persistent inflammation or complex disease. When faced with ongoing symptoms, the surgeon must decide whether to continue "the cooling off period" or proceed with a semi-elective procedure, given that additional time may or may not fully resolve the inflammation.

W. D. Buie (✉)
Foothills Medical Center, University of Calgary, Departments of Surgery and Oncology, Calgary, AB, Canada
e-mail: wdbuie@ucalgary.ca

M. E. Lipson
Peter Lougheed Centre, Alberta Health Services, University of Calgary, Calgary, AB, Canada
e-mail: melipson@ucalgary.ca

M. Boutros et al. (eds.), *Diverticulitis*, https://doi.org/10.1007/978-3-032-21720-2_19

Preoperative Assessment and Preparation

Prior to surgery, one must consider past surgical history, disease history, and other treatments that could signal complex or difficult operating conditions. Relevant history includes previous abdominal or pelvic surgery, previous bowel resections, history of radiation (remote or recent), or a diagnosis of inflammatory bowel disease. Ongoing intra-abdominal sepsis from abscess or fistula also complicates matters and increases the difficulty of the procedure owing to obscured or obliterated planes and compromised tissue quality [1]. The number of previous episodes of diverticulitis should also be solicited.

All patients should undergo an abdominopelvic CT scan to identify the diseased segment of bowel and to assist in preoperative planning. Although the sigmoid colon is typically involved, it is helpful to know whether the disease involves the rectosigmoid, mid sigmoid, upper sigmoid, or descending colon. In the latter situation, the splenic flexure will need to be mobilized to provide length for a tension-free anastomosis. CT will also identify any secondarily involved structures—including ureter, bladder, vagina, and small intestine, which will alter the surgical approach—in addition to incidental abdominal problems that may require management prior to surgery [1].

All patients should undergo a colonoscopy, after resolution of the acute attack, to rule out an underlying malignancy that may mimic chronic inflammation and fibrosis associated with previous attacks of diverticulitis [2–7]. Incidental colonic pathology may also be identified, which could require preoperative management or a change in intraoperative management.

The surgeon should assess each patient for comorbidities, including cardiopulmonary problems, diabetes, and hypertension that may affect postoperative recovery and outcomes. Routine bloodwork should be checked. Appropriate consultation should be arranged to risk-stratify patients and to help optimize or correct any reversible medical condition. A preoperative anesthesia consult may be appropriate to discuss options for postoperative pain control, including placement of an epidural catheter, TAP blocks, patient-controlled analgesia (PCA), bolus narcotics, and nonsteroidal anti-inflammatory drugs (NSAIDs).

Mechanical bowel preparation (MBP) with preoperative oral antibiotics is typically recommended for elective diverticular resection. When used in combination with oral antibiotics, MBP reduces the rates of SSI, anastomotic leak, readmission, and length of stay in comparison with other methods of bowel preparation [8–12]. Patients should also receive preoperative intravenous antibiotics administered within 60 minutes of the skin incision. The choice of antibiotics should be determined by the local patterns of resistance. There is no benefit to continuing antibiotics postoperatively in the absence of fecal contamination or persistent abscess.

All patients require DVT chemoprophylaxis with low-molecular-weight heparin and the addition of mechanical prophylaxis in high-risk patients as outlined in published guidelines [13].

Ureteric injuries in colorectal surgery are relatively uncommon, with estimates from large retrospective series and database studies varying between 0.24% and 1.9% [14–16]. They are more commonly associated with surgery for diverticular disease than for cancer [17, 18]. Prophylactic ureteric stents can be a useful adjunct to aid in the identification of the ureter during surgery, especially in complex cases where identification is expected to be challenging due to inflammation or fibrosis. Current guidelines suggest that ureteral stents may be used at the discretion of the surgeon, and that in less complicated cases, the risks may outweigh the benefits [1]. Despite what makes good common sense, there is no level one evidence demonstrating that prophylactic ureteric stents prevent or decrease iatrogenic ureteric injuries. However, they do aid in the intraoperative identification of ureteric injuries and a recent study demonstrated a trend toward increased use of stents in surgery for diverticulitis [19].

Though ureteral injuries are rare, the implications for the patient and surgeon are significant. Routine intraoperative identification of the left ureter should be undertaken in all diverticular cases as the anatomy is often distorted and the safety of the ureter is unclear [17]. While ureteral stents are believed to assist in early intraoperative identification of ureteric injuries, the majority of iatrogenic ureteric injuries are still recognized in the postoperative period [14, 18]. Besides adding to operative time, ureteral stents are not benign and come with risks including hematuria (typically self-limited), urinary tract infection, oliguria, secondary hydronephrosis from poststent obstruction, and ureteric injury during insertion [16, 17, 20]. Stent use may be limited by the availability of equipment or expertise, including easy access to urologic surgeons. Extra effort should be made to coordinate complex cases with urology in instances where ureteric stents might be particularly helpful [21].

Surgical technique plays an important role in ureteric identification and preservation. While open resection allows direct tactile feedback, identification of the ureter with minimally invasive techniques primarily relies on visual confirmation of its location and integrity, limiting the value of plain ureteric stents. Newer technologies to assist in ureteric identification during laparoscopy include lighted ureteric stents [20, 22]. Alternative strategies for ureteral identification with augmented reality employing infrared fluorescence and hyperspectral imaging are currently being investigated [17, 23].

Positioning

Surgery is performed in the lithotomy position under general anesthesia. The patient must be placed with their buttocks at the edge of the table to allow access to the anus for proctoscopy and reconstruction. The thighs should be level with the abdomen to facilitate access to the splenic flexure. For laparoscopic cases, the patient should be fixed to the operating table either with foam padding and tape, a strap across the chest, or with a bean bag to accommodate significant position changes, which aid with retraction and exposure. Both arms should be padded and tucked to permit dissection from either side of the patient, as required. A urinary catheter is inserted to decompress the bladder, aiding exposure during the pelvic dissection and helping to guide postoperative fluid management.

Open surgery also requires the lithotomy position with level thighs to allow for placement of the abdominal retractor of choice. Both arms can be placed perpendicular to the patient, provided they are well-padded and supported.

Surgical Principles and Operative Techniques

A number of principles are common to all diverticular surgeries and should be followed to ensure that the dissection proceeds safely and efficiently.

1. There are three distinct anatomic approaches to rectosigmoid resection for diverticular disease: medial to lateral, lateral to medial, and superior (flexure first). Surgeons should be familiar with all three approaches as each one has its own distinct advantages, making it preferable in specific situations regardless of the operative technique.
2. Surgical planes are typically identified away from significant fibrosis or chronic inflammation and followed back toward trouble; *"easy to hard"* and *"known to unknown."*
3. Work from all sides of the problem; *"circling like a wolf."* The most involved segment can often be reduced and isolated to a more reasonable segment that is clearly seen and safely divided. This will minimize the amount of bladder or vagina that is injured when dissecting a fistula.
4. Early identification of structures that are involved through inflammation (ureter, bladder, or vagina) helps to plan the optimal approach, minimizing collateral damage.
5. Often, the pelvis is obliterated with an inflamed and fixed sigmoid colon that is folded over the rectum. Identification of the lateral pelvic gutter on either side of the rectum allows entry into the pelvis and identification of the borders of the sigmoid colon, which facilitates dissection of the colon out of the pelvis prior to resection.

Operative Technique

Laparoscopic Approach

There is increasing level 1 evidence supporting the use of laparoscopic and minimally invasive techniques for the elective operative treatment of diverticulitis, and when the appropriate surgical expertise is available, a laparoscopic resection is considered the standard of care. When laparoscopic approaches are successful, they contribute to improved recovery, quicker return of bowel function, decreased length of stay, less adhesions, and decreased complications, including pulmonary, cardiovascular, and wound infections [24–29]. Long-term benefits include a decrease in incisional hernias and improved quality of life. However, surgeons must be flexible, incorporating hand-assisted laparoscopic surgery, hybrid approaches, and open surgery as necessary, choosing the most appropriate technique based on patient and disease factors. There should be a low threshold to convert to an open approach when confronted with a situation that makes laparoscopy unsafe, such as elevated body mass index, poor visibility, or severe fibrosis due to inflammation, adhesions, previous radiation, or unexpectedly complex disease. Recently reported conversion rates range anywhere from 5% to 20% depending on the series [25–28]. As expected, conversion from a minimally invasive to open technique is associated with slower return of bowel function, increased need for opioid analgesics, increased length of stay, and higher complication rates [27, 28].

Hand-Assisted Laparoscopic Approach

Hand-assisted laparoscopic surgery offers the benefits of both laparoscopy and open surgery and may facilitate safe resection while minimizing incisional morbidity in cases of smoldering diverticulitis or significant fibrosis [30]. Advantages include improved retraction of the abdominal viscera for better visibility, improved countertraction for dissection, and tactile feedback. This approach can be particularly useful when there is dense adhesive fibrosis of a relatively short segment of colon at the level of the pelvic brim. The tactile feedback available with a hand in the abdomen helps to guide finger dissection in the appropriate plane and allows a safer application of force than may be transmitted with laparoscopic instruments. We typically employ a lower midline or Pfannenstiel incision to facilitate placement of the gel port for access to the sigmoid colon around the level of the pelvic brim. When compared to open colectomy, hand-assisted surgery is associated with shorter hospital stay and lower complication rates [31].

The location of the hand port must be chosen carefully, as it should fulfill two functions. First, the chosen site must allow adequate visualization with the laparoscope and unrestricted use of the laparoscopic instruments. Ideally, the hand port site is also used for specimen extraction and preparation of the proximal colon for anastomosis. The port may be placed at the start of the procedure or, more commonly, when the area of difficulty is identified after the initial dissection is completed.

Hybrid Approach

The hybrid approach encourages laparoscopic mobilization where it is safe to do so, and conversion to an open approach for the most difficult or demanding portions of the resection. Laparoscopy can facilitate mobilization of the colon remote from the area of disease, such as the splenic flexure and transverse colon, to allow adequate length to create a tension-free anastomosis. The open incision can be limited to the lower midline or a Pfannenstiel, which is typically well tolerated and has less effect on postoperative respiratory muscle splinting.

Robotic Approach

Minimally invasive techniques have expanded to include the use of robotic-assisted surgery as a routine and standard approach to colon resection. The feasibility and safety of robotic-assisted sigmoidectomy has been demonstrated, and there is wide uptake and growing adoption of robotic technology worldwide in the treatment of almost every surgical disease including diverticular disease. The reported advantages include surgeon-controlled three-dimensional high-definition optics, a stable platform, and improved strength and articulation of instruments. Published series suggest that the conversion rate may be lower for robotic surgery when compared to laparoscopic surgery, but the series are small. The biggest disadvantages include the learning curve, longer operating times, and the significant increase in cost [30, 32]. Additional prospective studies are required to further assess the risks, benefits, and costs of this technique relative to laparoscopic surgery although surgeons and institutions have accepted this technology with wide spread adoption andimplementation [33].

Open Approach

Laparotomy, or open surgical technique, was for many years the standard against which other surgical approaches were measured and remains the technique of choice for the most difficult resections. Laparotomy may allow visualization and exposure not easily attainable with a minimally invasive approach. It permits immediate tactile feedback for dissection, including finger fracture, which may be the only safe method to separate densely adherent tissue secondary to inflammation and fibrosis. Open technique is the approach of choice in patients who lack adequate abdominal domain for laparoscopy owing to body habitus, abdominal wall defects, previous inflammatory conditions, or previous intra-abdominal surgery. It remains the default option when a surgeon is uncomfortable proceeding with a minimally invasive technique, and conversion should not be viewed as either failure or a complication. The procedure is performed through a midline incision from just above the umbilicus to the symphysis. The incision is extended superiorly if splenic flexure mobilization is required. It may be preceeded by a laparoscopic mobilization of the splenic flexure to decrease the size of the midline incision.

Minimally Invasive Technique: Technical Description

The intra-abdominal portion of the surgery is similar for all four techniques. The following is a detailed description of the minimally invasive technique:

The surgeon stands on the right side of the patient with his assistant to his left to control the camera. The monitor is located on the left side at the level of the left hip perpendicular to the surgeon's sight line. After suitable prepping and draping under general anesthesia with endotracheal intubation, the abdomen is accessed through a midline supra-umbilical incision under direct vision or through a Verres needle for insufflation with CO_2. We use a 10 mm supraumbilical port and two additional 5 mm ports placed under direct vision in the right lower and upper quadrants, spacing them one hand width apart. A third 5 mm port is placed in the left lower quadrant and located as necessary for countertraction. An additional 10 mm port should be available to convert one of the 5 mm ports to accept 10 mm instruments. The operative set should include atraumatic bowel graspers, endoscopic scissors, hook cautery, and the preferred energy device, either bipolar or ultrasonic energy devices. We also use a wound protector/retractor at our extraction site to decrease postoperative wound infection [34]. The operative table should be free to move into steep Trendelenburg, reverse Trendelenburg, and right and left lateral rotation, as required. Positioning depends on patient characteristics, anatomic differences, and the area of dissection.

Sigmoid Mobilization

The *medial approach* is commonly used in minimally invasive surgery.

Dissecting the Mesosigmoid Plane Following port placement, the omentum is lifted superiorly and placed above the transverse colon. The patient is placed in a slight Trendelenburg and rotated toward the right to move the small bowel out of the way to expose the medial aspect of the sigmoid mesentery. The sigmoid is lifted anteriorly, placing the mesentery under tension, and an incision is made 1–2 cm above the base of the right leaf of the sigmoid mesentery at the level of the sacral promontory. Although it is not necessary to perform a complete mesosigmoid dissection for benign disease, we recommend using this plane when possible, as it is bloodless, easy to dissect, and very familiar to surgeons performing colorectal surgery. The areolar plane between the mesosigmoid/mesorectal fascia and the retroperitoneal fascia is dissected sharply with cautery. While we prefer scissors, a hook is also appropriate.

Separating the Retroperitoneal Structures Dissection proceeds superiorly to the origin of the superior rectal vessels, inferiorly to the level of the sacral promontory, and laterally behind the mesosigmoid within the areolar tissue until the left ureter is identified and swept posteriorly. The ureter should be covered with a fine layer of investing fascia, and if clearly exposed, the dissection is too deep. The ureter is commonly identified as it crosses the bifurcation of the internal and external iliac vessels with its characteristic vermiculation. Explore this area carefully to reduce the amount of bleeding, as pooling may inhibit identification of important landmarks and structures. In situations of chronic inflammation and fibrosis, the surgeon may be forced unknowingly into the retroperitoneum, where the tissue is softer, causing dissection behind the ureter. In this instance, the ureter will be located on the underside of the elevated lateral peritoneum. Chronic inflammation may also cause the ureter to be pulled medially toward the midline, which may make it difficult to identify. The right ureter is usually lateral out of harm's way; however, in the case of significant retroperitoneal fibrosis, it may also be drawn medially and be subject to injury. The ureters must be identified prior to division of any significant structures. Similarly, the hypogastric nerves should be identified and preserved. They run over the aorta and coalesce into two nerves medial to the iliac vessels behind the investing fascia of the retroperitoneum. Once the plane is established posteriorly, the sigmoid is pulled medially, and any secondary adhesions between the sigmoid and the pelvic sidewall are taken down. The peritoneum is then opened sharply with cautery to connect with the mesosigmoid dissection.

In instances of significant inflammation, the sigmoid may be fused to the lateral side wall, making it difficult to identify and dissect the plane between the leaves of the peritoneum. Start the dissection superiorly away from trouble, where the peritoneal surfaces are easily identified. With inflammation, the planes are often preserved, as opposed to with malignancy, where the plane has been violated. Judicious use of traction and distraction of the peritoneal surfaces attacking the scarred area from all sides will reduce the dissection to a more manageable footprint. Often, the dissection can be performed with an inferior-to-superior approach. Make sure that the location of the ureter is known at all times. The ureter may have to be identified superiorly and followed inferiorly, dissecting structures off the medial surface. This is often the most difficult part of the dissection and may take considerable time. Inability to identify this plane safely or to ensure the integrity of the ureter are reasons to convert to a hand-assisted or an open approach.

The *lateral approach* is useful when there is considerable inflammation in the mesosigmoid with tethering and shortening of the mesentery, inhibiting the ability to provide tension for dissection, or when there are significant lateral adhesions.

The sigmoid is lifted anteriorly and medially to place the lateral leaf of the sigmoid mesentery under tension. Any secondary inflammatory adhesions present between the lateral pelvic sidewall and the sigmoid colon are released at this time. An incision is made in the peritoneum at the base of the mesentery. Following identification of the retroperitoneal fascia, the dissection is extended sharply with cautery in the areolar plane between the retroperitoneal fascia and the fascia of the mesosigmoid. The ureter and the remaining retroperitoneal structures are identified behind the retroperitoneal fascia and are preserved. The sigmoid sulcus, when present, is a reliable landmark for locating the left ureter. It is a pit-like depression at the base of the lateral leaf of the sigmoid mesentery, superior to the iliac bifurcation, which is directly anterior to the left ureter.

The dissection is completed posteriorly behind the mesosigmoid from the lateral to the medial side of the sigmoid mesentery, where the medial peritoneal leaf is incised, extending the peritoneal opening inferiorly to the sacral promontory and superiorly to the origin of the superior rectal vessels, and separating the mesosigmoid from the retroperitoneal structures sharply with cautery as outlined above. Similarly, the right ureter should be identified and preserved along with the hypogastric nerves.

The *superior approach* is less commonly used but may be necessary when there is significant inflammation in the upper sigmoid and the descending colon extending into the retroperitoneum, and when the splenic flexure will require mobilization. This approach centers around mobilization of the descending colon and splenic flexure first, as described below, to establish the dissection plane in normal tissue prior to approaching the area of retroperitoneal fibrosis and the base of the mesentery. Identification of this plane superiorly may assist in the dissection of the mesosigmoid as described above. The principles of dissection are applied, moving toward the area of difficulty with the identification and preservation of the ureters. It may be helpful to divide the descending colon early in an area of soft, pliable bowel proximal to the inflammation. This may improve traction and countertraction for the identification of the surgical planes.

Vascular Ligation

High ligation of the inferior mesenteric artery is not required for benign disease unless additional length is needed. Typically, the superior rectal artery is ligated just distal to the origin of the left colic artery, with ligation and division of the artery and vein. Vascular ligation may be accomplished with the application of an energy device, vascular clips, staples, or suture. All major vessels are doubly ligated for security. Although the artery and vein can be ligated together, we prefer to ligate them separately to preserve mobility.

It is not necessary to preserve the superior rectal vessels to improve rectal blood supply for anastomosis as there is no increase in complications such as anastomotic leak when comparing division versus preservation [35–38]. However, on occasion, the mesosigmoid plane may be obliterated with excessive fibrosis, making safe dissection impossible. In this situation, it may be best to dissect intramesenterically, staying anterior to the superior rectal vessel and leaving it intact [2, 36–38].

Splenic Flexure Mobilization

Typically, complete mobilization of the splenic flexure is not required if there is redundancy in the remaining descending and/or upper sigmoid colon. When part of the descending colon is resected due to involvement with inflammation or if the rectum has been damaged due to pelvic abscess or fistula, splenic flexure mobilization may be necessary to perform a tension-free anastomosis [39].

Lateral Dissection Mobilization of the splenic flexure to the midline is always the initial maneuver. The descending colon is retracted medially, and the peritoneum is incised just medial to the line of Toldt (the reflected edge of the retroperitoneal fascia) at the level of the upper sigmoid colon and continued proximally toward the splenic flexure. Sharp dissection with cautery is used to lift the left colon and its accompanying mesentery, which is rotated medially away from the retroperitoneum, with dissection progressing toward the splenic flexure, mobilizing the colon and rotating it toward the midline. Dissection too lateral and too deep may cause entry into the retroperitoneum, posterior to the kidney, into the retroperitoneal fat.

The dissection should be relatively bloodless, and the retroperitoneal investing fascia should be left intact, identifying and preserving the left gonadal vessels and the left ureter beneath it. Excessive bleeding implies an incorrect plane of dissection. Prior to completing mobilization of the splenic flexure, any attachments between the spleen and the colon are divided to avoid tearing of the splenic capsule. Avoid pulling downward on the splenic flexure, as this may also cause bleeding. The peritoneal incision is extended superiorly toward the splenic flexure approximately 1–2 cm lateral to the edge of the colon, medial to the reflected edge of the retroperitoneal fascia, and inferomedially to the spleen. The flexure is lifted medially to expose the retroperitoneal fascia along with the renocolic ligaments and the splenocolic ligaments, which are divided sharply with cautery or an energy device to release the splenic flexure from Gerota's fascia. The mobilization is continued medially, dividing the peritoneum superior to the colon and inferior to the lower border of the pancreas until the left colon is suspended on its mesentery at the midline. The omentum is separated from the left transverse colon with sharp dissection using cautery or an energy device until the left edge of the lesser sac is entered.

Superior Dissection The dissection can be started at the transverse colon. The omentum is lifted superiorly above the transverse colon. Beginning to the left of the middle colic vessels, the omentum is separated from the transverse colon by dividing the fusion plane with cautery and breaking into the lesser sac (Pauchet maneuver). The omentum is separated from any lateral attachments to the peritoneum at the splenic flexure. Care is needed to avoid putting traction on any attachments to the spleen. Next, the peritoneum at the inferior border of the pancreas is divided, lifting the colon and its mesentery off the retroperitoneum. The peritoneal incision is continued distally around the splenic flexure approximately 1–2 cm from the edge of the colon, continuing to lift the colon and its mesentery off the retroperitoneal (Gerota's) fascia. The dissection is continued inferiorly and medially, keeping the retroperitoneal fascia intact until the splenic flexure and descending colon are mobilized toward the midline.

Lengthening Maneuvers and Medial Dissection Following medialization of the descending colon, if additional length is required, a series of sequential steps can be undertaken. Provided the rectum is soft and pliable, it may be possible to mobilize the proximal rectum using the mesorectal plane. An additional two centimeters may be gained in this fashion by lifting the rectum out of the sacral hollow.

Additional measures include vascular mobilization, which is accomplished through a medial dissection. The inferior mesenteric artery is skeletonized and divided 1–2 cm from its origin. Care must be taken to preserve the marginal artery for the viability of the descending colon. The mesentery of the descending colon is lifted and the peritoneum incised lateral to the duodenal flexure/ligament of Treitz and posterior to the inferior mesenteric vein [40]. The plane between Gerota's fascia and the mesentery of the descending colon is developed with a combination of sharp and blunt dissection, both laterally and superiorly, to mobilize the entire descending colon to the flexure. The dissection is continued superiorly to the inferior border of the pancreas, where the inferior mesenteric vein is dissected, ligated, and divided [40]. This will provide an additional 5–10 cm in colonic mobility. Examine the distal descending colon for viability, as the resection margin may have to be revised. In this situation, be wary of using the upper sigmoid colon for the proximal anastomotic margin, as the blood supply will be tenuous.

Each of these maneuvers should be performed sequentially, testing the colon for adequate length after each maneuver to minimize any unnecessary manipulation of the colon and its blood supply.

Resection Margins

The distal resection margin should be at the level of the upper rectum to ensure that all of the sigmoid and its diverticula are removed. This prevents recurrent disease from retained sigmoid diverticula attached to the rectal stump [41, 42]. Once the proximal rectum is mobilized, a suitable region of soft rectum is chosen at the level of the sacral promontory where the tenia coli splay. The mesorectum is exposed, and the mesentery is divided using a pinch burn technique with an energy device. When dissecting laparoscopically, the instruments may be angulated; make sure that the mesentery is divided perpendicular to the bowel with no coning to ensure that the remaining bowel has adequate blood supply. Once cleared of mesentery, the rectum is divided at this level, perpendicular to its axis, with an endoscopic transverse stapler. This may take more than one firing. Occasionally, the upper rectum is involved with fibrosis due to chronic pelvic inflammation. In this case, the upper rectum will require mobilization with resection down to soft healthy tissue to ensure a safe anastomosis.

The proximal resection margin should be located in soft, disease-free colon without induration or muscular hypertrophy and with good blood supply. It is not necessary to remove all of the diverticula. Typically, the diseased segment is confined to the sigmoid such that the proximal resection margin is in the upper sigmoid or at the junction between the descending and sigmoid colon. Occasionally, the disease is located in the descending colon, which necessitates removing additional descending colon.

Specimen Extraction

Specimen extraction is performed through either a lower midline or Pfannenstiel incision or by enlarging the supra-umbilical port. A wound protector is placed to protect the wound and to serve as a retractor [34]. A suitable piece of soft proximal colon is identified in an area that is free from diverticula as outlined above. The colon is divided transversely, either with a stapler or between atraumatic bowel clamps, and the specimen is handed off.

Anastomosis

A full-thickness purse-string suture of polypropylene is placed in the proximal end of the colon, and a suitably sized anvil is introduced. The purse string is drawn tight such that the bowel edge is flush with the anvil's stem. Every attempt should be made to avoid the inclusion of individual diverticula in the staple line of the anastomosis. When present, the diverticulum can be sutured tightly to the stem using a second suture to pull it away from the staple line and include it in the resected tissue doughnut. At this point, the proximal margin with anvil in place is returned to the abdomen, the extraction incision is closed, and the abdomen is re-insufflated. If the supra-umbilical port is used for extraction, the closure is performed with two opposing sutures, which are used to resecure the Hasson trocar for re-insufflation (rather than tying the sutures immediately). The anastomosis is completed by introducing the stapler into the rectal stump, advancing the trocar through the rectal wall adjacent to the transverse staple line, and engaging the anvil. As the stapler is closed, the gun is withdrawn slightly so that the tissue at the top of the rectal stump is not under tension when the stapler is closed. After closing the stapler and just prior to firing, we wait about 30 seconds to let the tissue between the anvil and stapler equilibrate. If there is any question of tension on the anastomosis from attachments on the proximal colon, additional mobilization should be performed at this time. An air leak test is performed to ensure the integrity of the anastomosis using a rigid or flexible sigmoidoscope [1]. Any identified leaks between staples can be reinforced with suture, and the anastomosis retested. A significant air leak or visible mucosa requires complete anastomotic revision with resection, reanastomosis and retesting. The two tissue doughnuts are inspected for integrity and the presence of staples in the distaldoughnut. If no staples present then the anastomosis is at risk due to a strip of ischemic rectal wall between the transverse staple line and the circular staple line. The transverse and circular staple line should be reinforced with imbricating suture to prevent anastomotic leak.

Closure

The abdomen and port sites are closed in the usual fashion. Local anesthetic in the form of a TAP block or local infiltration is performed at this time [43].

Complex Disease

Fistula

Enteric fistulae are relatively common complications of diverticulitis where the infection penetrates into a neighboring pelvic structure. The most common structures include the urinary bladder, vagina, small intestine, colon, and skin. Rarely is the ureter or uterus involved.

Surgical principles include the following:

1. Resection of the affected segment of colon back to soft normal colonic tissue without muscular hypertrophy.
2. Preservation of the secondarily involved structure with minimal dissection, provided that malignancy has been ruled out; repair this structure as required.
3. Interposition of the omentum, if possible, between the repair and the new anastomosis to prevent recurrence. Mobilization of the omentum off the transverse colon with formation of a pedicle based on a major omental vessel may be required to reach the pelvis.

Colovesical Fistula

Typically, the fistula is located in the dome of the bladder. Occasionally, it may be posterior, closer to the trigone. Preoperative imaging should aid in identification and localization.

Patients typically present with either recurrent urinary tract infection or pneumaturia. Surgery is usually semi-elective, and recurrent urinary tract infection can be temporarily suppressed preoperatively with antibiotics if necessary. A colovesical fistula can be approached laparoscopically, hand-assisted, open, or hybrid, depending on disease factors (degree of inflammation, scarring, visibility), patient factors (body habitus, previous surgery), and the skill set of the surgeon [44]. It is easiest to divide the fistula prior to resection of the sigmoid.

The initial surgical approach to the fistula should be at a place where the natural plane is preserved. Dissection should proceed from all sides to minimize the intervening footprint and damage to the bladder. When using an open or hand port technique, a finger fracture can be very useful. Occasionally, the fistula may have closed over, and the bladder mucosa may not have to be entered. If the defect is small, the mucosa is not visible with a minimal defect in the muscular wall, then there is no need to repair the bladder, as it will close on its own. Larger defects in the muscular wall with or without visible bladder mucosa should be repaired in two layers using absorbable sutures to prevent the formation of a diverticulum. A standard sigmoid resection to include the fistula site with primary anastomosis is performed. Whenever possible, an omental pedicle should be placed between the anastomosis and the repair to minimize the chance of fistula recurrence.

Postoperatively, the urinary catheter should be retained for 1 week. If the hole has required suture repair, a retrograde cystogram is performed prior to removal of the catheter. In the absence of a repair, a cystogram is not required. One study suggests that a routine postoperative cystogram after surgery for enterovesical fistula may not be necessary for all patients if the bladder is drained for 1–2 weeks after bowel resection [45].

Colovaginal Fistula

Most (95%) colovaginal diverticular fistulas occur in the setting of a previous hysterectomy, as the uterus typically protects the vagina from contact with the colon [46]. The principles are similar to those for a colovesical fistula; dissect the surrounding attachments to reduce the footprint of the involved vagina to a minimum, in order to preserve as much vagina as possible. The remaining vaginal tissue should be soft and pliable to take a suture. Close the defect with an absorbable suture in a single layer. Again, whenever possible, interpose an omental pedicle.

Coloenteric Fistula

These fistulas are less common. Often, a number of small bowel loops may have walled off the area and require careful separation to expose the primary fistula site. Provided the small intestinal defect is less than 30% of the circumference, and the remaining small intestine is normal, primary repair can be performed. In the case of a larger defect or if there is questionable tissue integrity or the potential for luminal narrowing with repair, a formal wedge resection should be performed with either a handsewn or stapled anastomosis.

Stricture

Diverticular strictures are treated with primary resection back to normal tissue. When the stricture has prevented visualization of the mucosa to rule out concomitant malignancy, the colonic segment should be removed using oncologic principles. In addition, there is the option for endoscopic management in select cases [47].

Abscess

Occasionally, during dissection, a small residual abscess is present. These are usually sterile, but prior to resection, the abscess should be drained to prevent spillage and contamination. Dissect the surrounding structures systematically, preserving them as much as possible. Often, there is a significant amount of fibrosis due to chronic inflammation, which may preclude preservation, necessitating resection. In most cases the presence of a small abscess need not alter post operative wound management and the surgical incisions can be closed primarily. However, if there is any question of contamination of the surgical wound(s) many surgeons choose to only loosely approximate the skin with staples or suture to allow the wound to sit open with packing to facilitate drainage. With conscientious wound care these wounds subsequently heal by secondary intention avoiding the morbidity of a wound infection. When available a wound vac dressing may also be advantageous. A wound specialist or specialist wound care team can be a valuable resource in supporting these patients through their recovery.

Defunctioning Loop Ileostomy

All patients who are undergoing colorectal resection should have preoperative informed consent for a potential ostomy. While this is less likely to occur in an elective setting, the creation of a defunctioning loop ileostomy to protect a colorectal anastomosis depends on both patient factors and intraoperative findings [48, 49]. In the case of a positive leak test between staples, the anastomosis can be repaired with suture, imbricating the defect, and the anastomosis retested. However, if there is any question as to the integrity of the initial anastomosis, the anastomosis should be resected and revised. This should typically be possible without undue technical challenge in cases of a high colorectal anastomosis in the proximal rectum in patients with a typical pattern of sigmoid diverticular disease and a healthy pliable rectum. In the less frequent instance where the sigmoid colon has folded on itself and the inflammatory process has filled the pelvis secondarily involving the upper to mid rectum, one might find that a low anterior resection is required to carry the distal extent of the dissection into soft and healthy rectum to facilitate anastomosis. In this situation, re resection with further distal dissection to create a more distal anastomosis might prove quite challenging secondary to dissection in a hostile field. Consideration should be given to the creation of a defunctioning loop ileostomy. Persistent leakage following repair/revision or an inability to repair or revise an anastomosis mandates a defunctioning loop ileostomy plus or minus pelvic drainage.

The ability of an anastomosis to heal depends to a large extent on the quality of the intestine used for the anastomosis. While the proximal end can be resected back to a healthy, well-vascularized colon, additional resection on the rectal side creates a lower anastomosis with a higher risk of leak. A defunctioning loop ileostomy may be indicated in a situation where the consequences of a leak outweigh the presence of a stoma and a second operation for closure. However, primary anastomosis with a diverting ileostomy is still preferable to a Hartmann's procedure.

Patients with significant risk factors for anastomotic leak or decreased physiologic reserve with an inability to tolerate sepsis or re-laparotomy may also benefit from a defunctioning ileostomy. Risk factors for anastomotic leak include smoking, weight loss or poor nutrition, and chronic immunosuppression (e.g., steroids) [48, 49]. Defunctioning ileostomy does not prevent anastomotic leak but mitigates the clinical impact and reduces the risk of reoperation following an anastomotic leak.

Results

Studies suggest decreased postoperative complications and costs for procedures completed in a minimally invasive fashion versus open or converted cases [50, 51]. However, it is difficult to separate patient and disease factors from the decision to convert and the subsequent postoperative course. Evidence of patient-reported outcomes of bowel function and quality of life following elective resection for diverticular disease is accruing, but high-quality evidence is lacking [51–55]. It is difficult to know if statistically significant differences in quality of life or bowel function measures reflect meaningful real-world differences in patient quality of life. Following successful elective resection for diverticular disease, short-term risks include perioperative medical complications and anastomotic leak (1–10%), and short-to-medium-term risks include the need for re-intervention, which may occur in up to 15% of patients undergoing resection [53].

The risk of recurrent diverticulitis ranges from 4% to 11%, with a minority of patients requiring a second surgery [53, 56]. Current individualized approaches to sigmoid resection should weigh quality of life and the risk of repeated episodes of diverticulitis against the morbidity and possible complications of resection and the knowledge that a small subset of patients experience recurrence even after resection.

Conclusion

Despite the introduction of minimally invasive surgical techniques such as laparoscopic and robotic approaches, elective surgery for diverticular disease continues to present a dynamic challenge to general and colorectal surgeons. The inflammatory process can result in altered anatomy and distorted or abolished tissue planes, forcing a surgeon to marshal their anatomic knowledge to inform intraoperative decision making and to navigate what can be a very challenging operation. Surgical success requires sound preoperative planning and technical skill using an analytic and flexible approach to identify areas of safety and challenge throughout the dissection. The appropriate use of first principles including the three anatomic approaches (medial to lateral, lateral to medial, flexure first), beginning dissection in unaltered surgical planes ("easy to hard, known to unknown"), working around difficult areas of adhesion orinflammation to reduce the footprint ("circle like a wolf"), and identification and protection of critical structures including ureter, bladder, and vagina are critical consideration for operative success and good patient outcomes.

References

1. Feingold D, Steele SR, Lee S, et al. Practice parameters for the treatment of sigmoid diverticulitis. Dis Colon Rectum. 2014;57:284–94.
2. Brar MS, Roxin G, Yaffe PB, Stanger J, et al. Colonoscopy following nonoperative management of uncomplicated diverticulitis may not be warranted. Dis Colon Rectum. 2013;56(11):1259–64.
3. de Vries HS, Boerma D, Timmer R, van Ramshorst B, et al. Routine colonoscopy is not required in uncomplicated diverticulitis: a systematic review. Surg Endosc. 2014;28(7):2039–47.
4. Andrade P, Ribeiro A, Ramalho R, Lopes S, Macedo G. Routine colonoscopy after acute uncomplicated diverticulitis – challenging a putative indication. Dig Surg. 2017;34(3):197–202.
5. Suhardja TS, Norhadi S, Seah EZ, Rodgers-Wilson S. Is early colonoscopy after CT-diagnosed diverticulitis still necessary? Int J Color Dis. 2017;32(4):485–9.
6. Lau KC, Spilsbury K, Faoorque Y, Kariyawasam SB, et al. Is colonoscopy still mandatory after a CT diagnosis of left-sided diverticulitis: can colorectal cancer be confidently excluded? Dis Colon Rectum. 2011;54(10):1265–70.
7. Agarwal AK, Karanjawala BE, Maykel JA, Johnson EK, Steele SR. Routine colonic endoscopic evaluation following resolution of acute diverticulitis: is it necessary? World J Gastroenterol. 2014;20(35):12509–16.
8. Toneva GD, Deierhoi RJ, Morris M, et al. Oral antibiotic bowel preparation reduces length of stay and readmissions after colorectal surgery. J Am Coll Surg. 2013;216:756–62.
9. Ohman KA, Wan L, Guthrie T, et al. Combination of oral antibiotics and mechanical bowel preparation reduces surgical site infection in colorectal surgery. J Am Coll Surg. 2017;225:465–71.
10. Morris MS, Graham LA, Chu DI, Cannon JA, Hawn MT. Oral antibiotic bowel preparation significantly reduces surgical site infection rates and readmission rates in elective colorectal surgery. Ann Surg. 2015;261:1034–40.

11. Scarborough JE, Mantyh CR, Sun Z, Migaly J. Combined mechanical and oral antibiotic bowel preparation reduces incisional surgical site infection and anastomotic leak rates after elective colorectal resection: an analysis of colectomy-targeted ACS NSQIP. Ann Surg. 2015;262:331–7.
12. Kiran RP, Murray AC, Chiuzan C, Estrada D, Forde K. Combined preoperative mechanical bowel preparation with oral antibiotics significantly reduces surgical site infection, anastomotic leak, and ileus after colorectal surgery. Ann Surg. 2015;262:416–25.
13. Fleming F, Gaertner W, Ternent CA, Finlayson E, Herzig D, Paquette IM, Feingold DL, Steele SR. Clinical practice guidelines for the prevention of venous thromboembolic disease in colorectal surgery. Dis Colon Rectum. 2018;61:14–20.
14. Palaniappa NC, Telem DA, Ranasinghe NE, Divino CM. Incidence of iatrogenic ureteral injury after laparoscopic colectomy. Arch Surg. 2012;147:267–71.
15. Kutiyanawala MA, Scott ADN, Jameson J. Ureteric injuries during colorectal surgery: strategies for prevention. Color Dis. 1999;1:334–7.
16. Halabi WJ, Jafari MD, Nguyen VQ, et al. Ureteral injuries in colorectal surgery: an analysis of trends, outcomes, and risk factors over a 10-year period in the United States. Dis Colon Rectum. 2014;57:179–86.
17. Douissard J, Meyer J, Ris F, et al. Iatrogenic ureteral injuries and their prevention in colorectal surgery: results from a nationwide survey. Color Dis. 2019;21:595–602.
18. Coakley KM, Kasten KR, Sims SM, Prasad T, et al. Prophylactic ureteral catheters for colectomy: a National Surgical Quality Improvement Program-based analysis. Dis Colon Rectum. 2019;61:84–8.
19. Chiu AS, et al. Trends of ureteral stent usage in surgery for diverticulitis. J Surg Res. 2018;222:203–11.
20. Boyan WP Jr, Lavy D, Dinallo A, Otero J, et al. Lighted ureteral stents in laparoscopic colorectal surgery; a five-year experience. Ann Transl Med. 2017;5(3):44.
21. Mahmoud NN, Riddle EW. Minimally invasive surgery for complicated diverticulitis. J Gastrointest Surg. 2017;21:731–8.
22. Borowiec AM, Gill RS, Birch DW, Karmali S. The utility of lighted ureteral stents in laparoscopic colorectal resection: a survey of Canadian surgeons. Gastroenterology Res. 2011;4(4):143–8.
23. Osumi W, Yamamoto M, Taniguchi K, et al. Clinical experience with near-infrared ray catheter, a fluorescent ureteral catheter, on laparoscopic surgery for colon diverticulitis: a case report. Medicine (Baltimore). 2021;100(21):e26085. https://doi.org/10.1097/MD.0000000000026085. PMID: 34032744; PMCID: PMC8154449.
24. Purkayastha S, Constantinides VA, Tekkis PP, Athanasiou T, et al. Laparoscopic vs. open surgery for diverticular disease: a meta-analysis of nonrandomized studies. Dis Colon Rectum. 2006;49(4):446–63.
25. Klarenbeek BR, Veenhof AA, Bergamaschi R, et al. Laparoscopic sigmoid resection for diverticulitis decreases major morbidity rates: a randomized control trial. Ann Surg. 2009;249:39–44.
26. Gervaz P, Inan I, Perneger T, Schiffer E, Morel P. A prospective randomized single-blind comparison of laparoscopic versus open sigmoid colectomy for diverticulitis. Ann Surg. 2010;252:3–8.
27. Schwenk W, Haase O, Neudecker JJ, Muller JM. Short-term benefits for laparoscopic colorectal resection. Cochrane Database Syst Rev. 2005:CD003145.
28. Masoomi H, Buchberg B, Nguyen B, Tung V, Stamos MJ, Mills S. Outcomes of laparoscopic versus open colectomy in elective surgery for diverticulitis. World J Surg. 2011;35:2143–8.
29. Wu KL, Lee KC, Liu CC, Chen HH, Lu CC. Laparoscopic versus open surgery for diverticulitis: a systematic review and meta-analysis. Dig Surg. 2017;34(3):203–15. https://doi.org/10.1159/000450683. Epub 2016 Dec 10. PMID: 27941315.
30. Lee SW, Yoo J, Dujovny N, Sonoda T, et al. Laparoscopic vs. hand-assisted laparoscopic sigmoidectomy for diverticulitis. Dis Colon Rectum. 2006;49(4):464–9.
31. Benlice C, Costedio M, Stocchi L, Abbas MA, Gorgun E. Hand-assisted laparoscopic vs open colectomy: an assessment from the American College of Surgeons National Surgical Quality Improvement Program procedure-targeted cohort. Am J Surg. 2016;212:808–13.
32. Ogilvie JW Jr, Saunders RN, Parker J, Luchtefeld MA. Sigmoidectomy for diverticulitis – a propensity-matched comparison of minimally invasive approaches. J Surg Res. 2019;243:434–9.
33. Larkins K, Mohan H, Apte SS, Chen V, Rajkomar A, Larach JT, Smart P, Heriot A, Warrier S. A systematic review and meta-analysis of robotic resections for diverticular disease. Color Dis. 2022;24(10):1105–16. https://doi.org/10.1111/codi.16227. Epub 2022 Aug 9. PMID: 35723895.
34. Edwards JP, Ho AL, Tee MC, Dixon E, Ball CG. Wound protectors reduce surgical site infection: a meta-analysis of randomized controlled trials. Ann Surg. 2012;256(1):53–9.
35. Cirocchi R, Popivanov G, Binda GA, Henry BM, Toaszewski KA, Davies RJ, Di Saverio S. Sigmoid resection for diverticular disease – to ligate or to preserve the inferior mesenteric artery? Results of a systematic review and meta analysis. Color Dis. 2091;21:623–31.
36. Lehmann RK, Brounts LR, Johnson EK, Rizzo JA, Steele SR. Does sacrifice of the inferior mesenteric artery or superior rectal artery affect anastomotic leak following sigmoidectomy for diverticulitis? Am J Surg. 2011;201:623–7.
37. Tocchi A, Mazzoni G, Fornasari V, Miccini M, Daddi G, Tagliacozzo S. Preservation of the inferior mesenteric artery in colorectal resection for complicated diverticular disease. Am J Surg. 2001;182:162–7.

38. De Nardi P, Gassetta P. Does inferior mesenteric artery ligation affect outcome in elective colonic resection for diverticular disease? ANZ J Surg. 2018;88:E778–81.
39. Schlussel AT, Wiseman JT, Kelly JF, Davids JS, Maykel JA, Sturrock PR, Seeeney WB, Alavi K. Location if everything: the role of splenic flexure mobilization during colon resection for diverticulitis. Int J Surg. 2017;40:124–9.
40. Copaescu C, Barbulescu L, Tomulescu V. Laparoscopic mobilization of the splenic flexure as the first step of restorative colorectal resection. Chirurgia (Bucur). 2019;114:268–77.
41. Thaler K, Baig MK, Berho M, et al. Determinants of recurrence after sigmoid resection for uncomplicated diverticulitis. Dis Colon Rectum. 2003;46:385–8.
42. Benn PL, Wolff BG, Ilstrup DM. Level of anastomosis and recurrent colonic diverticulitis. Am J Surg. 1986;151:269–71.
43. Keller DS, Ermlich BO, Delaney CP. Demonstrating the benefits of transversus abdominis lane blocks on patient outcomes in laparoscopic colorectal surgery: review of 200 consecutive cases. J Am Coll Surg. 2014;219:1143–8.
44. Bastawrous AL, Landmann RG, Liu Y, Liu E, et al. Incidence, associated risk factors, and impact of conversion to laparotomy in minimally invasive sigmoidectomy for diverticular disease. Surg Endosc. 2019. https://doi.org/10.1007/s00464-019-06804-z. [Epub ahead of print].
45. de Groof EJ, Bruggeman AE, Buskens CJ, Tanis PJ, Bemelman WA. Selective use of cystogram following segmental bowel resection in patients with enterovesical fistula. Color Dis. 2019;21(9):1045–50. https://doi.org/10.1111/codi.14652. Epub 2019 May 13. PMID: 30993858.
46. Berger MB, Khandwala N, Fenner DE, Burney RE. Colovaginal fistulas: presentation, evaluation, and management. Female Pelvic Med Reconstr Surg. 2016;22(5):355–8. https://doi.org/10.1097/SPV.0000000000000289. PMID: 27171321; PMCID: PMC5002240.
47. Fejleh MP, Tabibian JH. Colonoscopic management of diverticular disease. World J Gastrointest Endosc. 2020;12(2):53–9. https://doi.org/10.4253/wjge.v12.i2.53. PMID: 32064030; PMCID: PMC6965002.
48. Platell C, Barwood N, Dorfmann G, Makin G. The incidence of anastomotic leaks in patients undergoing colorectal surgery. Color Dis. 2007;9:71.
49. Konishi T, Watanabe T, Kishimoto J, Nagawa H. Risk factors for anastomotic leakage after surgery for colorectal cancer: results of prospective surveillance. J Am Coll Surg. 2006;202:439.
50. Papageorge CM, Kennedy GD, Carchman EH. National trends in short-term outcomes following non-emergent surgery for diverticular disease. J Gastrointest Surg. 2016;20:1376–87.
51. Raskin ER, Keller DS, Gorrepati ML, Akiel-fu S, et al. Propensity-matched analysis of sigmoidectomies for diverticular disease. J Soc Laparoendosc Surg. 2019;23(1):e2018.00073.
52. Goldwag JL, Lyn RV, Wilson LR, Wilson MZ, Ivatury SJ. Effect of elective sigmoidectomy for diverticulitis on bowel function patient-reported outcomes. J Surg Res. 2019;241:135–40.
53. Bolkenstein HE, Consten ECJ, van der Palen J, van de Wall BJM, et al. Long-term outcome of surgery versus conservative management for recurrent and ongoing complaints after an episode of diverticulitis. Ann Surg. 2019;269(4):612–20.
54. Lin M, Raman SR. Evaluation of quality of life and surgical outcomes for treatment of diverticular disease. Clin Colon Rectal Surg. 2018;31:251–7.
55. Andeweg CS, Berg R, Staal JB, ten Broek RPG, et al. Patient-reported outcomes after conservative or surgical management of recurrent and chronic complaints of diverticulitis: systematic review and meta-analysis. Clin Gastroenterol Hepatol. 2016;14:183–90.
56. Choi KK, Martinolich J, Canete JJ, Valerian BT, et al. Elective laparoscopic sigmoid colectomy for diverticulitis – an updated look at recurrence after surgery. J Gastrointest Surg. 2019. https://doi.org/10.1007/s11605-018-04083-y. [Epub ahead of print].

Hartmann Reversal

20

Nicole D. Bouvy, V. R. W. Di Leonardo, and Neyla Boukhili

Introduction

Hartmann's procedure is one of many types of surgical approaches used in cases of complicated diverticulitis, namely Hinchey III or Hinchey IV. The diseased segment of colon, most commonly the sigmoid, is resected, and an end colostomy is created using the descending colon proximal to the segment, leaving the rectal stump closed. Despite the commonality of this procedure, it is not without significant complications. Colostomies are associated with a slew of surgical complications, including peristomal hernias in up to 58% [1], incisional hernias in up to 52% [2], peristomal skin complications (PSC) in 36–73% of patients [3], and stoma prolapse in 2% [4]. These complications are in addition to the significant impact that living with a stoma carries on patients' psychosocial health, including but not limited to poor body image perception, depression, sexual dysfunction, and low psychological adaptation [5].

N. D. Bouvy · V. R. W. Di Leonardo
Faculty of Health, Medicine and Life Sciences, Maastricht University, Maastricht, The Netherlands

Department of General Surgery, Maastricht University Medical Center, Maastricht, The Netherlands
e-mail: n.bouvy@mumc.nl

N. Boukhili (✉)
Department of Surgery, McGill University, Montreal, QC, Canada
e-mail: neyla.boukhili@mail.mcgill.ca

Hartmann's Reversal Rates and Reasons for Nonreversal

The first consideration for Hartmann's reversal is the determination of which patients fit the requirements for this procedure. Reversal rates for HP performed for an acute, severe diverticulitis are reported to range from 25% to 71% [6–9]. Many factors can impact the decision behind nonreversal, such as the morbidity associated with reversing the ostomy, the patient's age, and their general state of health and comorbidities. Hartmann reversal is associated with rates of morbidity and mortality as high as 47% and 16%, respectively, within the first 30 days after surgery [8]. Morbidities following Hartmann's reversal include cardiopulmonary complications, surgical site infections (SSI), urinary tract infections, anastomotic leaks, ostomy-related complications, wound dehiscence, ileus, and bleeding. The surgical decision to forego reversal appears correlated with patients' age, and increasing age is seemingly associated with decreased likelihood of undergoing reversal. Patients aged 70 years old and over with an American Society of Anesthesiologists (ASA) score of III or IV scarcely undergo Hartmann's reversal, whereas patients younger than 70 years old, with an ASA score of I or II, have a probability as high as 85% of undergoing reversal [8, 10]. The Charlson Comorbidity Index (CCI), a comorbidity screening tool, seems to be the most important predictor of intestinal restoration after Hartmann's rever-

M. Boutros et al. (eds.), *Diverticulitis*, https://doi.org/10.1007/978-3-032-21720-2_20

Table 20.1 Charlson Comorbidity Index score

Score	Description
1	Myocardial infarction history with ECG changes
	Congestive heart failure (i.e., exertional or paroxysmal nocturnal dyspnea responding to digitalis, diuretics, or afterload-reducing agents)
	Peripheral vascular disease (i.e., intermittent claudication or past bypass for chronic arterial insufficiency, history of gangrene or acute arterial insufficiency, or untreated thoracic or abdominal aneurysm ≥6 cm)
	CVA or TIA
	Dementia
	COPD
	Connective tissue disease
	Peptic ulcer disease (any history of treatment for ulcer disease or history of ulcer bleeding)
	Mild liver disease[a] (i.e., chronic hepatitis or cirrhosis without portal hypertension)
	Diabetes mellitus managed with medication without end-organ damage[a]
2	Hemiplegia
	Moderate to severe chronic kidney disease (i.e., moderate = urinary creatinine >3 mg/dL (0.27 mmol/L); severe = on dialysis, status post kidney transplant, uremia)
	Localized solid tumor[b]
	Leukemia
	Lymphoma
	Diabetes mellitus with end-organ damage (retinopathy, neuropathy, nephropathy)[a]
3	Moderate to severe liver disease[a] (i.e., cirrhosis and portal hypertension with or without variceal bleeding)
6	Metastatic tumor
	AIDS (not just HIV-positive)

Note: Add 1 point for every decade over 40 years of age, i.e., 50–59 years, 1 point; 60–69 years, 2 points, etc.
Abbreviations: *ECG* electrocardiogram, *CVA* cardiovascular accident, *TIA* transient ischemic attack, *COPD* chronic obstructive pulmonary disease, *AIDS* acquired immunodeficiency syndrome, *HIV* human immunodeficiency virus
[a]These are mutually exclusive; do not give points for both items, but choose the most severe option if applicable
[b]Exclude if >5 years since diagnosis

sal, followed by younger age and lower ASA score. A CCI score lower than 6 is associated with a 100% chance of Hartmann's reversal (Table 20.1) [11]. A more recent multivariate analysis showed that HR was less likely in patients aged >70 years, those with American Society of Anesthesiologists (ASA) class III or IV, elective surgery, those experiencing more than two HP-related complications, and those with a malignancy [12].

Timing of Hartmann Reversal

When considering Hartmann's reversal, it is crucial to select the appropriate timing of surgery. The timing of the surgery is not standardized, as evidenced by the mean interval between the initial Hartmann's procedure and reversal varying widely. Most patients are reversed at least 90–100 days after the initial procedure, and reversals earlier than 45 days are seldom performed. An early reversal (45–100 days) has similar rates of in-hospital mortality, transfusion, prolonged ileus, and other major complications compared to later reversals. Furthermore, it was associated with a lower chance of a prolonged length of hospital stay and hospital readmission [13].

Early reversal may be feasible in young and healthy patients, who are more likely to have recovered well from surgery without complications. In patients who are medically optimized and willing to undergo this procedure, surgeons should opt for an early Hartmann reversal. When determining the timing of the Hartmann reversal, there is a difference between optimal timing and feasible timing. In general practice, it is common to postpone Hartmann's reversal by 90 days, which explains the peak incidence as described. The rationale for postponing reversal by 90 days is solely based on current knowledge on the physiology of intra-abdominal adhesions [14].

One study showed that an interval between HP and reversal of >6 months was associated with a lower rate of complications [12]. Biologically, the formation of adhesions after initial HP is regarded as an inflammatory [15]. This process consists of different steps, starting with inflammation itself, followed by proliferation and remodeling. After about 90 days, the adhesions are thought to be optimally remodeled when one compares the strength of the adhesion versus the strength of normal tissue. It is thought that these adhesions become less dense and hostile after 90 days, hence the delay in reoperation. Adhesions that are not optimally remodeled have a significant negative impact on the quality of life of patients. Intra-abdominal adhesions are also associated with increased rates of iatrogenic bowel perforations during abdominal surgery, sepsis, incisional wound infections, and postoperative complications [16–18].

Based on a review of the literature, patients who are more likely to undergo an early reversal are generally younger, Caucasian, privately insured, and have less comorbidities [19]. Race and insurance factors may be a surrogate for socioeconomic differences in access to healthcare in specific countries. Hartmann's reversal is more commonly performed in wealthier patients from higher socioeconomic status than in underserved patients from lower socioeconomic status, although this difference has not been found to be statistically significant [20]. One recent study found timing of surgery did not affect the surgical complications rate or severity or the length of hospital stay [21].

Preoperative Preparation

Patients need to be optimized prior to surgery. Several strategies may lower perioperative morbidity. If applicable, patients should quit smoking, as smoking is associated with increased risk of complications such as wound infections, respiratory tract infections, other surgical site infections, and anastomotic leakage [22]. Patients should ideally quit smoking at least 8 weeks before surgery, as this has been shown to reduce postoperative respiratory complications by almost 50%, relative to active smoking (bronchospasm, respiratory failure, lung infection, pneumothorax, emphysema, etc.). Quitting smoking 4 weeks before surgery reduces respiratory complications by almost 25%. In contrast, smoking cessation less than 4 weeks prior to surgery does not reduce the risk of respiratory complications [23]. Another beneficial impact of early smoking cessation is improved wound healing [23]. Patients eligible for Hartman reversal should also be nutritionally optimized. A preoperative blood albumin level lower than 35 grams per liter is associated with increased postoperative complications; therefore, Hartmann reversal in patients with a poor nutritional status should be postponed [22]. Ideally, patients should not be overweight, as a BMI >30 kg/m^2 is also associated with an increased risk of surgical site infections [24].

Additional preoperative preparation to consider prior to Hartmann's reversal is preoperative optimization, which is also known as prehabilitation [25]. Overall, the aim of prehabilitation is to improve the preoperative condition of the patient and positively adjust modifiable risk factors for complications [26]. This can be done through aerobic exercise, inspiratory muscle training, and resistance training. A recent randomized clinical trial has shown that a multidisciplinary multimodal training prehabilitation program reduces postoperative complications in patients undergoing colorectal cancer surgery. We believe this can be applied to patients undergoing benign colorectal surgery as well [27]. The prehabilitation program starts 4 weeks prior to surgery and consists of exercise training, nutritional intervention, smoking cessation, and psychological support. Although this has been proven to be effective in a population of cancer patients undergoing surgery, we believe these results can be applied to patients undergoing Hartmann's reversal as well, or any abdominal surgery for that matter. The exercise training is guided by a physiotherapist and a sports physician, the nutritional intervention by a dietician, and the psychological support by a psychologist. Physical training consists of interval training for half an hour with a short warm-up at moderate intensity. Then, four intervals of high intensity intervals are completed by alternating moderate intensity activity and resistance training. Resistance training consists of strength training with increasing resistance over a 4-week course. Patients also receive instruction about breathing techniques to reduce the risk of pneumonia during hospital admission. Nutritional status is optimized through high-quality protein supplements consisting of 30 grams of protein, to establish an anabolic condition preoperatively. Supplementation of vitamins, especially vitamin D, may be beneficial due to its association with muscle mass and strength [28, 29]. To achieve smoking cessation, intensive counseling and nicotine replacement therapy should be offered to patients who are active smokers, as it highly impacts the postoperative course, as stated earlier.

When applied correctly, prehabilitation reduces pulmonary complications and overall postoperative morbidity. It also increases postoperative functional capacity relative to baseline, compared to patients without prehabilitation who show a decline in functional capacity postoperatively [25, 30, 31]. This increase in functional capacity is maintained for up to 5 days postoperatively, which is likely sufficient for patients to recover in a complication-free manner [32]. As is the case with other re-operative procedures, it is good practice to review the operative report of the original Hartmann's procedure case (particularly if done by a different surgeon). Surgeons may indicated the level of rectosigmoid transection and/or if the rectal stump was marked with a stitch. If a colonoscopy has not been done recently, it is often advised to perform a preoperative colonoscopy through the colostomy to ensure no additional pathology prior to bringing the patient to surgery. Similarly, the rectal stump can be evaluated endoscopically to get a sense of the stump height and to rule out concomitant pathology.

Surgical Procedure: Open or Laparoscopic?

Historically, Hartmann's procedure consisted of distal colonic resection with creation of an end colostomy using the proximal colon and closure of the residual rectal stump. This procedure was first described by Professor Henry Hartmann in 1921. Initially, he proposed HP as a primary treatment for obstructing cancers; however, more recently, the procedure has been widely applied for a variety of benign and malignant diseases of the colon, such as perforated diverticulitis. This chapter specifically speaks on Hartmann's reversal. Hartmann's reversal can be performed using a variety of approaches, including open, multiport, or single-port laparoscopy. Single-port access is usually the colostomy site. In the next section, we describe the surgical technique of laparoscopic Hartmann's reversal.

Laparoscopic Hartmann's reversal was first documented in 1993, and the procedure has shown many benefits compared to open reversal [33]. Since Hartmann's first reversal procedure, many researchers have reported various laparoscopic approaches and techniques. Patients are optimally positioned for transanal access. The following steps are important to achieve proper positioning:

- To prevent slipping during the procedure that could lead to nerve compression or hamper the creation of an anastomosis, antislipping measures are used to affix the patient to the operating table.
- Supine lithotomy position using stirrups with arms placed alongside the body, allowing the surgeon to be positioned on either side of the patient. Patients are put into a slight (usually 30°) Trendelenburg position and tilted to the right about 20°, causing the visceral organs to slide into the right upper quadrant of the abdomen.
- Urinary catheter insertion to ensure bladder decompression during the procedure, limiting the chance of iatrogenic bladder perforations.
- In some cases, the anesthesiologist and surgeon might decide to insert a nasogastric tube.

The surgical team consists of the head operating surgeon, one or two assistant surgeons, and a scrub nurse. Everyone should be positioned around the patient based on the team preference; however, usually the operating surgeon will stand on the right side of the patient. The assistant typically stands to the left of the surgeon, near the patient's right shoulder, holding both the laparoscope and a grasper. At some point during the procedure, either the surgeon or the assistant stands between the patient's legs in order to create an anastomosis. The scrub nurse stands close to the surgeon and the assistant.

The procedure follows the following steps:

- Temporary sealing of the colostomy
- Incision, open introduction of the first trocar
- With direct vision introduction of the other trocars, avoiding lesion of the epigastric vessels
- Exploration of the abdominal cavity
- Identification of the rectal stump
- Adhesiolysis
- Mobilization of the descending colon and, if necessary, mobilization of the splenic flexure
- Mobilization of the end colostomy
- Creation of the colorectal anastomosis

After temporarily sealing the end colostomy, for example, by using a sterilized stoma bag, the first incision is made away from the area of anticipated adhesions to allow exploration of the abdominal cavity without iatrogenic injuries. The preferred site for camera inversion is the right hypochondrium area, where the first trocar is inserted into the abdominal cavity using an open technique. All other trocars are inserted under direct laparoscopic visualization to prevent injury. Care should be taken to avoid injury to the epigastric vessels. After insertion of the first trocar, pneumoperitoneum, a pressure of 12 mm Hg can be established. An additional 5–12 mm trocars are inserted at the midclavicular line, umbilical level, and right lower quadrant. Additional trocars can be placed to facilitate pelvic adhesiolysis in the supraumbilical and suprapubic locations as needed. Although we mention quite specific trocar locations, these may need to be adjusted based on body habitus and prior surgical history (e.g., patients with a history of open cholecystectomy might have upper abdominal adhesions, therefore the first trocar may not be inserted in the right hypochondrium). Trocar size may vary, but must be at least 10–12 mm to accommodate repositioning of a 10 mm camera.

After exploring the abdominal cavity and visualizing the patient's anatomy and possible adhesions, adhesions are taken down and the colostomy is mobilized. The colostomy is sutured closed using a purse-string technique. Insertion of a stapler anvil into the lumen of the proximal colon might be done at this step or later during the procedure. The former end colostomy, which is now the sealed descending colon, needs to be freed from various planes, such as cutaneous, subcutaneous, and muscular planes, whilst also taking care not to make an injury to the colonic wall. The previously established pneumoperitoneum allows for exposure of the correct plane of dissection. Special care needs to be taken to not harm the mesentery of the colon.

After reestablishing the pneumoperitoneum, adhesiolysis of intra-abdominal adhesions should be performed. This step can be very difficult depending on the density, extent, and nature of the adhesions. Only the adhesions that interfere with the surgical procedure should be dissected. Particularly, adhesions hindering access to the pelvis, adhesions hindering atraumatic mobilization of the descending colon, and adhesions that might lead to obstruction. Adhesiolysis can generally be performed laparoscopically to achieve hemostasis, with or without an ultrasonic or bipolar vessel sealant device. Monopolar cautery should be avoided to minimize the risk of iatrogenic bowel injury. To avoid bleeding, it is important to dissect along the anatomically correct tissue planes, which is facilitated by pneumodissection, gentle traction, and contraction using atraumatic graspers. Once the adhesions are dissected, the abdomen should be explored again to get a clear overview, determine whether the adhesiolysis was sufficient to achieve adequate exposure of the relevant anatomy, and rule out any iatrogenic injury to the bowel.

Next, the rectal stump is identified. The exact location of the rectal stump is based on the level of transection during the original Hartmann's procedure and the extent of adhesions related to postoperative complications that might have occurred after that initial procedure. An endorectal bougie is inserted, allowing transanal manipulation of the rectal stump, which can facilitate its identification and mobilization. Identification of the rectal stump can be difficult when the rectal stump is low, especially when rectal transection has been completed at or below the peritoneal reflection.

After the rectal stump is identified, it needs to be mobilized. The method of mobilization depends on the length of the rectal stump. When the rectum is short, only anterior dissection should be performed. Posterior dissection is generally not necessary nor recommended, as it can result in injury to the sympathetic plexus (hypogastric nerves and hypogastric plexus). When the rectal stump is long and includes a segment of sigmoid, complete circumferential mobilization of the Hartmann's pouch is performed. When the stump is too long or stenotic (from prior inflammation or scarring), the stump can be stapled and shortened by transecting it down to the preferred length.

Following mobilization of the rectal stump, the descending colon is mobilized. To facilitate a tension-free colorectal anastomosis, the splenic flexure may also need to be mobilized. This step may have previously been done during the initial Hartmann procedure to create a tension-free stoma, however this is uncommon. The decision for mobilization of the descending colon before or after colostomy takedown is based on the surgeon's preference. In order to mobilize the descending colon, the left mesocolon needs to be detached from Toldt's fascia and the anterior surface of the pancreas. It may be necessary to divide the left colic artery, originating from the inferior mesenteric artery, for improved mobility. Cranially, the phreno-colic ligament and attachments of the omentum to the transverse colon may need to be dissected. The left ureter should be protected from injury, and it is not necessary to identify or dissect it during this procedure. Every effort should be made to avoid retroperitoneal dissection due to possible iatrogenic injury to the ureter. Following all the above bowel-lengthening maneuvers, the descending colon should be moved down toward the rectal stump in preparation for the anastomosis.

Note: Usually, the anvil is not inserted until this point of the procedure; however, it is possible for it to be used in freeing the colostomy from the abdominal wall prior to this point. We will continue the description of the procedure, assuming the anvil is inserted at this time.

The anvil is inserted into the lumen of the descending colon after it is trimmed back to a well-vascularized region to limit the possibility of postoperative anastomotic leakage due to ischemia. After insertion of the anvil, the colon is again closed using a purse-string suture and returned to the abdominal cavity. Subsequently, there is placement of a wound protector that can be capped, and then reestablishment of the pneumoperitoneum takes place. The circular stapler is inserted transanally with the tip of the circular stapler facing the anterior wall of the rectal stump to prevent injury to the sympathetic plexus. The spike is then carefully deployed through the rectal wall to avoid injury to anterior strictures such as the posterior vaginal wall. The anvil is then connected to the spike of the stapler. It is important to confirm the correct orientation of the bowel and the mesentery, as well as ensure no other structure is caught in the stapler prior to closing and firing. After firing the stapler, the anastomosis needs to be tested to limit the chance of postoperative complications. Two widely applied methods are checking the colonic donuts to ensure roundness and intactness, and an air leak test. Perfusion of the anastomosis can be checked with indocyanine green, which is a fluorescent dye. This is described in more detail later (*Specific Surgical Techniques and Their Impact on Outcome*).

The trocars are then removed under direct vision, with fascial closure for 10–12 mm incisions. The colostomy site is closed in layers. Local infiltration with an analgesic such as ropivacaine may be done to reduce postoperative pain [34, 35].

When the relatively new single-port approach is considered, the colostomy is mobilized first.

The anvil for the circular stapler is inserted into the proximal descending colon (either to the end or to the side) and closed with a purse-string suture, after which the descending colon is returned into the abdominal cavity. This allows the surgeon to enter the abdominal cavity, too. A small wound protector with a cap is placed over the prior colostomy site to establish pneumoperitoneum. The rest of the procedure is described: adhesiolysis, mobilization of both the descending colon and rectal stump, and ultimately creation of an anastomosis. The main difference between a multiport and single-port laparoscopic approach is the access. The multiport laparoscopic approach utilizes multiple trocars, while the single-port technique uses the colostomy site as the only access port for all laparoscopic instruments [36].

The open approach differs greatly. During an open procedure, a midline incision is made to access the abdominal cavity. This incision can be extended cranially if needed. The subsequent steps are similar to the laparoscopic approach.

Specific Surgical Techniques and Their Impact on Outcome

We will discuss several perioperative techniques and their impact on the postoperative outcomes of patients undergoing Hartmann's reversal.

The creation of an anastomosis must adhere to certain rules. The most important rules are that an anastomosis should always be tension-free and should always be well perfused.

When creating a tension-free anastomosis during Hartmann's reversal, the splenic flexure may need to be mobilized. Although one may always consider mobilizing the splenic flexure, the benefits may not always outweigh the risks of this additional surgical step. This is because mobilizing the splenic flexure is an independent risk factor for anastomotic leakage [37], justifying reluctance toward routine mobilization of the splenic flexure.

Adequate perfusion of the anastomosis is also critical. There is a question as to whether the inferior mesenteric artery should be ligated or preserved, and if ligated, whether high or low ligation should be performed. This ligation can either be a high tie, where the entire inferior mesenteric artery is ligated, thus ligating all of its branches, or a low tie, where the inferior mesenteric artery is ligated below the furcation of the left colic artery, therefore preserving it. A meta-analysis has shown ambivalent results; when randomized and nonrandomized trials are combined, neither technique was superior, with a 7% versus 11% rate of anastomotic leakage in the IMA ligation versus IMA preservation group, a difference without statistical significance [38–40]. However, the only randomized trial in this meta-analysis demonstrated an 8% versus 29% anastomotic leak rate in the IMA preservation versus ligation group, a statistically significant difference in favor of preservation [41]. More recent literature suggests no difference in anastomotic leak rates between ligation and preservation of the inferior mesenteric artery and even shows a slight preference for ligation [42–44]. Sometimes ligation of the inferior mesenteric artery may be necessary. If ligation is performed, the best option seems to be a low-tie ligation of the inferior mesenteric artery, since the low-tie ligation has a lower rate of anastomotic leakage (3.3% vs. 9.0%) [45]. This is likely because of better perfusion of the colorectal anastomosis. A more recent meta-analysis showed a slight, nonsignificant difference for low-tie ligation over high-tie ligation [46]. In the literature, there also seems to be a preference for preservation of the superior rectal artery, one of the branches of the inferior mesenteric artery, which gets ligated in a high-tie and a low-tie ligation of the inferior mesenteric artery. Preservation of the superior rectal artery during the initial Hartmann procedure seems to be associated with lower rates of anastomotic leak [47]. In conclusion, when debating whether or not ligation of the inferior mesenteric artery should be performed, it seems best to preserve the artery whenever possible to allow better perfusion of the anastomosis during Hartmann's reversal.

Recently, there has been a rising interest in assessing the perfusion of intestinal anastomoses intraoperatively using fluorescence imaging. The most frequently used dye is indocyanine green

(ICG), which can be seen in real-time during surgery. When the anastomosis seems to be inadequately perfused, the level of the anastomosis can be changed during surgery. This has shown to reduce anastomotic leakages from an average of 7.5–10% to 3–3.5%, which is statistically significant and clinically relevant, as prevention of anastomotic leakage is of paramount importance [48–50]. An updated meta-analysis states that the weighted mean rate of change in surgical plan based on ICG-FA was 9.6% (95% CI 7.3–11.8) and varied from 0.64% to 28.75%. Using ICG-FA was associated with significantly lower odds of AL (OR 0.452; 95% CI 0.366–0.558) and complications (OR 0.747; 95% CI 0.592–0.943) [51]. Furthermore, when the fluorescent dye is used to assess perfusion, the incidence of postoperative anastomotic leakage is considerably reduced [52].

Finally, a patient with a colorectal anastomosis at the rectum has a chance of recurrent diverticulitis in the descending colon, and no chance of recurrent diverticulitis in the rectum. The rationale behind the above statement is that the rectum has a continuous, circular muscularis propria layer and is therefore not prone to developing diverticulosis, whereas the descending colon is prone to diverticulosis because of its taeniae coli and therefore could be prone to developing (recurrent) diverticulitis.

Perioperative and Short-Term Postoperative Parameters and Complications

In general, laparoscopic Hartmann reversal is favored over open Hartmann reversal. Several studies, including meta-analyses and systematic reviews, provide evidence in favor of laparoscopic surgery. We will review the literature surrounding laparoscopic versus open Hartmann reversal below.

Firstly, the mean operating time is shorter in laparoscopy than in open reversal. Although the mean operating time within one group varies greatly, statistical analysis shows a shorter operation time during laparoscopy, ranging from roughly 100 to 290 minutes. There is also an average difference of 24 minutes in favor of laparoscopy in recent literature, indicating a shorter operating time when Hartmann's reversal is performed laparoscopically [24, 53]. This difference is due in part to the increasing experience in laparoscopy of surgeons worldwide. High-volume surgeons (more than 40 resections per year) tend to approach a Hartmann reversal more often via laparoscopy than laparotomy [54]. The estimated blood loss in a laparoscopic reversal is lower as well, which, on average, differs by 100 mL of blood loss in favor of a laparoscopic Hartmann reversal compared with an open reversal [53–56]. Patients undergoing laparoscopy return to a normal diet 1.5 days earlier than patients who underwent open reversal, which is on average after 4 days [55, 57]. Time to flatus is also faster in the laparoscopy group in comparison with the open reversal group, which, on average, is 3 days postoperatively [55, 57]. Patients are discharged up to several days earlier when they have a laparoscopic reversal in comparison to open reversal [23, 55, 57–59]. Patients operated by a high-volume surgeon tend to be discharged earlier, and these patients have a lower 90-day mortality when compared to patients operated by a low-volume surgeon [54].

Regarding complications, the laparoscopic Hartmann reversal is also favored [60, 61]. A laparoscopic Hartmann reversal tends to have less overall short-term and long-term morbidity, anastomotic failures postoperatively, cardiopulmonary complications, postoperative hemorrhages, wound dehiscence, urinary tract infections, reoperations, and sepsis compared to open reversal (Table 20.2) [53, 56, 59].

Reoperation rates appear similar between the groups and therefore do not favor either of the two mentioned approaches [60, 61]. Reoperation occurs in about 5% of patients regardless of which approach was used for the Hartmann reversal [53]. Mortality is a little under 1% after reversal and does not differ between the groups [53].

Table 20.2 Overview of subjects favoring laparoscopic or open Hartmann reversal

In favor of laparoscopic reversal	In favor of open reversal
Shorter operation time	Better surgical view during the operation
Shorter hospital stay	–
Lower estimated blood loss	–
Faster return to normal diet postoperatively	–
Faster time to flatus	–
Less wound infections	–
Less anastomotic failure	–
Less cardiopulmonary complications	–
Less hemorrhages	–
Less wound dehiscence	–
Less urinary tract infections	–
Fewer reoperations	–
Less sepsis	–

Long-Term Postoperative Complications: What to Monitor?

When considering long-term postoperative complications, it is important to focus on postoperative complications and the impact on the quality of life.

One of the reasons to reverse the initial Hartmann procedure is to improve the quality of life of patients with a colostomy [6]. Colostomies are associated with parastomal hernias, stoma prolapse, skin irritation from difficulties with pouching, dehydration, fistulae; all of which often require medical or surgical reintervention [62]. Hartmann's reversal can be complicated by incisional hernias, regardless of the indication for colostomy [60]. A higher BMI, as well as a history of stoma prolapse, parastomal hernia, hypertension, and a reversed colostomy, are associated with an increased risk of incisional hernias [63, 64]. Meaning, all of Hartmann's reversal patients are at increased risk of incisional hernia. A reverse colostomy is also a risk factor for surgical site infections, posing a five times higher risk of surgical site infections than their ileostomy counterparts [65].

Another frequent postoperative complication after abdominal surgery is the formation of adhesions. Adhesions are less likely to occur after laparoscopic surgery than open surgery, occurring in 48% versus 73% of patients, respectively [66]. Adhesions may not be symptomatic, and adhesive bowel obstruction may be managed conservatively. When a Hartmann's reversal is done laparoscopically, the average incidence of symptomatic adhesions leading to small bowel obstruction is 4.6% after 2 years and 10.7% after 5 years. In addition, adhesions in patients that require surgical intervention only occur in 1.2% after 2 years and 2.6% after 5 years [67].

The quality of life of patients before and after colostomy reversal is subject to research. Global Quality of Life scores improve after stoma reversal, particularly the quality of life due to increased physical functioning, less sleeplessness, less fatigue, less appetite loss, less nausea and vomiting, less flatulence, less constipation, and less diarrhea [68]. Finally, sexual interest improves in men as well as women after colostomy reversal [68].

Conclusion

If the patient is fit enough to undergo a second surgery, Hartmann reversal should be considered and can dramatically improve a patient's quality of life with acceptable morbidity rates. Given the re-operative nature of this procedure, Hartmann reversal can be technically challenging, and the surgeon should be adequately prepared for a potentially complex case.

References

1. Antoniou SA, Agresta F, Garcia Alamino JM, et al. European Hernia Society guidelines on prevention and treatment of parastomal hernias. Hernia. 2018;22(1):183–98. https://doi.org/10.1007/s10029-017-1697-5. Epub 2017 Nov 13. PMID: 29134456.
2. Loire M, Bridoux V, Mege D, et al. Long-term outcomes of Hartmann's procedure versus primary anastomosis for generalized peritonitis due to perforated diverticulitis: follow-up of a prospective multicenter randomized trial (DIVERTI). Int J Color Dis. 2021;36(10):2159–64. https://doi.org/10.1007/s00384-021-03962-2. Epub 2021 Jun 4. PMID: 34086087.

3. D'Ambrosio F, Pappalardo C, Scardigno A, et al. Peristomal skin complications in ileostomy and colostomy patients: what we need to know from a public health perspective. Int J Environ Res Public Health. 2022;20(1):79. https://doi.org/10.3390/ijerph20010079. PMID: 36612395; PMCID: PMC9819694.
4. Krishnamurty DM, Blatnik J, Mutch M. Stoma complications. Clin Colon Rectal Surg. 2017;30(3):193–200. https://doi.org/10.1055/s-0037-1598160. Epub 2017 May 22. PMID: 28684937; PMCID: PMC5498161.
5. Ayaz-Alkaya S. Overview of psychosocial problems in individuals with stoma: a review of literature. Int Wound J. 2019;16(1):243–9. https://doi.org/10.1111/iwj.13018. Epub 2018 Nov 4. PMID: 30392194; PMCID: PMC7948730.
6. Vonk-Klaassen SM, de Vocht HM, den Ouden ME, Eddes EH, Schuurmans MJ. Ostomy-related problems and their impact on quality of life of colorectal cancer ostomates: a systematic review. Qual Life Res. 2016;25(1):125–33.
7. Horesh N, Rudnicki Y, Dreznik Y, Zbar AP, Gutman M, Zmora O, et al. Reversal of Hartmann's procedure: still a complicated operation. Tech Coloproctol. 2018;22(2):81–7.
8. Moro-Valdezate D, Royo-Aznar A, Martin-Arevalo J, Pla-Marti V, Garcia-Botello S, Leon-Espinoza C, et al. Outcomes of Hartmann's procedure and subsequent intestinal restoration. Which patients are most likely to undergo reversal? Am J Surg. 2019;218:918–27.
9. van de Wall BJ, Draaisma WA, Schouten ES, Broeders IA, Consten EC. Conventional and laparoscopic reversal of the Hartmann procedure: a review of literature. J Gastrointest Surg. 2010;14(4):743–52.
10. Royo-Aznar A, Moro-Valdezate D, Martin-Arevalo J, Pla-Marti V, Garcia-Botello S, Espin-Basany E, et al. Reversal of Hartmann's procedure: a single-centre experience of 533 consecutive cases. Color Dis. 2018;20(7):631–8.
11. Charlson ME, Pompei P, Ales KL, MacKenzie CR. A new method of classifying prognostic comorbidity in longitudinal studies: development and validation. J Chronic Dis. 1987;40(5):373–83.
12. Kang JH, Kang BM, Yoon SN, et al. Analysis of f actors affecting reversal of Hartmann's procedure and post-reversal complications. Sci Rep. 2020;10(1):16820. https://doi.org/10.1038/s41598-020-73791-w. PMID: 33033297; PMCID: PMC7545186.
13. Resio BJ, Jean R, Chiu AS, Pei KY. Association of timing of colostomy reversal with outcomes following Hartmann procedure for diverticulitis. JAMA Surg. 2019;154:218–24.
14. Maciver AH, McCall M, James Shapiro AM. Intra-abdominal adhesions: cellular mechanisms and strategies for prevention. Int J Surg. 2011;9(8):589–94.
15. Moris D, Chakedis J, Rahnemai-Azar AA, Wilson A, Hennessy MM, Athanasiou A, et al. Postoperative abdominal adhesions: clinical significance and advances in prevention and management. J Gastrointest Surg. 2017;21(10):1713–22.
16. ten Broek RP, Issa Y, van Santbrink EJ, Bouvy ND, Kruitwagen RF, Jeekel J, et al. Burden of adhesions in abdominal and pelvic surgery: systematic review and met-analysis. BMJ. 2013;347:f5588.
17. ten Broek RP, Strik C, Issa Y, Bleichrodt RP, van Goor H. Adhesiolysis-related morbidity in abdominal surgery. Ann Surg. 2013;258(1):98–106.
18. Strik C, Stommel MWJ, Hol JC, van Goor H, Ten Broek RPG. Quality of life, functional status and adhesiolysis during elective abdominal surgery. Am J Surg. 2018;215(1):104–12.
19. Horesh N, Lessing Y, Rudnicki Y, Kent I, Kammar H, Ben-Yaacov A, et al. Considerations for Hartmann's reversal and Hartmann's reversal outcomes-a multicenter study. Int J Color Dis. 2017;32(11):1577–82.
20. Seetharam S, Paige J, Horgan PG. Impact of socioeconomic deprivation and primary pathology on rate of reversal of Hartmann's procedure. Am J Surg. 2003;186(2):154–7.
21. Horesh N, Lessing Y, Rudnicki Y, et al. Timing of colostomy reversal following Hartmann's procedure for perforated diverticulitis. J Visc Surg. 2020;157(5):395–400. https://doi.org/10.1016/j.jviscsurg.2020.01.005. Epub 2020 Jan 15. PMID: 31954631.
22. Fleming FJ, Gillen P. Reversal of Hartmann's procedure following acute diverticulitis: is timing everything? Int J Color Dis. 2009;24(10):1219–25.
23. Pierre S, Rivera C, Le Maitre B, Ruppert AM, Bouaziz H, Wirth N, et al. Guidelines on smoking management during the perioperative period. Anaesth Crit Care Pain Med. 2017;36(3):195–200.
24. Brathwaite S, Latchana N, Esemuede I, Harzman A, Husain S. Risk factors for surgical site infection in open and laparoscopic Hartmann closure: a multivariate analysis. Surg Laparosc Endosc Percutan Tech. 2017;27(1):51–3.
25. Hughes MJ, Hackney RJ, Lamb PJ, Wigmore SJ, Christopher Deans DA, Skipworth RJE. Prehabilitation before major abdominal surgery: a systematic review and meta-analysis. World J Surg. 2019;43(7):1661–8.
26. van Rooijen S, Carli F, Dalton SO, et al. Preoperative modifiable risk factors in colorectal surgery: an observational cohort study identifying the possible value of prehabilitation. Acta Oncol. 2017;56(2):329–34.
27. van Rooijen S, Carli F, Dalton S, et al. Multimodal prehabilitation in colorectal cancer patients to improve functional capacity and reduce postoperative complications: the first international randomized controlled trial for multimodal prehabilitation. BMC Cancer. 2019;19(1):98.
28. Mithal A, Bonjour JP, Boonen S, et al. Impact of nutrition on muscle mass, strength, and performance in older adults. Osteoporos Int. 2013;24(5):1555–66.
29. Salles J, Chanet A, Giraudet C, et al. 1,25(OH)2-vitamin D3 enhances the stimulating effect of leucine and insulin on protein synthesis rate through Akt/PKB and mTOR mediated pathways in murine

C2C12 skeletal myotubes. Mol Nutr Food Res. 2013;57(12):2137–46.
30. Moran J, Guinan E, McCormick P, et al. The ability of prehabilitation to influence postoperative outcome after intra-abdominal operation: a systematic review and meta-analysis. Surgery. 2016;160(5):1189–201.
31. van Rooijen SJ, Molenaar CJL, Schep G, et al. Making patients fit for surgery: introducing a four pillar multimodal prehabilitation program in colorectal cancer. Am J Phys Med Rehabil. 2019;98:888–96.
32. Mans CM, Reeve JC, Elkins MR. Postoperative outcomes following preoperative inspiratory muscle training in patients undergoing cardiothoracic or upper abdominal surgery: a systematic review and meta analysis. Clin Rehabil. 2015;29(5):426–38.
33. Gorey TF, O'Connell PR, Waldron D, Cronin K, Kerin M, Fitzpatrick JM. Laparoscopically assisted reversal of Hartmann's procedure. Br J Surg. 1993;80(1):109.
34. Yang PF, Morgan MJ. Laparoscopic versus open reversal of Hartmann's procedure: a retrospective review. ANZ J Surg. 2014;84(12):965–9.
35. Leroy J, Costantino F, Cahill RA, et al. Technical aspects and outcome of a standardized full laparoscopic approach to the reversal of Hartmann's procedure in a teaching centre. Color Dis. 2011;13(9):1058–65.
36. de Ruijter WM, van Loon YT, Wasowicz DK, et al. Reversal of Hartmann's procedure utilizing single-port laparoscopy: an attractive alternative to laparotomy. Surg Endosc. 2016;30(5):1894–901.
37. Nowakowski M, Malczak P, Mizera M, et al. The safety of selective use of splenic flexure mobilization in sigmoid and rectal resections-systematic review and meta-analysis. J Clin Med. 2018;7(11):392.
38. Cirocchi R, Trastulli S, Farinella E, et al. Is inferior mesenteric artery ligation during sigmoid colectomy for diverticular disease associated with increased anastomotic leakage? A meta-analysis of randomized and non-randomized clinical trials. Color Dis. 2012;14(9):e521–9.
39. Cirocchi R, Marchetti F, Mari G, et al. Inferior mesenteric artery ligation level in rectal cancer surgery: still no answer-a systematic review and meta-analysis. Langenbeck's Arch Surg. 2023;408(1):286. https://doi.org/10.1007/s00423-023-03022-z.
40. Reyaz I, Reyaz N, Salah QM, et al. Comparison of high ligation versus low ligation of the inferior mesenteric artery (IMA) on short-term and long-term outcomes in sigmoid colon and rectal cancer surgery: a meta-analysis. Cureus. 2023;15(5):e39406. https://doi.org/10.7759/cureus.39406.
41. Tocchi A, Mazzoni G, Fornasari V, Miccini M, Daddi G, Tagliacozzo S. Preservation of the inferior mesenteric artery in colorectal resection for complicated diverticular disease. Am J Surg. 2001;182(2):162–7.
42. Lehmann RK, Brounts LR, Johnson EK, Rizzo JA, Steele SR. Does sacrifice of the inferior mesenteric artery or superior rectal artery affect anastomotic leak following sigmoidectomy for diverticulitis? A retrospective review. Am J Surg. 2011;201(5):623–7.
43. De Nardi P, Gazzetta P. Does inferior mesenteric artery ligation affect outcome in elective colonic resection for diverticular disease? ANZ J Surg. 2018;88(11):E778–E81.
44. Cirocchi R, Popivanov G, Binda GA, et al. Sigmoid resection for diverticular disease – to ligate or to preserve the inferior mesenteric artery? Results of a systematic review and meta-analysis. Color Dis. 2019;21(6):623–31.
45. Zeng J, Su G. High ligation of the inferior mesenteric artery during sigmoid colon and rectal cancer surgery increases the risk of anastomotic leakage: a meta-analysis. World J Surg Oncol. 2018;16(1):157.
46. Yang Y, Wang G, He J, Zhang J, Xi J, Wang F. High tie versus low tie of the inferior mesenteric artery in colorectal cancer: a meta-analysis. Int J Surg. 2018;52:20–4.
47. Sohn M, Schlitt HJ, Hornung M, et al. Preservation of the superior rectal artery: influence of surgical technique on anastomotic healing and postoperative morbidity in laparoscopic sigmoidectomy for diverticular disease. Int J Color Dis. 2017;32(7):955–60.
48. van den Bos J, Al-Taher M, Schols RM, van Kuijk S, Bouvy ND, Stassen LPS. Near-infrared fluorescence imaging for real-time intraoperative guidance in anastomotic colorectal surgery: a systematic review of literature. J Laparoendosc Adv Surg Tech A. 2018;28(2):157–67.
49. Watanabe J, Ishibe A, Suwa Y, et al. Indocyanine green fluorescence imaging to reduce the risk of anastomotic leakage in laparoscopic low anterior resection for rectal cancer: a propensity score-matched cohort study. Surg Endosc. 2020;34:202–8.
50. Blanco-Colino R, Espin-Basany E. Intraoperative use of ICG fluorescence imaging to reduce the risk of anastomotic leakage in colorectal surgery: a systematic review and meta-analysis. Tech Coloproctol. 2018;22(1):15–23.
51. Emile SH, Khan SM, Wexner SD. Impact of change in the surgical plan based on indocyanine green fluorescence angiography on the rates of colorectal anastomotic leak: a systematic review and meta-analysis. Surg Endosc. 2022;36(4):2245–57. https://doi.org/10.1007/s00464-021-08973-2. Epub 2022 Jan 13.
52. Wada T, Kawada K, Takahashi R, et al. ICG fluorescence imaging for quantitative evaluation of colonic perfusion in laparoscopic colorectal surgery. Surg Endosc. 2017;31(10):4184–93.
53. Guerra F, Coletta D, Del Basso C, Giuliani G, Patriti A. Conventional versus minimally invasive Hartmann takedown: a meta-analysis of the literature. World J Surg. 2019;43:1820–8.
54. Aquina CT, Probst CP, Becerra AZ, et al. The impact of surgeon volume on colostomy reversal outcomes after Hartmann's procedure for diverticulitis. Surgery. 2016;160(5):1309–17.
55. Mazeh H, Greenstein AJ, Swedish K, et al. Laparoscopic and open reversal of Hartmann's procedure–a comparative retrospective analysis. Surg Endosc. 2009;23(3):496–502.

56. Celentano V, Giglio MC, Bucci L. Laparoscopic versus open Hartmann's reversal: a systematic review and meta-analysis. Int J Color Dis. 2015;30(12):1603–15.
57. De'angelis N, Brunetti F, Memeo R, et al. Comparison between open and laparoscopic reversal of Hartmann's procedure for diverticulitis. World J Gastrointest Surg. 2013;5(8):245–51.
58. Brathwaite S, Kuhrt M, Yu L, Arnold M, Husain S, Harzman AE. Retrospective evaluation of laparoscopic versus open Hartmann's reversal: a single-institution experience. Surg Laparosc Endosc Percutan Tech. 2015;25(5):e156–8.
59. Arkenbosch J, Miyagaki H, Kumara HM, Yan X, Cekic V, Whelan RL. Efficacy of laparoscopic-assisted approach for reversal of Hartmann's procedure: results from the American College of Surgeons National Surgical Quality Improvement Program (ACS-NSQIP) database. Surg Endosc. 2015;29(8):2109–14.
60. Medellin Abueta A, Senejoa NJ, Pedraza Ciro M, et al. Laparoscopic Hartmann's reversal has better clinical outcomes compared to open surgery: an international multicenter cohort study involving 502 patients. Health Sci Rep. 2022;5(5):e788. https://doi.org/10.1002/hsr2.788. PMID: 36090626; PMCID: PMC9434380.
61. Kong JC, Guerra GR, Prabhakaran S, et al. Is laparoscopic Hartmann's reversal a safe option? A systematic review and meta-analysis. World J Color Surg. 2020;9(4):57–63. https://doi.org/10.4103/1941-8213.305888.
62. Geng HZ, Nasier D, Liu B, Gao H, Xu YK. Meta-analysis of elective surgical complications related to defunctioning loop ileostomy compared with loop colostomy after low anterior resection for rectal carcinoma. Ann R Coll Surg Engl. 2015;97(7):494–501.
63. Chen Q, Itani KMF. Incidence, recurrence and risk factors of hernias following stoma reversal. Am J Surg. 2017;214(2):232–8.
64. Amelung FJ, de Guerre L, Consten ECJ, et al. Incidence of and risk factors for stoma-site incisional herniation after reversal. BJS Open. 2018;2(3):128–34.
65. Liang MK, Li LT, Avellaneda A, Moffett JM, Hicks SC, Awad SS. Outcomes and predictors of incisional surgical site infection in stoma reversal. JAMA Surg. 2013;148(2):183–9.
66. Okabayashi K, Ashrafian H, Zacharakis E, et al. Adhesions after abdominal surgery: a systematic review of the incidence, distribution and severity. Surg Today. 2014;44(3):405–20.
67. Bensley RP, Schermerhorn ML, Hurks R, et al. Risk of late-onset adhesions and incisional hernia repairs after surgery. J Am Coll Surg. 2013;216(6):1159–67 e1–12.
68. Sandra-Petrescu F, Weiss C, Post S, Runkel N, Kienle P. Quality of life and timing of stoma closure in patients with rectal cancer undergoing low anterior resection with diverting stoma: a Multicenter longitudinal observational study. Dis Colon Rectum. 2016;59(4):281–90.

Functional Outcomes After Diverticulitis Surgery

21

Cameron W. Hunt, Liliana G. Bordeianou, and Jon M. Harrison

Introduction

Epidemiology

According to the Centers for Disease Control and Prevention, the number of inpatient discharges for diverticular disease increased from 233,000 in 1997 to 314,000 in 2006 [1]. Between 1998 and 2005, age-adjusted admissions for acute diverticulitis increased 26%, with incidence rates increasing primarily in younger age groups (18–44 and 45–64 years of age). Importantly, admission rates for the youngest age group increased by 82% and elective operations by 73% [2]. During this same time period, the number of elective operations for diverticulitis in all age groups increased by 38%, while overall mortality from population-adjusted admission for acute diverticulitis, surgical mortality, and likelihood of colostomy formation from elective surgery decreased [2]. In spite of increasing admission rates and improved surgical outcomes, there is on-going controversy surrounding the timing between non-operative treatment and intervention for an acute episode of diverticulitis.

C. W. Hunt · J. M. Harrison
Department of Surgery, Massachusetts General Hospital, Boston, MA, USA
e-mail: cwhunt@mgh.harvard.edu; jmharrison@partners.org

L. G. Bordeianou (✉)
Department of Surgery, Massachusetts General Hospital and Harvard Medical School, Boston, MA, USA
e-mail: lbordeianou@mgh.harvard.edu

Treatment

When treating an acute episode of diverticulitis, four principles dictate care. These include symptom alleviation, recurrence prevention, fidelity to elective over emergency procedures, and maintenance of intestinal continuity [3]. Non-operative treatment, through dietary changes and lifestyle alterations, can also be used to treat acute uncomplicated diverticulitis and some forms of complicated diverticulitis [4]. Non-operative management can also be used for patients with perforated diverticulitis [5] and small abscesses (less than 3 cm) can be managed expectantly [6–8].

Since the adoption of computed tomography (CT)-guided percutaneous drainage for abscesses in the 1980s, patients previously treated with emergent/urgent colectomy can now be treated with interventional radiology (IR) abscess drainage [9]. Urgent surgery, however, is still recommended in patients with diffuse peritonitis, sepsis, and in instances where a suspicion of colon cancer cannot be excluded, as well as for patients where non-operative therapy fails [4, 9].

For patients with a medically managed episode of acute, uncomplicated diverticulitis, the literature regarding definitive treatment is less clear. Until 2000, the American Society of Colon

M. Boutros et al. (eds.), *Diverticulitis*, https://doi.org/10.1007/978-3-032-21720-2_21

and Rectal Surgeons (ASCRS) recommended elective sigmoid resection after two episodes of diverticulitis in order to prevent recurrence, emergency operation, and/or colostomy [10]. For context, historic series estimated a 33% recurrence rate after an initial attack of uncomplicated diverticulitis [11, 12], but more recent studies have estimated recurrence rates to be slightly lower, between 13% and 23% [13–16]. Following an index episode of diverticulitis, one study estimated the risk of requiring emergency surgery with stoma formation to be 1 in 2000 patient-years of follow-up [11], meaning 18 patients would require elective colectomy to prevent 1 emergent operation due to recurrent diverticulitis [15]. Since the chances of lethal complications from an expectant approach are low, this supports an in-depth discussion between the surgeon and the patient—with emphasis directed toward quality of life (QoL)-related issues after an episode of diverticulitis.

Accordingly, the 2020 clinical practice guidelines from the ASCRS recommend an individualized approach when considering elective resection after recovery from an acute episode of uncomplicated diverticulitis [4]. This individualized approach considers: risks of surgery, overall patient satisfaction, attack severity, chronic or recurring symptoms, and effects of recurrent attacks on lifestyle (individual and professional) [4]. Similar international guidelines emphasize a case-by-case approach to elective resection following an acute episode of uncomplicated diverticulitis [17–20].

Impact on Function and Quality of Life

With the current guidelines recommending resection for "persistent residual symptoms related or attributed to prior attacks" and the potential "lifestyle limitations" [4], it is important to understand how QoL is impacted by diverticular disease. Following an episode of diverticulitis, patients may suffer from cramping, abdominal pain, bloating, distension, diarrhea, and constipation [21]. As a result, these symptoms lead to reduced social functioning, emotional functioning, and QoL when compared with controls [21]. One of the earliest studies to evaluate how diverticular disease impacts QoL was conducted in the United Kingdom and compared patients with symptomatic diverticulitis to healthy controls [22]. This study used a 32-item questionnaire initially validated on patients with inflammatory bowel disease to assess four areas: gastrointestinal symptoms, systemic symptoms, emotional function, and social function [23], and demonstrated significantly lower QoL scores in all four areas for patients suffering from symptomatic diverticulitis [22].

Quality of Life Measures

Impacts of diverticulitis on QoL should be assessed through verified instruments, which can be broadly separated into three categories: those assessing general QoL, disease-related QoL, or disease-specific QoL (Table 21.1). Instruments assessing general QoL can be used to measure the heavy burdens that cancer, chronic inflammatory diseases, and disorders involving chronic pain place on patients, their families, and the decisions they make [27]. Health-related quality of life (HRQOL) aims to estimate the impacts of these burdens by collecting subjective experiences of physical, social, and emotional health, to assess overall well-being [27]. Additionally, clinicians can use HRQOL to assess functional capacity and disease severity when individualizing a treatment plan.

Table 21.1 Quality of life indices

QoL category	Disease-related QoL		Disease-specific QoL
Index	GIQLI	FIQoL	DV-QoL
Citation	Eypasch et al. [24]	Rockwood et al. [25]	Spiegel et al. [26]
Number of items	36	29	17
Categories (items)	Symptoms (19) Physical state (7) Emotions (5) Social functioning (4) Medical treatment (1)	Lifestyle (10) Coping/behavior (9) Depression/self-perception (7) Embarrassment (3)	Physical symptoms (5) Concerns (cognitions) (3) Emotions (4) Behavioral changes (5)
Scoring per item	0 least desirable 4 most desirable	1 alteration present most of the time 4 alteration present none of the time	–
Maximum score	144	4 (per category)	–

QoL quality of life, *FIQoL* Fecal Incontinence Quality of Life, *GIQLI* Gastrointestinal Quality of Life Index, *DV-QoL* Diverticulitis Quality of Life

General Quality of Life

Medical Outcomes Study Short-Form 36 (SF-36)

This 36-item instrument is used to assess eight health concepts: (1) limitations to physical activities from health problems, (2) limitations to usual role activities from health problems, (3) bodily pain, (4) general health perceptions, (5) limitations to usual role activities from emotional problems, (6) limitations to social activities from physical or emotional problems, (7) general mental health, and (8) vitality/energy [28]. Each of the eight concepts is transformed to a 0–100 scale [28]. Overall, higher scores indicate less disability and 100 represents the lowest pain and highest HRQOL [28]. A Physical Component Summary (PCS-36) can be calculated from the first four health concepts, and a Mental Component Summary (MCS-36) can be calculated from the last four. After its construction from the Medical Outcomes Study, McHorney et al. [29] conducted analyses to demonstrate item-internal consistency, item-discriminant validity, and reliability coefficients.

Cleveland Global Quality of Life Questionnaire (CGQL)

Developed as an alternative to the SF-36, this instrument can assess three clinical elements: (1) current QoL, (2) current quality of health, and (3) current energy level [30]. Each is rated on a scale of 0 (worst) to 10 (best), which gives a sum of 30 that can be divided by 30 to give the CGQL score (range 0–1) [30]. This instrument was originally designed to assess HRQOL in patients with ulcerative colitis and Crohn's disease [30, 31]. Kiran et al. [30] demonstrated internal consistency and a significant correlation with the SF-36.

Disease-Related Quality of Life

Gastrointestinal Quality of Life Index (GIQLI)

This 36-item questionnaire was developed by an international board of experts to measure QoL in patients with gastrointestinal disease and explores five main domains: (1) symptoms (19 items), (2) physical state (7 items), (3) emotions (5 items), (4) social functioning (4 items), and (5) medical treatment (1 item) [24]. Each question is scored from 0 (least desirable) to 4 (most desirable), and the five domains each receive a specific domain score [24, 32]. The most desirable, maximum summed score is 144 [24]. Eypasch et al. [24] developed the GIQLI through three phases, including data collection from 70 patients with gastrointestinal diseases, validation against generic measures of QoL, and testing in patients with stable gastrointestinal diseases along with patients who underwent surgery. Although also commonly used in upper gastrointestinal surgery, the GIQLI has been used to measure QoL in patients undergoing colon surgery [33].

Fecal Incontinence Quality of Life Scale (FIQoL)

This 29-item instrument measures QoL issues associated with fecal incontinence through four categories: (1) lifestyle (10 items), (2) coping/behavior (9 items), (3) depression/self-perception (7 items), and (4) embarrassment (3 items) [25]. Each of the four categories receives a scaled category score between 1 (alteration present most of the time) and 4 (alteration present none of the time) [25]. Psychometric evaluation demonstrated test/retest reliability, internal reliability, and convergent validity through a significant correlation with subscales in the SF-36 [25].

Disease-Specific Quality of Life

Diverticulitis Quality of Life Index (DV-QoL)

This 17-item instrument aims to provide a disease-targeted HRQOL measure for four condition-related concepts: (1) physical symptoms (5 items), (2) concerns (3 items), (3) emotions (4 items), and (4) behavioral changes (5 items) [26]. Each concept provides separate scores, as well as a total DV-QoL score when summed [26]. The DV-QoL was developed through a focus group of patients with symptomatic uncomplicated diverticular disease (SUDD), and validated through a high correlation with the SF-36 in a sample of 197 patients [26].

Since its validation, Polese et al. [34] used the DV-QoL to successfully evaluate QoL in patients who underwent elective laparoscopic sigmoid resection for uncomplicated diverticulitis. This study tracked patients treated surgically, patients treated medically, and healthy volunteers, and collected DV-QoL and SF-36 scores for patients before and after their treatment [34]. In addition to confirming a significant correlation between DV-QoL scores and SF-36 scores, when compared to medically treated patients, this study found that surgically treated patients presented significantly higher improvement between pre- and post-treatment DV-QoL scores in the "concerns" and "behavioral changes" sections [34].

Consensus on Quality of Life Instruments

Patient-reported outcomes (PROs) are gaining more recognition by health care providers and organizations [35], and even for diverticular disease, there are many existing instruments to measure related symptoms—including those mentioned above. A battery of recommended validated instruments could foster a common language of patient-reported symptoms, allowing for accurate interpretation of patient perceived symptom severity, and comparison of treatment options through meta-analyses and systematic reviews [36–38]. The Pelvic Floor Disorders Consortium (PFDC) laid the framework for this common language through evidence-based consensus of the best available validated instruments for five symptom categories related to pelvic floor disorders: fecal incontinence, urinary incontinence, constipation, lower urinary tract symptoms, and sexual dysfunction [36–38]. This consensus resulted in a battery of recommended instruments named the IMPACT (*I*nitial *M*easurement of *Pa*tient Reported Pelvic Floor *C*omplaints *T*ool), which allows for a common initial patient assessment through 35 questions for men and 45 for women [36–38]. By incorporating this single tool agreed upon by the PFDC, clinicians can gather relevant long-term data through validated scoring for these key symptoms of diverticular disease.

Functional Outcomes After Elective Resection for Diverticulitis

Functional outcomes following elective resection for an acute episode of diverticulitis can be separated into bowel function, genitourinary function, and sexual function. Related to bowel function, outcomes can be sorted by general bowel function (Table 21.2), gastrointestinal QoL (Table 21.3), persistent symptoms, and incontinence (Table 21.4).

Table 21.2 Studies on general bowel function following elective resection for diverticulitis

General bowel function			
Citation	Surgery	Mean post-operative follow-up time	Main finding
Ambrosetti et al. [39]	Elective laparoscopic sigmoidectomy	40 months	93% of patients considered bowel function unchanged or better than before 87% of patients considered the results satisfying, good, or excellent
Thorn et al. [40]	Elective colonic resection	48 months	78% of patients classified post-operative bowel function as good 22% of patients classified post-operative bowel function as fair to worse

Table 21.3 Studies on gastrointestinal quality of life following elective resection for diverticulitis

Gastrointestinal quality of life			
Citation	Surgery	Mean post-operative follow-up time	Main finding
Pasternack et al. [41]	Laparoscopic-assisted sigmoidectomy	40 months	Mean patient GIQLI scores increased from 95 points pre-operative to 114 points post-operative
Forgione et al. [42]	Elective laparoscopic sigmoidectomy	3 months 6 months 12 months	Mean patient GIQLI scores increased from 99.5 points pre-operative, to 113.5 points by 3 months, 112.8 points by 6 months, and 111.5 points by 12 months

GIQLI Gastrointestinal Quality of Life Index

Table 21.4 Studies on persistent symptoms and incontinence following elective resection for diverticulitis

Persistent symptoms and incontinence			
Citation	Surgery	Mean post-operative follow-up time	Main finding
Egger et al. [43]	Elective sigmoid resection (laparotomy or laparoscopy)	33 months	25% of patients reported persistent symptoms
Levack et al. [44]	Elective or emergent sigmoid colectomy and intestinal continuity (laparoscopic or open)	50.1 months	On the MBFI, 19.6% of patients reported fecal urgency and 20.8% of patients reported incomplete evacuation
Turoldo et al. [45]	Elective or urgent resection	66 months	On the MBFI, 4.25% of patients reported fecal urgency and 17.0% of patients reported incomplete evacuation

MBFI Memorial Bowel Function Index

Bowel Function

The majority of patients who undergo elective resection for an acute episode of diverticulitis have unchanged or improved bowel function postoperatively (Table 21.2). This is supported by a study of patients who underwent elective laparoscopic sigmoidectomy after a mean of 110 days following a CT-proven acute episode of diverticulitis [39]. After 40 months of post-surgery follow-up, 93% of patients considered their bowel function unchanged or better than before, while 87% of patients considered their results satisfying, good, or excellent [39]. It is important to note that in this study, nearly all patients (93%) had suffered two previous attacks of diverticulitis [39]. Another study focused on patients who underwent elective colonic resection for diverticulitis, with 68% of these patients having suffered three or more previous attacks of diverticulitis [40]. After 48 months of post-surgery follow-up, the authors found that 78% of patients classified their post-operative bowel function (stool characteristics, number of bowel movements per week, constipation, continence, and abdominal symptoms) as good, while 22% of patients classified it as fair to worse [40].

The majority of patients who undergo elective resection for an acute episode of diverticulitis have objective improvement on the GIQLI (Table 21.3). This is supported by data wherein, after a mean of 40 months following laparoscopic-assisted sigmoidectomy for diverticulitis, retrospectively collected GIQLI scores revealed an increase from 58% of patients that reported a GIQLI score above 100 points before surgery to 83% of patients that reported a GIQLI score above 100 points after surgery [41]. Additionally, mean GIQLI scores increased significantly from 95 to 114 points [41]. This is further evidenced by a prospective study that tracked functional impacts of elective laparoscopic sigmoidectomy for diverticulitis in 46 patients and found that 78% of patients reported a relevant increase of 10 points between pre-operative and post-operative GIQLI scores [42]. This translated to a mean GIQLI score improvement from 99.5 points at a pre-operative check, to 113.5 points by 3 months, 112.8 points by 6 months, and 111.5 points by 12 months [42]. Additional encouraging results included GIQLI scores that increased more than 20% in 41% of patients, GIQLI scores that increased more than 50% in 9% of patients, and the finding that the most significant GIQLI improvements were observed in patients with the lowest pre-operative scores [42].

A fraction of patients who undergo elective resection for an acute episode of diverticulitis have persistent symptoms (Table 21.4). One study focused on outcomes in patients who underwent elective sigmoid resection (47% laparotomy, 53% laparoscopy) [43]. After 33 months of follow-up, 25% of patients reported persistent symptoms related to painful constipation, painful abdominal distension, frequent painful diarrhea, or abdominal cramps [43]. The authors found that neither the presence of complications nor the surgical technique, laparotomy or laparoscopy, was significantly related to these persistent symptoms [43].

A fraction of patients who undergo elective resection for an acute episode of diverticulitis suffer from incontinence (Table 21.4). One study looked at patients after a mean of 50.1 months following elective or emergent sigmoid colectomy (laparoscopic or open procedures) [44]. Using separate assessment tools, patients reported their symptoms. On the Memorial Bowel Function Index (MBFI) [46], 19.6% of patients reported fecal urgency and 20.8% of patients reported incomplete evacuation, while on the Fecal Incontinence Severity Index (FISI) [47], 24.8% of patients reported clinically relevant fecal incontinence (Table 21.5) [44]. On the FIQoL, 21.6% of patients reported using anti-diarrheal medication "most of the time" or "always" [44]. In this study, 55% of patients had suffered more than two previous attacks of diverticulitis [44]. This is also supported in the longer term, in a study that focused on outcomes following elective and urgent surgeries for diverticulitis [45]. After 66 months of follow-up, the results revealed two main findings sorted by instrument: on the MBFI (Table 21.5), 4.25% of patients indicated fecal urgency, 17.0% indicated incomplete evacuation, and 23.4% indicated lifestyle/diet modification, while on the SF-36, 85.1% of patients indicated they were in good health [45]. Ultimately, the findings were encouraging, since 91.4% of patients in this study reported they would agree to go through with surgery again [45].

Post-surgical incontinence after elective resection for diverticulitis is an important discussion point for disease-related and general QoL. In one study, after 50 months of follow-up from surgery for colon cancer or diverticulitis, 25% of patients reported that bowel dysfunction limited their normal life functions more than once a month [48]. Within this group of patients, lower bowel function scores on the Bowel Disorder Score (BDS) (Table 21.5) significantly predicted lower scores on the FIQoL and the Short Form 12, an abbreviated version of the SF-36 [48]. Additionally, these results are supported by findings that scores on the FISI (Table 21.5) were significantly correlated with scores on the FIQoL [56].

Table 21.5 Quality of life instrument summaries

Bowel function instruments	
Memorial Bowel Function Index (MBFI) [46]	The MBFI is an 18-item questionnaire originally designed for patients who underwent sphincter-preserving surgery for rectal cancer, and measures symptoms of urgency, incomplete emptying, frequency, fecal incontinence, and lifestyle modifications.
Fecal Incontinence Severity Index (FISI) [47]	The FISI is an instrument assessing fecal incontinence, and is scored out of a cumulative weighted score of 0 to 61—where 0 indicates no incontinence, and 61 indicates incontinence to gas, liquid, mucus, and solid stool at least twice a day.
Bowel Disorder Score (BDS) [48]	The BDS is an instrument measuring bowel function, and includes questions regarding frequency, fecal incontinence, urgency, stool soiling, liquid stool, use, and limitations of life.
Genitourinary and sexual function instruments	
International Prostate Symptom Score (IPSS) [49]	The IPSS is an instrument originally designed to assess bladder function in men after cancer surgery, and consists of seven items concerning bladder emptying, frequency, intermittency, urgency, weak stream, straining, and nocturia.
International Index of Erectile Function 5 (IIEF-5) [50]	The IIEF-5 is a 5-item abridged version of the original IIEF, and is an instrument designed to detect the presence and severity of erectile dysfunction through questions regarding erectile function, orgasmic function, sexual desire, intercourse satisfaction, and overall satisfaction.
Urinary Distress Inventory (UDI) [51]	The UDI is an instrument assessing urinary distress through six domains examining lower urinary tract symptoms, incontinence, and detrusor overactivity in women.
Additional quality of life instruments	
Stoma Care Quality of Life Index (SQLI) [52]	The SQLI is a 34-item questionnaire used to assess stoma-related QoL, and is divided into three sections: (1) QoL: psychological well-being, physical well-being, body image, pain, sexual activity, nutrition, social concerns, (2) satisfaction of medical care: patient satisfaction, improvement, experience, and (3) self-efficacy: self-efficacy, help and advice.
EuroQol Visual Analogue Scale (EQ-VAS) [53]	The EQ-VAS is a single-term analog scale that measures the "value" of current health.
EuroQol—5 Dimension (EQ-5D) [53]	The EQ-5D is a five-item instrument that measures the "societal value" of current health.
European Organization for Research and Treatment of Cancer (EORTC) Quality of Life Questionnaire—C30 (QLQ-C30) [54]	The QLQ-C30 is an instrument originally piloted in patients with lung cancer, and focuses on three domains: (1) functional: physical, role, cognitive, emotional, social, (2) symptom: fatigue, pain, nausea, and vomiting, and (3) global health.
European Organization for Research and Treatment of Cancer (EORTC) Quality of Life Questionnaire—C38 (QLQ-CR38) [55]	The QLQ-CR38 is a 38-item colorectal cancer-specific QoL instrument focusing on side effects of various treatment modalities, body image, sexuality, and future perspective, and has been tested in colorectal cancer patients.

A subset of patients who undergo elective resection for an acute episode of diverticulitis suffer from new post-surgical abdominal symptoms. After 40 months of post-surgery follow-up, 9.3% of patients who underwent elective laparoscopic sigmoidectomy described new post-surgical abdominal symptoms [39]. Importantly, these persistent symptoms are not exclusive to the post-operative course following elective resection for diverticulitis and may be observed at higher rates following a non-operatively treated acute episode of diverticulitis. Specifically, after a mean of 25 months of follow-up from non-operative management for acute diverticulitis, 69% of patients suffered new, recurrent, short-lived abdominal pain with a median duration of 4 h and a rate of 4.8 episodes per month [57].

Genitourinary and Sexual Function

Although there are few studies focusing on the impact of surgery for diverticulitis on urinary and sexual function, the current evidence indicates that surgery does not lead to functional impairment. In addition to being one of the few prospective studies focusing on the impact of surgery for diverticulitis on bowel function, Forgione et al. [42] is one of the few studies examining the impact of surgery for diverticulitis on urinary and sexual function. This study used the International Prostate Symptom Score (IPSS) [49] to assess urinary function and the International Index of Erectile Function 5 (IIEF-5) [50] to assess sexual potency in men, and the Urinary Distress Inventory (UDI) [51] to assess urinary function along with a modified section from the GIQLI to assess sexual function in women (Table 21.5) [42]. After elective laparoscopic sigmoidectomy for diverticulitis, results from this prospective study revealed that men and women did not demonstrate significant alterations in urinary or sexual functioning from baseline (pre-operative) to 3, 6, and 12 months postoperatively [42].

Following elective colonic resection for diverticulitis, between 78% and 83% of patients classified their results as good with respect to bowel function [39, 41], up to 25% of patients suffered persistent symptoms [43], and between 17.0% and 20.8% of patients reported on-going stooling difficulties [44, 45]. With regard to genitourinary and sexual function, patients who underwent elective operative treatment for diverticulitis did not demonstrate impairments within 1 year following surgery [42]. These results indicate that following elective resection for diverticulitis, many patients may experience improved bowel function and unimpaired genitourinary and sexual function, but some may still experience persistent gastrointestinal symptoms, incontinence, or new abdominal pain. A measure like the IMPACT, which queries aspects of urinary symptoms and sexual function, can objectively measure clinical improvement across these domains or be used for future studies [36–38].

Stoma Formation and Quality of Life

Patients undergoing urgent or emergent diverticulitis surgery are significantly more likely to undergo staged resection (Hartmann's procedure) with stoma formation, which significantly impacts QoL [58]. Compared to the 90% of patients who undergo reversal following a proximal diverting ileostomy for primary resection and anastomosis, 44% of patients who undergo a Hartmann's procedure for diverticulitis never undergo reversal and are left with a terminal stoma [58].

Patients who undergo surgery for an acute episode of diverticulitis with stoma formation may experience alterations in lifestyle and sexual function. Not specific to diverticulitis patients, studies have found that approximately 80% of stoma patients experience significant lifestyle changes, and more than 40% experience problems with their sex lives [59]. A European study spanning 16 countries and including 4739 patients who underwent surgery that resulted in a stoma (the majority with a colostomy from carcinoma) assessed QoL through the Stoma Care Quality of Life Index (SQLI) (Table 21.5) [52]. Physical well-being and sexual activity (assessed through one question: "sexual activity sufficient to meet your needs?") received the lowest average score immediately following surgery, but rose along with the average SQLI scores at 3, 6, 9, and 13 months postoperatively [52].

Evidence also supports that patients who undergo surgery for an acute episode of diverticulitis with end colostomy formation suffer from decreases in the value of their current health. Vermeulen et al. [60] conducted a study at five teaching hospitals for patients who underwent emergent surgery for perforated diverticulitis by comparing patients who underwent Hartmann's procedure or primary anastomosis against healthy control patients. After 71 months of post-surgery follow-up, the results indicated similar EQ-VAS and EQ-5D QoL scores [53] (Table 21.5) between primary anastomosis patients and healthy controls, but significantly lower QoL scores in Hartmann's procedure patients compared to healthy controls [60]. In addition, from the QLQ-C30 [54] and QLQ-CR38 [55] (Table 21.5), the results revealed significantly better scores for primary anastomosis patients compared to Hartmann's procedure patients on five scales: global health status, physical function, fatigue, dyspnea, and body image [60].

Staged resection leading to stoma formation is more common for patients operated on for diverticulitis in the acute setting, and almost half of patients who undergo a Hartmann's procedure are left with an end ileostomy or colostomy [58]. Stoma management after an episode of diverticulitis poses a substantial burden to patients in multiple domains of life. Therefore, when possible, maintaining intestinal continuity should remain a priority.

Outcomes for Specific Disease Features of Diverticulitis

Certain patterns of presentation for diverticulitis, pre-operative symptoms, and complications can either increase or decrease the potential that patients will benefit from elective surgery. These cases can include patients suffering from recurring, chronic, ongoing diverticulitis-related symptoms (Table 21.6), pre-operative symptoms suggestive of irritable bowel syndrome (IBS) (Table 21.7), fistulae complicating diverticulitis (Table 21.8), and stricture (Table 21.9).

Chronic, Recurring, or Ongoing Symptoms

Patients with chronic, recurring, or ongoing disease-related symptoms following a non-operatively treated episode of diverticulitis have the chance to benefit greatly from favorable outcomes after elective resection for diverticulitis (Table 21.6).

A retrospective study by van de Wall et al. [61] studied patients who underwent elective resection for recurring or persistent complaints after an episode of diverticulitis, where 36% of these patients had two or three in-hospital episodes of diverticulitis prior to resection, and the remaining 64% of patients had at least one. After 33 months of follow-up, results from a visual analogue scale (VAS) questionnaire revealed improved general QoL in 89.3% of patients, reduced abdominal pain in 87.5% of patients, reduced discomfort from abnormal defecation in 77.1% of patients, and reduced fatigue in 75.2% of patients [61].

Table 21.6 Studies on surgical outcomes for patients suffering from chronic, recurring, or ongoing symptoms of diverticulitis

Chronic, recurring, or ongoing symptoms			
Citation	Surgery	Mean post-operative follow-up time	Main finding
van de Wall et al. [61]	Elective resection	33 months	On the VAS questionnaire, 89.3% of patients reported improved general QoL, and 87.5% reported reduced abdominal pain
van de Wall et al. [62]	Elective sigmoidectomy	6 months	Mean patient GIQLI score was significantly higher in the surgical treatment group compared to medical treatment group (mean difference 14.2) 23% of medical treatment patients underwent elective resection for ongoing complaints
Bolkenstein et al. [63]	Elective sigmoidectomy	5 years	Patient GIQLI scores remained significantly elevated from van de Wall et al. 2017 [62] 46% of medical treatment patients underwent elective resection for ongoing complaints

VAS visual analog scale, *GIQLI* Gastrointestinal Quality of Life Index

Table 21.7 Studies on surgical outcomes for patients suffering from pre-operative symptoms suggestive of irritable bowel syndrome

Pre-operative symptoms suggestive of IBS			
Citation	Surgery	Mean post-operative follow-up time	Main finding
Thorn et al. [40]	Elective colonic resection	48 months	Pre-operative functional symptoms suggestive of IBS significantly predicted less successful functional outcomes
Ambrosetti et al. [39]	Elective laparoscopic sigmoidectomy	40 months	83% of the 13% of patients who considered their final result as mediocre had a pre-operative history indicative of an irritable colon

IBS irritable bowel syndrome

Table 21.8 Studies on surgical outcomes for patients suffering from fistulae complicating diverticulitis

Symptoms of colovesical fistulae complicating diverticulitis			
Citation	Surgery	Mean post-operative follow-up time	Main finding
Engledow et al. [64]	Laparoscopic surgery	2 years	No recurrences of diverticulitis or fistulation after laparoscopic resection for colovesical or colovaginal fistulae complicating diverticulitis
Menenakos et al. [65]	Laparoscopic surgery	5.1 years	No recurrences of diverticulitis after laparoscopic surgery for colovesical or colovaginal fistulae complicating diverticulitis

Table 21.9 Studies on surgical outcomes for patients suffering from stricture complicating diverticulitis

Symptoms of stricture complicating diverticulitis			
Citation	Surgery	Mean post-operative follow-up time	Main finding
Venara et al. [66]	Elective sigmoidectomy (half laparotomy and half laparoscopy)	78 days	Mean post-operative GIQLI score similar to healthy patients 91% of patients reported satisfaction with their surgical resection

GIQLI Gastrointestinal Quality of Life Index

Another systematic review and meta-analysis by Andeweg et al. [67] reviewed 21 studies that measured patient QoL and other PROs after medical or surgical treatment for recurrent or chronic complaints of diverticulitis, and the results showed that these patients had significantly higher SF-36 scores after elective resection compared to medical treatment. A lower percentage of patients indicated suffering from gastrointestinal symptoms after elective laparoscopic resection (9%) compared to patients after medical treatment (36%), and similarly, a lower percentage of patients indicated chronic abdominal pain after elective laparoscopic resection (11%) compared to after medical treatment (38%) [67].

Last, a randomized controlled trial, the DIRECT study [62, 63], collected data from patients presenting with recurring complaints (more than two episodes of diverticulitis within 2 years) or ongoing complaints (diverticulitis-related complaints lasting more than 3 months) after an acute episode of diverticulitis at 24 teaching hospitals and 2 academic hospitals in the Netherlands. This study randomized 53 patients to the surgical treatment group (elective sigmoidectomy) and 56 patients to the medical treatment group (lifestyle monitoring, supplementary fiber, analgesics, and laxatives) [62, 63]. After 6 months of follow-up, the surgical treatment group demonstrated significantly higher GIQLI scores than the medical treatment group (mean difference 14.2), along with significantly better EQ-5D scores (Table 21.5), VAS-pain scores, and SF-36 physical scores [62], all of which remained persistently elevated at 5 years [63]. Additionally, the number of medically treated patients who underwent elective resection for ongoing complaints climbed from 23% at 6 months [62] to 46% at 5 years [63].

Irritable Bowel Syndrome

Patients who suffer from symptoms suggestive of IBS before elective resection for diverticulitis have an increased chance of worse post-operative outcomes (Table 21.7). IBS-suggestive symptoms include emptying difficulties, low abdominal pain, mucus in stool, altered bowel habits, irregular frequency, and stool formation [40]. After 4 years of follow-up for elective resection for diverticulitis, pre-operative functional symptoms suggestive of IBS significantly predicted less successful functional outcomes [40]. Similarly, after 40 months of follow-up for elective laparoscopic sigmoidectomy to treat diverticulitis, 83% of the 13% of patients who considered their final result as mediocre had a pre-operative history indicative of an irritable colon [39]. For these patients, it is important to recognize symptoms that may result from IBS in addition to diverticulitis, which may be more likely to persist after surgery [3].

Fistulizing Disease

Patients who recover after an acute episode of diverticulitis complicated by fistulae can experience benefits from surgery through symptom relief in bowel function, genitourinary function, and sexual function (Table 21.8) [68]. Fistulae complicate 2–4% of patients presenting with complicated diverticulitis, with the most common being colovesical fistulae (colon-bladder; approximately 60%) and colovaginal fistulae (colon-vagina; approximately 30%) [69]. Less commonly, diverticulitis may be complicated by other forms of fistula, including: coloenteric (colon-small bowel), colocutaneous (colon-skin), colouterine (colon-uterus), and colosalpingal (colon-fallopian tube) [70]. Certain groups of patients are more at risk for fistula formation, including patients treated non-operatively with CT-guided percutaneous drainage for an acute episode of diverticulitis complicated by abscesses. In this subset, patients can have up to a 25% increased chance of fistulae [71]. Additionally, colocutaneous fistulae most often occur in patients who have previously undergone an operation for diverticulitis [72, 73], while the majority of women presenting with diverticular fistulae of the female genital tract (colovesical and colovaginal) have previously undergone a hysterectomy [74, 75].

Presenting symptoms from a colovesical fistula secondary to diverticulitis include urinary frequency, dysuria, pneumaturia, fecaluria, pyuria, and hematuria [73]. For treatment, multiple studies have found that colonic resection can relieve symptoms with safe and feasible post-operative outcomes [64, 65, 69]. One study found no recurrence of diverticulitis or fistulation after 2 years in patients treated with laparoscopic resection for a colovesical or colovaginal fistula [64]. A second study found that primary anastomosis for patients with diverticulitis complicated by fistulae resulted in acceptable morbidity (uncomplicated post-operative course in 69% of patients) without mortality [69]. Notably, out of patients who underwent primary resection and anastomosis for colovesical or colovaginal fistulae of diverticular origin, 44% of patients without a protecting ileostomy suffered from leakage, compared to 7.1% of patients who received a defunctioning ileostomy [76]. Since patients with fistulae may have an increased chance of anastomotic leakage, this highlights the importance of considering diversion [76]. A final study evaluating surgical results after resection of fistulae found that elective laparoscopic colectomy is feasible and safe for these patients [65]. In their cohort, researchers found that elective laparoscopic surgery led to one conversion to an open procedure, 27.7% morbidity, no mortality, one fistula recurrence within a 5.1-year follow-up, and no recurrences of diverticulitis within the 5.1-year follow-up [65].

Presenting symptoms of a fistula to the female genital tract include vaginal discharge of feces, vaginal discharge of gas, purulent vaginal discharge, and abdominal pain [73, 74]. One study reviewed patients who had undergone surgery for diverticulitis complicated by fistulae to the female genital tract, and found that only 28% of patients experienced morbidity and no patients experienced mortality, pointing to a safe outcome in the majority of patients [74].

Diverticular Stricture

Patients with stricture secondary to diverticulitis may also benefit from elective resection for diverticulitis (Table 21.9). Although diverticular stricture occurs in less than 1% of patients with diverticular disease, it can lead to diarrhea, constipation, bowel obstruction, and abdominal pain [66, 77]. Additionally, stricture can prevent thorough endoscopic exploration of the colon and the ability to rule out malignancy [66], and one cohort analysis of 291 patients admitted for acute diverticulitis described stenosis as an indication for elective sigmoid resection [68]. More recently, Venara et al. [66] studied the impact of elective sigmoidectomy in patients diagnosed with sigmoid stricture, where half of the resections were performed by laparotomy and the other half by laparoscopy. After 78 days of follow-up, the results revealed a mean GIQLI score of 122 points in available patients [66]. Complications occurred in 31% of patients, but 91% of patients were satisfied with their surgical intervention [66]. The authors conclude that surgery for sigmoid stricture resulted in an acceptable complication rate and a QoL similar to healthy patients, and should therefore be recommended to allow for symptom relief and endoscopic exploration in patients with stricture secondary to diverticular disease [66].

In summary, patients suffering from recurrent and ongoing diverticulitis-related complaints following an acute episode of diverticulitis demonstrated significant QoL improvements following resection [61–63, 67], while patients presenting with pre-operative symptoms suggestive of IBS had an increased risk for less favorable outcomes following elective resection [39, 40]. In patients with diverticulitis complicated by fistulae, fistulae to the bladder can severely affect urinary function [73], fistulae to the female genital tract can lead to purulent vaginal discharge [73, 74], and fistulae to the small bowel can lead to deterioration of bowel function [70]. Since surgical treatment for all these forms of fistulae resulted in acceptable morbidity, mortality, and low rates of recurrence for both fistulae and diverticulitis [64, 65, 69, 74], patients with fistulae complicating diverticulitis have the potential to benefit greatly from resection. In patients with diverticulitis complicated by stricture, surgery can relieve symptoms and allow for endoscopic exploration while resulting in acceptable complication rates and QoL similar to healthy patients [66].

Technical Factors

Technical factors during elective resection for diverticulitis can impact functional and QoL outcomes based on time to recovery, persistent symptoms, and rate of recurrences. These technical factors include a laparoscopic approach versus an open approach, the amount of colon resected, and stapled versus hand-sewn anastomosis.

Laparoscopic Versus Open Approach

Since its application in colorectal surgery, laparoscopy has overall improved patient outcomes [78]. Retrospective studies have revealed that compared to open resection, laparoscopic resection for diverticulitis results in lower morbidity, earlier diet advancement, improved minor complication rate, and shorter hospital stay [79–83]. In 2009, a randomized controlled trial confirmed the utility of laparoscopy by directly comparing laparoscopic and open sigmoid resection for diverticular disease through the SF-36 [84]. Short-term results of laparoscopic resection demonstrated significantly improved QoL, shorter hospitalization, less pain [84], and a 27% reduction in major morbidity (compared to open resection) at 6 months [85]. Accordingly, the most recent practice guidelines from the ASCRS recommend a minimally invasive approach as the preferred approach for elective colonic resection for diverticulitis [4].

In the immediate post-operative period, laparoscopic colon resection offers a more rapid return of bowel function than open colonic resection. Post-operative studies focusing on laparoscopic versus open elective colectomy for diverticulitis have found that the average time for return of bowel function is shorter in laparoscopically treated patients [86–90]. One particular retrospective study focused on elective laparoscopic anterior resection for complicated and recurrent sigmoid diverticulitis, and demonstrated a significantly shorter time for passage of first flatus in patients operated on with a laparoscopic technique (mean of 2.63 days) compared to patients operated on with an open technique (mean of 4.65 days) [86].

In addition, studies have demonstrated short-term QoL benefits to laparoscopic sigmoid resection through the GIQLI. Pasternack et al. [41] evaluated disease-related QoL after elective laparoscopic-assisted sigmoidectomy for diverticular disease by retrospectively collecting GIQLI scores. After 40 months of follow-up, the authors found a significant improvement in post-operative GIQLI scores (mean of 114 points) compared to pre-operative GIQLI scores (mean of 95 points) [41]. Additionally, a prospective study by Roscio et al. [91] studied the disease-related QoL after elective laparoscopic sigmoid colectomy for diverticulitis by comparing GIQLI scores before and after surgery [91]. After a follow-up between 6 and 12 months, the authors found a significant improvement in post-operative scores (mean of 129.6 points) compared to mean pre-operative scores (mean of 97.1 points) [91].

When compared head-to-head with open resection, there is mixed evidence supporting a difference in QoL between patients who underwent laparoscopic versus open sigmoid resection for diverticulitis in the elective setting [92–94]. A Cochrane review by Abraha et al. [95] compared laparoscopic and open resection for acute sigmoid diverticulitis through three randomized trials (392 patients), and found mixed results for QoL outcomes. Specifically, one study suggested improved QoL in the laparoscopic group 6 weeks after elective surgery through the SF-36 [85], however, evidence from the other two trials (measured through QLQ-C30 (Table 21.5) [93] and the GIQLI [92]) showed little or no difference in QoL improvement when comparing the laparoscopic and open elective resection groups. Outside of this review, one study compared QoL in patients who underwent elective laparoscopic sigmoid colectomy versus elective open sigmoid colectomy for diverticulitis [94]. After 40.5 months of follow-up, the results showed similar GIQLI scores between the two groups, although significantly more laparoscopic resection patients were satisfied with their cosmetic result than open resection patients (97% vs. 63%) [94]. Thus, although the QoL outcomes of the two approaches may be similar beyond 30 months, there are still many short-term benefits and improved cosmesis with the laparoscopic approach.

Beyond comparing laparoscopic and open resection, studies have begun comparing QoL outcomes between different laparoscopic techniques. One study evaluated the QoL in patients after single-port laparoscopic resection for the treatment of diverticular disease [96]. After 6 months of follow-up, the authors found significant improvements in overall GIQLI scores when comparing post-operative scores (mean of 110.8 points) to pre-operative scores (mean of 102.0 points)—with significant improvements in the following domains: symptoms, physical, and emotions [96]. Another study directly compared the outcomes of single-incision laparoscopic sigmoidectomy and four-port laparoscopic sigmoidectomy for recurrent diverticulitis, and single-incision patients indicated significantly better cosmetic results than multiport patients [97].

Length of Resected Segment

Studies have found that the length of colon resected during surgery for diverticulitis is correlated with decreased recurrence and improved patient satisfaction, potentially due to better function from colorectal anastomosis instead of colocolonic anastomosis [39]. A review of 501 consecutive patients who had resection with primary anastomosis found that significantly more patients recurred after resection when the sigmoid colon was the distal margin (12.5%) compared to the rectum (6.7%) [98]. Supporting this further, another study included patients who underwent surgical treatment, where 27.2% of patients reported ongoing abdominal pain, and the authors found that there was a significant difference between the length of colon resected in symptomatic patients (mean of 17.6 cm) compared to asymptomatic patients (mean of 19.3 cm) [99]. In another study with patients who underwent elective laparoscopic sigmoidectomy for diverticulitis, after 40 months of follow-up, the 87% of patients who considered their final result excellent/good had a longer average length of resected colon (mean of 23.2 cm) than the 13% of patients who considered their final result mediocre (mean of 20.1 cm); suggesting a short length of resected colon was associated with worse post-operative satisfaction [39].

Type of Anastomosis

While the studies focusing on functional outcomes after hand-sewn versus stapled anastomosis during surgery for diverticulitis are limited, a retrospective study of patients who underwent elective left hemicolectomy with primary anastomosis to the proximal rectum for complicated sigmoid diverticulitis compared patients with hand-sewn anastomoses to patients with stapled anastomoses [100]. Short-term outcomes were assessed 6 months after surgery, and found that there was no post-operative mortality, and morbidity was not significantly different between the two groups [100]. Functional outcomes were better for patients with a hand-sewn anastomosis, with a higher percentage of patients with stapled anastomoses reporting constipation (28% vs. 9%) and dyschezia (39% vs. 18%), and a higher percentage of patients with hand-sewn anastomoses reporting normal stool consistency (79% vs. 43%) [100].

Improved immediate post-operative outcomes, short-term disease-related QoL, and long-term QoL favor patients who undergo laparoscopic resection over open resection for diverticulitis. Decreased rates of recurrence and post-operative symptoms coupled with increased patient satisfaction favor anastomosis to the upper rectum rather than the distal sigmoid colon. Short-term functional outcomes, through lower rates of constipation and higher rates of normal stool consistency, favor hand-sewn over stapled anastomoses.

Long-Term Outcomes

Patients who undergo elective resection for diverticulitis are often able to recover to a similar QoL compared to patients who undergo non-operative treatment for less severe stages of diverticular disease in the long-term (over 5 years). For studies that found similar long-term outcomes in disease-related [101] or general QoL [102, 103] (Table 21.10) in non-operative treatment patients versus elective resection patients, there were pre-existing differences between the patient groups. While the non-operative groups were primarily composed of lower Hinchey score patients with a shorter history of diverticular disease, the resection groups were primarily composed of higher Hinchey score patients with a more extensive history of diverticular disease [101–103].

The majority of patients who undergo surgery for an acute episode of diverticulitis do not experience impaired disease-related QoL or general QoL when compared to patients treated non-operatively in the long-term. Recovery of disease-related QoL was demonstrated through a study in the Czech Republic that compared patients treated non-operatively for Hinchey I diverticulitis (fasting, increased fiber, antibiotics, and/or endoscopic hemostasis) versus surgically for

Table 21.10 Studies on long-term outcomes following resection for diverticulitis

Citation	Mean post-treatment follow-up time	Diverticular features in medically treated group	Diverticular features in surgically treated group	Conclusion at follow-up
Adamova [101]	7 years	Hinchey I patients	Hinchey I, II, and III patients	Similar GIQLI scores in both groups
Koo et al. [103]	5 years	5% with a history of diverticular disease	70% with a history of diverticular disease	Similar impairments in SF-36 QoL domains in both groups
Bargellini et al. [102]	8.3 years	35% Hinchey II, III, and IV patients	Elective surgical treatment: 64% Hinchey II, III, and IV patients Emergency surgical treatment: 100% Hinchey II, III, and IV patients	CGQL scores for "current quality of health" were significantly worse in patients who underwent emergency surgery, but were otherwise similar

GIQLI Gastrointestinal Quality of Life Index, *CGQL* Cleveland Global Quality of Life questionnaire

Hinchey I, II, and III patients (primary anastomosis) [101]. After 7 years of follow-up, the authors found similar GIQLI scores between the two groups [101].

Recovery of general QoL is demonstrated through two studies [102, 103]. In the first study, patients under 50 years of age who were treated non-operatively or surgically (both elective and emergent) completed the SF-36 after 5 years of follow-up, and the results indicated overall similar impairments in all SF-36 QoL domains [103]. Importantly, there was a pre-existing difference in disease history, since 70% of patients treated surgically had a history of diverticular disease treated non-operatively for a mean of 4.3 years, with an average of three previous hospital admissions from recurrent attacks, while only 5% of patients treated non-operatively had a history of diverticular disease [103].

Another study focused on patients who underwent medical treatment (antibiotic therapy or percutaneous drainage), elective surgery (laparoscopic left colectomy), or emergency surgery (Hartmann's procedure, open colonic resection and colostomy, laparoscopic exploration, or left colectomy without stoma) [102]. After 8.3 years of follow-up, the authors found that while CGQL scores for "current quality of health" were worse for patients who had undergone emergency surgery, scores between the groups were otherwise similar [102]. Again, disease severity varied among the three groups, with patients suffering from Hinchey II, III, or IV diverticulitis comprising 35% of the medical treatment group, 64% of the elective surgery group, and 100% of the emergency surgery group [102].

While patients who undergo elective resection for diverticulitis often have more recurrences and/or more severe Hinchey scores than patients who undergo non-operative treatment, surgery provides these patients with the chance to return to an acceptable QoL post-procedurally. For patients suffering from a disease burden substantial enough to justify surgery, long-term studies support surgical intervention to improve disease-related and general QoL.

Conclusion and Summary

Management of diverticulitis requires a thoughtful discussion regarding many domains related to disease severity, recurrences, complicating features, and, most importantly, patient preference. Decisions are heavily influenced by QoL, and patients should choose elective resection to prevent the burden of future episodes of similar severity and/or frequency, specifically when this burden is heavy enough to justify those that come with surgery (short-term morbidity, recovery, and new or persistent symptoms) [3].

For outcomes after elective colonic resection for diverticulitis, most patients indicate improved bowel function, but there is the potential for post-operative abdominal pain and persistent symptoms. Studies indicate that while the majority of patients classify their bowel function results as good following surgery, between 10% and 25% of patients experience new or persistent abdominal pain and symptoms following diverticulitis surgery. Patients who undergo operative treatment for diverticulitis do not demonstrate impaired genitourinary or sexual function within 1 year following surgery.

- Patients who undergo stoma formation during surgery for diverticulitis are at an increased risk for lower QoL as well as changes in lifestyle and sexual activity. Therefore, during surgery for diverticulitis, intestinal continuity should be maintained when possible.

The role of surgery in improving QoL is more clearly demonstrated in patients who have been shown to benefit more or less from operative treatment.

- Specifically, patients suffering from recurrent episodes of diverticulitis (two or more within 2 years) and ongoing symptoms (lasting more than 3 months after an episode) may benefit more from surgical treatment than non-operative treatment, eliminating the potential for long-term sequelae. After undergoing elective resection, these patients show improved general QoL in the short-term, improved general QoL compared to patients that underwent medical treatment, and improved general and disease-specific gastrointestinal QoL compared to medically treated patients in the long-term.
- Patients who have pre-operative symptoms suggestive of IBS (difficulty emptying, low abdominal pain, mucus in stool, etc.) may benefit less often from surgical treatment. These patients have an increased risk of less favorable post-operative outcomes, and the presence of these symptoms may be predictive of decreased patient satisfaction in the short-term.
- Patients with fistulae secondary to diverticulitis suffer additional symptoms that complicate diverticulitis, and these patients may benefit more from surgical treatment relieving these symptoms. Colovesical fistulae severely affect urinary function, colovaginal fistulae can lead to purulent vaginal discharge, and coloenteric fistulae can lead to deterioration of bowel function. Surgical treatment in these patients can relieve these symptoms and results in acceptable rates of morbidity, mortality, and recurrence.
- Patients with diverticular stricture also suffer additional symptoms (diarrhea, constipation, bowel obstruction, etc.), and may benefit more from surgical treatment, relieving these symptoms and allowing for thorough endoscopic exploration of the colon to rule out malignancy (prevented by bowel obstruction). Patients who undergo elective sigmoidectomy for diverticulitis complicated by sigmoid stricture demonstrate acceptable patient satisfaction and disease-related gastrointestinal QoL scores comparable to healthy subjects.

Additionally, there are technical factors that can impact patient outcomes following elective resection after an acute episode of diverticulitis.

- When comparing laparoscopic and open colonic resection, the laparoscopic approach can improve QoL immediately following surgery. Relative to open colonic resection, the laparoscopic approach results in lower morbidity, earlier diet advancement, improved minor complication rate, and a shorter hospital stay. In addition, although the laparoscopic approach may not improve post-operative QoL significantly relative to the open approach, it may provide a cosmetic benefit.
- When comparing colorectal anastomoses completed with the rectum as the distal margin to colocolonic anastomoses completed with the sigmoid colon as the distal margin, colorectal anastomosis is preferable due to a lower risk of recurrence and improved QoL. Colorectal anastomosis is correlated with decreased rates of recurrence, increased patient satisfaction, and less persistent abdominal pain.

- When comparing hand-sewn and stapled anastomoses following primary resection for diverticulitis, hand-sewn anastomoses may improve functional outcomes. These improved outcomes in patients with hand-sewn anastomoses may be attributable to lower rates of constipation and dyschezia, and higher rates of normal stool consistency, relative to patients with stapled anastomoses.

Interestingly, while patients who undergo elective resection for diverticulitis often have experienced a heavy disease burden worsened by more recurrences and a more severe Hinchey score than patients who undergo non-operative treatment, studies support that in the long-term (beyond 5 years) these patients demonstrate general and disease-specific QoL levels similar to patients treated non-operatively.

In summary, following an index acute episode of diverticulitis, the chances of mortality from an expectant approach are low. For this group of patients who suffer from continued recurrences, as well as patients with ongoing symptoms and patients who develop complications secondary to diverticulitis, surgery offers significantly improved symptom relief and improved QoL. Additionally, surgical management has the potential to decrease patient anxiety associated with recurrences, but this must also be balanced with operative risk. An understanding of the research focusing on PROs after elective resection for diverticulitis allows for an engaged discussion surrounding elective resection, and for an appropriately informed weighing of current QoL against the promising prospects and risks that must be considered when planning next steps after an acute episode of diverticulitis.

References

1. Centers for Disease Control and Prevention. National Hospital Discharge Survey (NHDS) Publications and Reports. 2015. http://www.cdc.gov/nchs/nhds/nhds_publications.htm. Accessed 25 Mar 2019.
2. Etzioni DA, Mack TM, Beart R, Kaiser AM. Diverticulitis in the United States: 1998-2005: changing patterns of disease and treatment. Ann Surg. 2009;249:210–7.
3. Regenbogen SE, Hardiman KM, Hendren S, Morris AM. Surgery for diverticulitis in the 21st century: a systematic review. JAMA Surg. 2014;149:292–303.
4. Hall J, Hardiman K, Lee S, et al. The American Society of Colon and Rectal Surgeons clinical practice guidelines for the treatment of left-sided colonic diverticulitis. Dis Colon Rectum. 2020;63:728–47.
5. Dharmarajan S, Hunt SR, Birnbaum EH, Fleshman JW, Mutch MG. The efficacy of nonoperative management of acute complicated diverticulitis. Dis Colon Rectum. 2011;54:663–71.
6. Brandt D, Gervaz P, Durmishi Y, Platon A, Morel P, Poletti PA. Percutaneous CT scan-guided drainage vs. antibiotherapy alone for Hinchey II diverticulitis: a case-control study. Dis Colon Rectum. 2006;49:1533–8.
7. Siewert B, Tye G, Kruskal J, et al. Impact of CT-guided drainage in the treatment of diverticular abscesses: size matters. AJR Am J Roentgenol. 2006;186:680–6.
8. Jeffrey R, Federle MP, Tolentino CS. Periappendiceal inflammatory masses: CT-directed management and clinical outcome in 70 patients. Radiology. 1988;167:13–6.
9. Morris AM, Regenbogen SE, Hardiman KM, Hendren S. Sigmoid diverticulitis: a systematic review. JAMA. 2014;311:287–97.
10. Wong WD, Wexner SD, Lowry A, et al. The Standards Task Force. The American Society of Colon and Rectal Surgeons. Practice parameters for the treatment of sigmoid diverticulitis—supporting documentation. Dis Colon Rectum. 2000;43:290–7.
11. Janes S, Meagher A, Frizelle FA. Elective surgery after acute diverticulitis. Br J Surg. 2005;92:133–42.
12. Stollman N, Raskin JB. Diverticular disease of the colon. Lancet. 2004;363:631–9.
13. Hall JF, Roberts PL, Ricciardi R, et al. Long-term follow-up after an initial episode of diverticulitis: what are the predictors of recurrence? Dis Colon Rectum. 2011;54:283–8.
14. Eglinton T, Nguyen T, Raniga S, Dixon L, Dobbs B, Frizelle FA. Patterns of recurrence in patients with acute diverticulitis. Br J Surg. 2010;97:952–7.
15. Anaya DA, Flum DR. Risk of emergency colectomy and colostomy in patients with diverticular disease. Arch Surg. 2005;140:681–5.
16. Broderick-Villa G, Burchette RJ, Collins JC, Abbas MA, Haigh PI. Hospitalization for acute diverticulitis does not mandate routine elective colectomy. Arch Surg. 2005;140:576–83.
17. Kruis W, Nguyen GP, Leifeld L. German guidelines. J Clin Gastroenterol. 2016;50(Suppl 1):S47–9.
18. Schultz JK, Yaqub S, Oresland T. Management of diverticular disease in Scandinavia. J Clin Gastroenterol. 2016;50(Suppl 1):S50–2.
19. Binda GA, Cuomo R, Laghi A, et al. Practice parameters for the treatment of colonic diverticular disease: Italian Society of Colon and Rectal Surgery (SICCR) guidelines. Tech Coloproctol. 2015;19:615–26.

20. Andersen JC, Bundgaard L, Elbrond H, Laurberg S, Walker LR, Stovring J. Danish national guidelines for treatment of diverticular disease. Dan Med J. 2012;59:C4453.
21. Reddy VB, Longo WE. The burden of diverticular disease on patients and healthcare systems. Gastroenterol Hepatol (N Y). 2013;9:21–7.
22. Bolster LT, Papagrigoriadis S. Diverticular disease has an impact on quality of life—results of a preliminary study. Color Dis. 2003;5:320–3.
23. Guyatt G, Mitchell A, Irvine EJ, et al. A new measure of health status for clinical trials in inflammatory bowel disease. Gastroenterology. 1989;96:804–10.
24. Eypasch E, Williams JI, Wood-Dauphinee S, et al. Gastrointestinal quality of life index: development, validation and application of a new instrument. Br J Surg. 1995;82:216–22.
25. Rockwood TH, Church JM, Fleshman JW, et al. Fecal Incontinence Quality of Life Scale: quality of life instrument for patients with fecal incontinence. Dis Colon Rectum. 2000;43:9–17.
26. Spiegel B, Reid MW, Bolus R, W, et al. Development and validation of a disease-targeted quality of life instrument for chronic diverticular disease: the DV-QOL. Qual Life Res. 2015;24:163–79.
27. Borgaonkar MR, Irvine EJ. Quality of life measurement in gastrointestinal and liver disorders. Gut. 2000;47:444–54.
28. Ware J, Sherbourne CD. The MOS 36-item short-form health survey (SF-36). I. Conceptual framework and item selection. Med Care. 1992;30:473–83.
29. McHorney CA, Ware J, Lu JF, Sherbourne CD. The MOS 36-item Short-Form Health Survey (SF-36): III. Tests of data quality, scaling assumptions, and reliability across diverse patient groups. Med Care. 1994;32:40–66.
30. Kiran RP, Delaney CP, Senagore AJ, et al. Prospective assessment of Cleveland Global Quality of Life (CGQL) as a novel marker of quality of life and disease activity in Crohn's disease. Am J Gastroenterol. 2003;98:1783–9.
31. Scarpa M, Ruffolo C, D'Inca R, et al. Health-related quality of life after ileocolonic resection for Crohn's disease: long-term results. Inflamm Bowel Dis. 2007;13:462–9.
32. Schwenk W, Neudecker J, Haase O, Raue W, Strohm T, Muller JM. Comparison of EORTC quality of life core questionnaire (EORTC-QLQ-C30) and gastrointestinal quality of life index (GIQLI) in patients undergoing elective colorectal cancer resection. Int J Color Dis. 2004;19:554–60.
33. Maartense S, Dunker MS, Slors J, et al. Laparoscopic-assisted versus open ileocolic resection for Crohn's disease: a randomized trial. Ann Surg. 2006;243:143–53.
34. Polese L, Bressan A, Savarino E, et al. Quality of life after laparoscopic sigmoid resection for uncomplicated diverticular disease. Int J Color Dis. 2018;33:513–23.
35. McLeod LD, Coon CD, Martin SA, Fehnel SE, Hays RD. Interpreting patient-reported outcome results: US FDA guidance and emerging methods. Expert Rev Pharmacoecon Outcomes Res. 2011;11:163–9.
36. Bordeianou LG, Anger JT, Boutros M, et al. Measuring pelvic floor disorder symptoms using patient-reported instruments: proceedings of the consensus meeting of the pelvic floor consortium of the American Society of Colon and Rectal Surgeons, the International Continence Society, the American Urogynecologic Society, and the Society of Urodynamics, Female Pelvic Medicine and Urogenital Reconstruction. Dis Colon Rectum. 2020;63:6–23.
37. Bordeianou LG, Anger JT, Boutros M, et al. Measuring pelvic floor disorder symptoms using patient-reported instruments: proceedings of the consensus meeting of the pelvic floor consortium of the American Society of Colon and Rectal Surgeons, the International Continence Society, the American Urogynecologic Society, and the Society of Urodynamics, Female Pelvic Medicine and Urogenital Reconstruction. Female Pelvic Med Reconstr Surg. 2020;26:1–15.
38. Bordeianou LG, Anger J, Boutros M, et al. Measuring pelvic floor disorder symptoms using patient-reported instruments: proceedings of the consensus meeting of the pelvic floor consortium of the American Society of Colon and Rectal Surgeons, the International Continence Society, the American Urogynecologic Society, and the Society of Urodynamics, Female Pelvic Medicine and Urogenital Reconstruction. Tech Coloproctol. 2020;24:5–22.
39. Ambrosetti P, Francis K, Weintraub D, Weintraub J. Functional results following elective laparoscopic sigmoidectomy after CT-proven diagnosis of acute diverticulitis evaluation of 43 patients and review of the literature. J Gastrointest Surg. 2007;11:767–72.
40. Thorn M, Graf W, Stefansson T, Pahlman L. Clinical and functional results after elective colonic resection in 75 consecutive patients with diverticular disease. Am J Surg. 2002;183:7–11.
41. Pasternak I, Wiedemann N, Basilicata G, Melcher GA. Gastrointestinal quality of life after laparoscopic-assisted sigmoidectomy for diverticular disease. Int J Color Dis. 2012;27:781–7.
42. Forgione A, Leroy J, Cahill RA, et al. Prospective evaluation of functional outcome after laparoscopic sigmoid colectomy. Ann Surg. 2009;249:218–24.
43. Egger B, Peter MK, Candinas D. Persistent symptoms after elective sigmoid resection for diverticulitis. Dis Colon Rectum. 2008;51:1044–8.
44. Levack MM, Savitt LR, Berger DL, et al. Sigmoidectomy syndrome? Patients' perspectives on the functional outcomes following surgery for diverticulitis. Dis Colon Rectum. 2012;55:10–7.
45. Turoldo A, Bortul M, Ceglar S, Dobrinja C, de Manzini N. Does sigmoidectomy for diverticu-

lar disease have a negative impact on patients' quality of life and bowel function? Ann Ital Chir. 2016;87:564–71.
46. Temple LK, Bacik J, Savatta SG, et al. The development of a validated instrument to evaluate bowel function after sphincter-preserving surgery for rectal cancer. Dis Colon Rectum. 2005;48:1353–65.
47. Rockwood TH, Church JM, Fleshman JW, et al. Patient and surgeon ranking of the severity of symptoms associated with fecal incontinence: the fecal incontinence severity index. Dis Colon Rectum. 1999;42:1525–32.
48. Magdeburg J, Glatz N, Post S, Kienle P, Rickert A. Long-term functional outcome of colonic resections: how much does faecal impairment influence quality of life? Color Dis. 2016;18:O405–13.
49. Pocard M, Zinzindohoue F, Haab F, Caplin S, Parc R, Tiret E. A prospective study of sexual and urinary function before and after total mesorectal excision with autonomic nerve preservation for rectal cancer. Surgery. 2002;131:368–72.
50. Rosen RC, Cappelleri JC, Smith MD, Lipsky J, Pena BM. Development and evaluation of an abridged, 5-item version of the International Index of Erectile Function (IIEF-5) as a diagnostic tool for erectile dysfunction. Int J Impot Res. 1999;11:319–26.
51. Jones L. The use of validated questionnaires to assess female sexual dysfunction. World J Urol. 2002;20:89–92.
52. Marquis P, Marrel A, Jambon B. Quality of life in patients with stomas: the Montreux Study. Ostomy Wound Manage. 2003;49:48–55.
53. Lamers LM, McDonnell J, Stalmeier P, Krabbe P, Busschbach J. The Dutch tariff: results and arguments for an effective design for national. Health Econ. 2006;15:1121–32.
54. Aaronson NK, Ahmedzai S, Bergman B, Bullinger M, Cull A, Duez NJ, et al. The European Organization for Research and Treatment of Cancer QLQ-C30: a quality-of-life instrument for use in international clinical trials in oncology. J Natl Cancer Inst. 1993;85:365–76.
55. Sprangers MA, te Velde A, Aaronson NK. The construction and testing of the EORTC colorectal cancer-specific quality of life questionnaire module (QLQ-CR38). European Organization for Research and Treatment of Cancer Study Group on Quality of Life. Eur J Cancer. 1999;35:238–47.
56. Bordeianou L, Rockwood T, Baxter N, Lowry A, Mellgren A, Parker S. Does incontinence severity correlate with quality of life? Prospective analysis of 502 consecutive patients. Color Dis. 2008;10:273–9.
57. Simpson J, Neal KR, Scholefield JH, Spiller RC. Patterns of pain in diverticular disease and the influence of acute diverticulitis. Eur J Gastroenterol Hepatol. 2003;15:1005–10.
58. Salem L, Anaya DA, Roberts KE, Flum DR. Hartmann's colectomy and reversal in diverticulitis: a population-level assessment. Dis Colon Rectum. 2005;48:988–95.
59. Nugent KP, Daniels P, Stewart B, Patankar R, Johnson CD. Quality of life in stoma patients. Dis Colon Rectum. 1999;42:1569–74.
60. Vermeulen J, Gosselink MP, Busschbach JJV, Lange JF. Avoiding or reversing Hartmann's procedure provides improved quality of life after perforated diverticulitis. J Gastrointest Surg. 2010;14:651–7.
61. van de Wall B, Draaisma WA, van Iersel JJ, Consten ECJ, Wiezer MJ, Broeders I. Elective resection for ongoing diverticular disease significantly improves quality of life. Dig Surg. 2013;30:190–7.
62. van de Wall B, Stam MAW, Draaisma WA, et al. Surgery versus conservative management for recurrent and ongoing left-sided diverticulitis (DIRECT trial): an open-label, multicentre, randomised controlled trial. Lancet Gastroenterol Hepatol. 2017;2:13–22.
63. Bolkenstein HE, Consten ECJ, van der Palen J, et al. Long-term outcome of surgery versus conservative management for recurrent and ongoing complaints after an episode of diverticulitis: 5-year follow-up results of a multi center randomized controlled trial (DIRECT-Trial). Ann Surg. 2019;269:612–20.
64. Engledow AH, Pakzad F, Ward NJ, Arulampalam T, Motson RW. Laparoscopic resection of diverticular fistulae: a 10-year experience. Color Dis. 2007;9:632–4.
65. Menenakos E, Hahnloser D, Nassiopoulos K, Chanson C, Sinclair V, Petropoulos P. Laparoscopic surgery for fistulas that complicate diverticular disease. Langenbecks Arch Surg. 2003;388:189–93.
66. Venara A, Toque L, Barbieux J, et al. Sigmoid stricture associated with diverticular disease should be an indication for elective surgery with lymph node clearance. J Visc Surg. 2015;152:211–5.
67. [Andeweg CS, Berg R, Staal JB, ten Broek RPG, van Goor H. Patient-reported outcomes after conservative or surgical management of recurrent and chronic complaints of diverticulitis: systematic review and meta-analysis. Clin Gastroenterol Hepatol 2016;14:183–190.
68. Klarenbeek BR, Samuels M, van der Wal MA, van der Peet DL, Meijerink WJ, Cuesta MA. Indications for elective sigmoid resection in diverticular disease. Ann Surg. 2010;251:670–4.
69. Vasilevsky CA, Belliveau P, Trudel JL, Stein BL, Gordon PH. Fistulas complicating diverticulitis. Int J Color Dis. 1998;13:57–60.
70. Tracy L, Baker M, Pigazzi A. Colouterine fistula masquerading as a complex adnexal mass: a case report. J Reprod Med. 2016;61:87–91.
71. Devaraj B, Liu W, Tatum J, Cologne K, Kaiser AM. Medically treated diverticular abscess associated with high risk of recurrence and disease complications. Dis Colon Rectum. 2016;59:208–15.
72. Fazio VW, Church JM, Jagelman DG, et al. Colocutaneous fistulas complicating diverticulitis. Dis Colon Rectum. 1987;30:89–94.

73. Colcock BP, Stahmann FD. Fistulas complicating diverticular disease of the sigmoid colon. Ann Surg. 1972;175:838–46.
74. Hjern F, Goldberg SM, Johansson C, Parker SC, Mellgren A. Management of diverticular fistulae to the female genital tract. Color Dis. 2007;9:438–42.
75. Woods RJ, Lavery IC, Fazio VW, Jagelman DG, Weakley FL. Internal fistulas in diverticular disease. Dis Colon Rectum. 1988;31:591–6.
76. Smeenk RM, Plaisier PW, van der Hoeven JAB, Hesp WL. Outcome of surgery for colovesical and colovaginal fistulas of diverticular origin in 40 patients. J Gastrointest Surg. 2012;16:1559–65.
77. Sugihara K, Muto T, Morioka Y, Asano A, Yamamoto T. Diverticular disease of the colon in Japan. A review of 615 cases. Dis Colon Rectum. 1984;27:531–7.
78. Fowler DL, White SA. Laparoscopy-assisted sigmoid resection. Surg Laparosc Endosc. 1991;1:183–8.
79. Kwon S, Billingham R, Farrokhi E, et al. Adoption of laparoscopy for elective colorectal resection: a report from the Surgical Care and Outcomes Assessment Program. J Am Coll Surg. 2012;214:909–918.e1.
80. Alves A, Panis Y, Slim K, Heyd B, Kwiatkowski F, Mantion G. French multicentre prospective observational study of laparoscopic versus open colectomy for sigmoid diverticular disease. Br J Surg. 2005;92:1520–5.
81. Dwivedi A, Chahin F, Agrawal S, et al. Laparoscopic colectomy vs. open colectomy for sigmoid diverticular disease. Dis Colon Rectum. 2002;45:1309–15.
82. Lacy AM, Garcia-Valdecasas JC, Delgado S, et al. Laparoscopy-assisted colectomy versus open colectomy for treatment of non-metastatic colon cancer: a randomised trial. Lancet. 2002;359:2224–9.
83. Senagore AJ, Duepree HJ, Delaney CP, Dissanaike S, Brady KM, Fazio VW. Cost structure of laparoscopic and open sigmoid colectomy for diverticular disease: similarities and differences. Dis Colon Rectum. 2002;45:485–90.
84. Klarenbeek BR, Veenhof AA, Bergamaschi R, et al. Laparoscopic sigmoid resection for diverticulitis decreases major morbidity rates: a randomized control trial: short-term results of the Sigma Trial. Ann Surg. 2009;249:39–44.
85. Klarenbeek BR, Bergamaschi R, Veenhof AAFA, et al. Laparoscopic versus open sigmoid resection for diverticular disease: follow-up assessment of the randomized control Sigma trial. Surg Endosc. 2011;25:1121–6.
86. Lu C, Ho Y. Elective laparoscopic surgical management of recurrent and complicated sigmoid diverticulitis. Tech Coloproctol. 2008;12:201–6.
87. Faynsod M, Stamos MJ, Arnell T, Borden C, Udani S, Vargas H. A case-control study of laparoscopic versus open sigmoid colectomy for diverticulitis. Am Surg. 2000;66:841–3.
88. Berthou JC, Charbonneau P. Elective laparoscopic management of sigmoid diverticulitis. Results in a series of 110 patients. Surg Endosc. 1999;13:457–60.
89. Liberman MA, Phillips EH, Carroll BJ, Fallas M, Rosenthal R. Laparoscopic colectomy vs traditional colectomy for diverticulitis. Outcome and costs. Surg Endosc. 1996;10:15–8.
90. Dean PA, Beart RW, Nelson H, Elftmann TD, Schlinkert RT. Laparoscopic-assisted segmental colectomy: early Mayo Clinic experience. Mayo Clin Proc. 1994;69:834–40.
91. Roscio F, Grillone G, Frattini P, De Luca A, Girardi V, Scandroglio I. Effectiveness of elective laparoscopic treatment for colonic diverticulitis. JSLS. 2015;19:e2014.00120.
92. Gervaz P, Mugnier-Konrad B, Morel P, Huber O, Inan I. Laparoscopic versus open sigmoid resection for diverticulitis: long-term results of a prospective, randomized trial. Surg Endosc. 2011;25:3373–8.
93. Raue W, et al. Laparoscopic sigmoid resection for diverticular disease has no advantages over open approach: midterm results of a randomized controlled trial. Langenbecks Arch Surg. 2011;396:973–80.
94. Seitz G, Seitz EM, Kasparek MS, Königsrainer A, Kreis ME. Long-term quality-of-life after open and laparoscopic sigmoid colectomy. Surg Laparosc Endosc Percutan Tech. 2008;18:162–7.
95. Abraha I, Binda GA, Montedori A, Arezzo A, Cirocchi R. Laparoscopic versus open resection for sigmoid diverticulitis. Cochrane Database Syst Rev. 2017;11:CD009277.
96. Vestweber B, Vestweber K-H, Paul C, Rink AD. Single-port laparoscopic resection for diverticular disease: experiences with more than 300 consecutive patients. Surg Endosc. 2016;30:50–8.
97. D'Hondt M, Pottel H, Devriendt D, et al. SILS sigmoidectomy versus multiport laparoscopic sigmoidectomy for diverticulitis. JSLS. 2014;18:e2014.00319.
98. Benn PL, Wolff BG, Ilstrup DM. Level of anastomosis and recurrent colonic diverticulitis. Am J Surg. 1986;151:269–71.
99. Munson KD, Hensien MA, Jacob LN, Robinson AM, Liston WA. Diverticulitis. A comprehensive follow-up. Dis Colon Rectum. 1996;39:318–22.
100. Sielezneff I, Malouf AJ, Pirro N, Cesari J, Brunet C, Sastre B. Short-term functional outcome following elective surgery for complicated sigmoid diverticular disease: sutured or stapled end-to-end anastomosis to the proximal rectum? Color Dis. 2001;3:23–7.
101. Adamova Z. Comparison of long-term quality of life in patients with diverticular disease. Are there any benefits to surgery? Cent Eur J Med. 2012;7:571–7.
102. Bargellini T, Martellucci J, Tonelli P, Valeri A. Long-term results of treatment of acute diverticulitis: still lessons to be learned? Updat Surg. 2013;65:125–30.
103. Koo V, Strange J, Lam CY, Epanomeritakis M. Young patients with diverticular disease: a preliminary quality of life study. Int J Surg. 2007;5:244–9.

Management of the Immunosuppressed Patient

22

Ahmed Alkhamis and Neyla Boukhili

Introduction

Diverticular disease is a common colorectal problem and is reflected by the worldwide prevalence drastically increasing over the past several decades. While it was previously thought that 20% of patients with diverticulosis would have one or more acute episodes of diverticulitis during their lifetime, current estimates are more conservative, between 4% and 5% [1, 2]. In the United States alone, there are over 300,000 admissions for diverticulitis, resulting in 1.5 million days of inpatient care [3] and 1.5 million outpatient visits each year [4].

While there is some consensus regarding the timing and type of operation for diverticulitis in the immunocompetent (IMC) population, these remain controversial in the immunosuppressed (IMS) population. Immunosuppressed patients typically include solid organ transplant recipients and patients who are on chronic corticosteroid therapy or other immunomodulators, but may include other medical conditions as well (Table 22.1). The management of diverticulitis in the IMS population is becoming increasingly relevant because the indications for immunosuppressants are continuously expanding, and IMS patients are living longer as healthcare improves.

Immunosuppressed patients are suspected to have a higher incidence of diverticulitis (approximately 1% compared to 0.02% in the IMC) [1], as well as more virulent disease. Immunosuppressed patients are also suspected to have more complicated recurrences that warrant a more aggressive surgical management algorithm [5]. Consequently, current acute diverticulitis guidelines recommend that surgeons should maintain a low threshold for operative intervention in the emergency setting and strongly consider elective colectomy after a single episode of uncomplicated diverticulitis in the IMS patients. The World Society of Emergency Surgery (WSES) guidelines recommend planning sigmoid resection after an episode of acute left-sided colonic diverticulitis treated conservatively [6], while the American Society of Colon and Rectal Surgeons (ASCRS) recommended individualized approach regarding surgical resection [7]. The European Association of Endoscopic Surgery (EAES) and the Society of American Gastrointestinal and Endoscopic Surgeons (SAGES) do recommend surgical resection after an episode of complicated diverticulitis in IMS patients as they are at high risk of for early, frequent, and severe relapses after a complicated episode [8]. However, these recommendations are mostly based on small single-center studies.

A. Alkhamis (✉)
Kuwait University, Health Science Center, Jabriya, State of Kuwait
e-mail: ahmed.alkhamis@ku.edu.kw

N. Boukhili
Department of Surgery, McGill University, Montreal, QC, Canada
e-mail: neyla.boukhili@mail.mcgill.ca

M. Boutros et al. (eds.), *Diverticulitis*, https://doi.org/10.1007/978-3-032-21720-2_22

Table 22.1 Definition of immunosuppression

IMS definitions	Underlying diseases
Immunosuppressive therapy (e.g., azathioprine, cyclosporine, mycophenolate, tacrolimus, tumor necrosis factor (TNF) antigens, methotrexate)	Solid organ transplant patients Rheumatoid arthritis cancer Lupus erythematous
Chronic systemic corticosteroid treatment	Chronic obstructive pulmonary disease Inflammatory bowel disease Myasthenia gravis Wegner granulomatosis
Congenital or acquired immunodeficiency	HIV/AIDS
End-stage renal failure	On hemodialysis Peridialysis
Chemotherapeutic agents (e.g., Doxorubicin, Taxol, cyclophosphamide, Platinum, 5-Fluorouracil, Gemcitabine)	Visceral and hematological malignancies

IMS immunosuppressed

Furthermore, some studies have recently challenged these aggressive treatment strategies, with data showing similar outcomes and recurrence rates compared to IMS patients, particularly if the first episode of acute diverticulitis was uncomplicated. In addition, there is conflicting data regarding the safety of elective resection in this subpopulation compared to the IMC patients. Chapter 2 will review the epidemiology and management of diverticulitis in the IMS patient.

Definition of Immunosuppressants

Defining what constitutes the state of immunosuppression is challenging, and to date, there is no clear consensus. The various study definitions of IMS used in the diverticulitis literature may partly explain the inconsistent results between studies. This is likely because the optimal immunological effect of various immunosuppressive therapies, where the patient is deemed to be in an adequate state of immunosuppression, is not well defined and is dependent on various pharmacological factors, including the dose, frequency, and duration of the drug being administered. In addition, common medical conditions such as chronic renal failure and collagen vascular disease have been shown to put the body in a similar immunosuppressive status at certain disease severity [9, 10]. Very few studies have attempted to evaluate outcomes according to various kinds of IMS, in part due to the large sample size that would be required for such an undertaking. Defining what constitutes immunosuppressive status has become even more complicated since recent data has shown significant variability in the morbidity associated with different classes of immunosuppressants following an acute episode of colonic diverticulitis [11].

In general terms, we can define IMS patients as those who have undergone a solid organ transplant (such as lung, heart, liver, kidney, and pancreatic transplants) or patients on regular immunosuppressive medications like corticosteroids, chemotherapy, or biologic factors. In addition, patients with a history of collagen vascular disease or chronic renal failure on dialysis or peridialysis status should be included (Table 22.1). A 1-time pulse or a limited short course (duration of ≤10 days) of an immunosuppressive medication should not be included in the definition of IMS status.

Disease Presentation

Patients with IMS exhibit a distinct disease epidemiology, frequently presenting with more complicated disease courses and an increased likelihood of requiring surgical intervention during their initial admission. This heightened severity is attributed to several interconnected pathophysiological mechanisms. A dampened immune response in IMS patients can lead to a delayed or attenuated inflammatory reaction [12], masking typical symptoms and consequently delaying presentation to medical care. This delay allows the disease process to advance unchecked, resulting in more extensive and severe complications [12]. Furthermore, the underlying immune dysfunction and the often-associated comorbidities can impair wound healing, contributing to poorer surgical outcomes and a higher risk of postoperative complications [13].

In all patients presenting with suspected diverticulitis, a focused history and physical examination should be performed. A physical examination, including left iliac fossa pain (with or without local peritoneal signs), fever, and leukocytosis, without generalized peritonitis or hemodynamic instability, is typically consistent with acute uncomplicated diverticulitis. The diagnosis can be confirmed via computed tomography (CT) of the abdomen and pelvis, with findings most often consistent with diverticulosis with associated wall thickening and fat stranding. It is of utmost importance to realize, contrary to IMC patients, that IMS patients' clinical examinations can be frequently unreliable, so a low threshold should be set for surgical intervention with more liberal use of imaging.

Management of the Index Episode

As mentioned earlier, it is important to recognize that IMS patients tend to have an insidious onset of symptoms that is more severe compared to IMC patients. Therefore, surgeons should have a low threshold to keep patients in a monitored setting if surgical intervention is unnecessary upon assessment and then institute urgent surgical intervention when needed.

When emergency surgery was indicated, IMS patients were less likely to undergo reconstruction procedures without a stoma compared to IMC patients, and Hartmann's procedure was the procedure of choice in most centers [4, 14, 15]. However, where contamination is limited, a valid and safe alternative surgical option to Hartmann's was primary anastomosis with a diverting stoma. This latter approach has recently gained popularity, specifically among colorectal surgical specialists [15].

On another note, urgent colectomy is typically required for any patient who presents with diffuse peritonitis or whose nonoperative management of an acute episode fails, regardless of the patient's immune status. Unfortunately, data shows that in the emergency setting, IMS patients have higher mortality rates compared to IMC patients after colectomy [5, 16–19]. A recent retrospective review of the American College of Surgeons National Surgical Quality Improvement Program (NSQIP) prospectively maintained database (n = 26,987), reported IMS patients' mortality rate to be four times higher than IMC patients following emergency colectomy (16% vs. 4%) [5]. Similar trends were also identified by Reshef et al. [16, 18] case matched control study of 102 patients, which found the IMS patients mortality rates following emergency colectomy to be 19% compared to none in the IMC patients. As for postoperative morbidity, data appears inconsistent, with some showing worse [5, 18, 20–22] and others showing similar outcomes compared to IMC patients [14, 15, 19, 23]. However, the overall trends, regardless of the statistical significance, point toward worse morbidity in the IMS population following emergency colectomy. The NSQIP data review found major postoperative morbidity (e.g., cardiorespiratory event, renal insufficiency, thromboembolic event, return to the operating room, deep and organ space infection, urinary tract infection, and wound dehiscence) to be higher in the IMS compared to IMC patients (48% vs. 28%). Reshef et al. [16, 18] case control study reported similar outcomes, with overall morbidity being 52% compared to 24% in the IMC patients.

More progressive surgical approaches are currently being trialed. Two recent randomized controlled trials following perforated diverticulitis with purulent or fecal peritonitis in IMC patients reported better perioperative outcomes following primary anastomosis with diverting loop ileostomy, compared to Hartmann's [21, 22, 24, 25]. The studies found similar mortality rates between the two techniques, but the rate of stoma reversal was significantly higher in the primary anastomosis group compared to the Hartmann's. This data could indicate a decreased indication of the Hartmann's procedure for the general population, regardless of how complicated the disease. It is important to consider the applicability of these findings to the IMS population because this group remains understudied, as former study did not specify the inclusion of IMS patients, and the latter only included immunocompetent patients.

Role of Elective Surgery

A history of complicated diverticulitis, such as stricture, fistula, or obstruction, is an indication for elective resection after resolution of the acute episode, regardless of the immunological status. In addition, a history of large paracolic (>4 cm) or successfully treated pelvic abscess with or without percutaneous drainage are relative indications for elective resection. Without surgery, the risk of recurrence can be as high as 40% [7]. (*For more discussion on elective surgery for recurrent diverticulitis, refer to* Chap. 17).

For IMC patients with uncomplicated disease, a decision analysis model has demonstrated no increase in colostomy or mortality rates when elective resection was offered following the first compared to the fourth episode of uncomplicated diverticulitis [23, 26]. In fact, it is not unreasonable to elect for nonoperative management even after the fourth episode. The decision to operate should be individualized to each patient in relation to risk of surgery, overall medical condition, severity of the attack, the presence or absence of "smoldering" subclinical disease, and the effect of recurrence on patient quality of life. As for IMS patients, the data regarding the most appropriate timing and type of surgical intervention are less clear. Even though IMS patients were more likely to experience failure of nonoperative management at the index episode of acute diverticulitis, it appears that the rate of overall complications and the need for emergency surgery in subsequent episodes is not significantly different compared to IMC patients [1, 24, 25, 27, 28]. This has placed recommending elective sigmoidectomy for IMS after the index uncomplicated episode into question. Conversely, a study by Klarenbeek et al. [26, 29] showed that IMS therapy, having collagen vascular disease, or chronic renal failure was associated with perforation on the recurrent episode, favoring elective colectomy.

There is a paucity of data in the literature regarding mortality and morbidity following elective colectomy for diverticulitis in the IMS patients. The recent clinical practice guideline task force of the American Society of Colon and Rectal Surgeons advised surgeons to individualize decisions regarding surgical resection after the first uncomplicated attack as data regarding surgical resection are not compelling and whether the specific cause of immunosuppression, such as organ transplant, end-stage renal disease, and connective tissue disease, should influence treatment recommendations is unknown [7].

Performing an elective resection potentially allows IMS patients to avoid recurrence. Some data has shown that when recurrence occurs, it is more severe and more closely associated with increased risk of emergency colectomy and its inherited complications, compared to IMC patients. Furthermore, there is data showing no significant difference in both morbidity and mortality between IMS and IMC patients following elective resection [5, 7, 16, 18]. At optimal medical condition, performing an elective resection is relatively safe for the prevention of significant morbidity and mortality from an episode that may occur in the emergency settings. However, a recent NSQIP review reported a small yet significant increase in major morbidity and wound dehiscence following elective colectomy for diverticulitis in the IMS compared to IMC patients [14]. This is an indication that an elective resection might not be without risks, as we previously thought.

It appears that reconstruction with primary anastomosis with or without a protective stoma is the procedure of choice if an elective procedure is appropriate [5, 15]. The choice to divert or not should be based on patient fragility status, degree of immunosuppression and medical comorbidities. It is likely appropriate and safer to divert the patient if the immunosuppressant(s) cannot be withheld 2–4 weeks (depending on the half-life of the immunosuppressive drug) before and after surgery.

At present, it is difficult to generate a single recommendation that fits all immunosuppressed patients regarding the indication for elective colectomy, so surgeons and patients should consider the entire clinical picture.

Outcomes by Type of Immunosuppression

Biondo et al. [1] investigated outcomes of colonic diverticulitis according to the type of immunosuppressive agent used. Of 192 patients, 76 patients (39.3%) had emergency colectomy. Patients who had chronic corticosteroid therapy were significantly more likely to need emergency surgery compared to transplant, malignant neoplasm, chronic renal failure, or other immunosuppressants. There was no significant difference in postoperative mortality or complications between the groups. Kvasnovsky et al. [27] (31) systematic review and meta-analysis evaluated diverticular disease complications following various drugs, including corticosteroids, and reported a ninefold increase in the odds of perforation and abscess formation (OR 9.08, 95% CI 3.49–23.99) ($p < 0.01$). Halabi et al. [28] (32) evaluated 2616 kidney transplant patients who had colorectal resections for various medical conditions but predominantly diverticular disease. They found that kidney transplant status significantly increased the risk of having postoperative acute renal failure. However, there was no significant difference in postoperative morbidities and mortality. Brandl et al. [29] (33) compared 15 immunosuppressed patients (for solid organ transplant, autoimmune disease, or cerebral metastasis) to 212 immunocompetent patients following emergency admission for acute diverticulitis. They reported significantly higher postoperative morbidity, longer hospital stay, higher use of the intensive care unit, and in-hospital mortality in IMS patients. Cronley et al. [30] (34) looked into human immunodeficiency virus (HIV) patients who were hospitalized for acute diverticulitis and found that HIV+ status increased just under four times the risk of in-hospital death (OR 3.94, 95% CI 1.52–10.2) compared to the general population, although they received less surgical interventions (OR 0.74, 95% CI 0.57–0.95). Samdani et al. [31] (35) investigated whether chemotherapy is associated with increased risk and severity of recurrent diverticulitis. Of 131 patients, chemotherapy compared to no chemotherapy patients were more likely to undergo emergency surgery (75% vs. 23.5%, $p = 0.03$). When surgical resection was undertaken, they were more likely to be diverted (100% vs. 25%, $p = 0.03$) and more likely to have postoperative complications (100% vs. 9.1%, $p < 0.01$). However, there were no significant differences in terms of the severity of acute diverticulitis at index admission, failure of nonoperative management, and frequency of recurrence.

Summary

A challenging factor that limits the generalizability of the study results is the broad spectrum of inclusion criteria for the IMS genre and the nearly impossible task of ranking patients based on immunosuppression status. It is especially challenging if they are using the same category of immunosuppressants (Table 22.1). This significant heterogeneity has contributed to the conflicting data and uncertainty regarding the best management of colonic diverticulitis in the IMS population.

Patients with complicated diseases that were successfully managed with nonoperative management with or without percutaneous drain should proceed with elective resection, like IMC patients. As for patients with uncomplicated diseases at the index episode, which was successfully managed nonoperatively, it is likely reasonable to recommend close surveillance and recommend surgical resection as necessary. It would be appropriate to institute surgical resection if there is a concern that a further episode may have negative impacts on the patient's future quality of life or medical status due to the patient's co-existing medical conditions or overall frailty. Hartmann's procedure or resection and primary anastomosis with diverting stoma appear to be the most appropriate surgical options. The decision between the two procedures should be made based on the degree of contamination and the patient's physiological status at the time of operation. In the elective settings, resection and primary anastomosis with or without stoma appear to be the most appropriate option.

References

1. Biondo S, Trenti L, Elvira J, Golda T, Kreisler E. Outcomes of colonic diverticulitis according to the reason of immunosuppression. Am J Surg. 2016;212(3):384–90.
2. Delveus H, Lanzing G, Sahli H, Rönnow CF, Dahlbäck C, Buchwald P. Diverticulosis and risk of diverticulitis in 10 years; a Swedish retrospective observational study. Scand J Gastroenterol. 2024;59(4):433–6. https://doi.org/10.1080/00365521.2023.2301345. Epub 2024 Jan 11. PMID: 38206087.
3. Kozak LJ, DeFrances CJ, Hall MJ. National hospital discharge survey: 2004 annual summary with detailed diagnosis and procedure data. Vital Health Stat 13. 2006;162:1–209.
4. Shaheen NJ, Hansen RA, Morgan DR, Gangarosa LM, Ringel Y, Thiny MT, et al. The burden of gastrointestinal and liver diseases, 2006. Am J Gastroenterol. 2006;101(9):2128–38.
5. Al-Khamis AKJ, Torabi N, Demian M, Kezouh A, Gordon PH, Boutros M. Operative management of acute diverticulitis in immunosuppressed compared to immunocompetent patients: a systematic review. World J Surg Proced. 2015;5(1):155–66.
6. Sartelli M, Weber DG, Kluger Y, et al. 2020 update of the WSES guidelines for the management of acute colonic diverticulitis in the emergency setting. World J Emerg Surg. 2020;15(1):32. https://doi.org/10.1186/s13017-020-00313-4. PMID: 32381121; PMCID: PMC7206757.
7. Hall J, Hardiman K, Lee S, et al. Prepared on behalf of the Clinical Practice Guidelines Committee of the American Society of Colon and Rectal Surgeons. The American Society of Colon and Rectal Surgeons clinical practice guidelines for the treatment of left-sided colonic diverticulitis. Dis Colon Rectum. 2020;63(6):728–47.
8. Francis NK, Sylla P, Abou-Khalil M, et al. EAES and SAGES 2018 consensus conference on acute diverticulitis management: evidence-based recommendations for clinical practice. Surg Endosc. 2019;33(9):2726–41. https://doi.org/10.1007/s00464-019-06882-z. Epub 2019 Jun 27. PMID: 31250244; PMCID: PMC6684540.
9. Espi M, Koppe L, Fouque D, Thaunat O. Chronic kidney disease-associated immune dysfunctions: impact of protein-bound uremic retention solutes on immune cells. Toxins (Basel). 2020;12(5):300. https://doi.org/10.3390/toxins12050300. PMID: 32384617; PMCID: PMC7291164.
10. Hamilton CD. Immunosuppression related to collagen-vascular disease or its treatment. Proc Am Thorac Soc. 2005;2(5):456–60. https://doi.org/10.1513/pats.200508-091JS. PMID: 16322600; PMCID: PMC2713334.
11. Samdani T, Pieracci FM, Eachempati SR, Benarroch-Gampel J, Weiss A, Pietanza MC, et al. Colonic diverticulitis in chemotherapy patients: should operative indications change? A retrospective cohort study. Int J Surg. 2014;12(12):1489–94.
12. Tartaglia D, Cremonini C, Annunziata E, et al. WIRES-T for Acute Diverticulitis Study Group. Acute diverticulitis in immunocompromised patients: evidence from an international multicenter observational registry (Web-based International Register of Emergency Surgery and Trauma, Wires-T). Tech Coloproctol. 2023;27(9):747–57. https://doi.org/10.1007/s10151-023-02758-6. Epub 2023 Feb 7.
13. Beyene RT, Derryberry SL Jr, Barbul A. The effect of comorbidities on wound healing. Surg Clin North Am. 2020;100(4):695–705. https://doi.org/10.1016/j.suc.2020.05.002. Epub 2020 Jun 17. PMID: 32681870.
14. Al-Khamis A, Abou Khalil J, Demian M, Morin N, Vasilevsky CA, Gordon PH, et al. Sigmoid colectomy for acute diverticulitis in immunosuppressed vs immunocompetent patients: outcomes from the ACS-NSQIP database. Dis Colon Rectum. 2016;59(2):101–9.
15. Golda T, Kreisler E, Mercader C, Frago R, Trenti L, Biondo S. Emergency surgery for perforated diverticulitis in the immunosuppressed patient. Color Dis. 2014;16(9):723–31.
16. Reshef A, Stocchi L, Kiran RP, et al. Case-matched comparison of perioperative outcomes after surgical treatment of sigmoid diverticulitis in solid organ transplant recipients versus immunocompetent patients. Color Dis. 2012;14(12):1546–52.
17. Hwang SS, Cannom RR, Abbas MA, Etzioni D. Diverticulitis in transplant patients and patients on chronic corticosteroid therapy: a systematic review. Dis Colon Rectum. 2010;53(12):1699–707.
18. Pourfarziani V, Mousavi-Nayeeni SM, Ghaheri H, et al. The outcome of diverticulosis in kidney recipients with polycystic kidney disease. Transplant Proc. 2007;39(4):1054–6.
19. Hesterberg R, Muller F, Schmidt WU, Moslein G, Lammers B. Sigmoid diverticulitis in immunosuppressive drug therapy. Der Chirurg. 1994;65(10):873–6.
20. de'Angelis N, Esposito F, Memeo R, et al. Emergency abdominal surgery after solid organ transplantation: a systematic review. World J Emerg Surg. 2016;11(1):43.
21. Bridoux V, Regimbeau JM, Ouaissi M, et al. Hartmann's procedure or primary anastomosis for generalized peritonitis due to perforated diverticulitis: a prospective multicenter randomized trial (DIVERTI). J Am Coll Surg. 2017;225(6):798–805.
22. Lambrichts DVP, Vennix S, Musters GD, et al. Hartmann's procedure versus sigmoidectomy with

primary anastomosis for perforated diverticulitis with purulent or faecal peritonitis (LADIES): a multicentre, parallel-group, randomised, open-label, superiority trial. Lancet Gastroenterol Hepatol. 2019;4:599–610.
23. Salem L, Veenstra DL, Sullivan SD, Flum DR. The timing of elective colectomy in diverticulitis: a decision analysis. J Am Coll Surg. 2004;199(6):904–12.
24. Sugrue J, Lee J, Warner C, et al. Acute diverticulitis in renal transplant patients: should we treat them differently? Surgery. 2018;163(4):857–65.
25. Larson ES, Khalil HA, Lin AY, et al. Diverticulitis occurs early after lung transplantation. J Surg Res. 2014;190(2):667–71.
26. Klarenbeek BR, Samuels M, van der Wal MA. Indications for elective sigmoid resection in diverticular disease. Ann Surg. 2010;251(4):670–4. https://doi.org/10.1097/SLA.0b013e3181d3447d. PMID: 20224374.
27. Kvasnovsky CL, Papagrigoriadis S, Bjarnason I. Increased diverticular complications with nonsteriodal anti-inflammatory drugs and other medications: a systematic review and meta-analysis. Color Dis. 2014;16(6):O189–96. https://doi.org/10.1111/codi.12516. PMID: 24320820.
28. Halabi WJ, Jafari MD, Nguyen VQ, et al. Colorectal surgery in kidney transplant recipients: a decade of trends and outcomes in the United States. Am Surg. 2013;79(10):1026–33. PMID: 24160793.
29. Brandl A, Kratzer T, Kafka-Ritsch R, et al. Diverticulitis in immunosuppressed patients: a fatal outcome requiring a new approach? Can J Surg. 2016;59(4):254–61. https://doi.org/10.1503/cjs.012915. PMID: 27240131; PMCID: PMC4961488.
30. Cronley K, Wenzke J, Hussan H, et al. Diverticulitis in HIV-infected patients within the United States. HIV Med. 2016;17(3):216–21. https://doi.org/10.1111/hiv.12304. Epub 2015 Aug 18. PMID: 26283564.
31. Samdani T, Pieracci FM, Eachempati SR, et al. Colonic diverticulitis in chemotherapy patients: should operative indications change? A retrospective cohort study. Int J Surg. 2014;12(12):1489–94. https://doi.org/10.1016/j.ijsu.2014.10.032. Epub 2014 Nov 7. PMID: 25448673; PMCID.

23 Shared Decision-Making in Recurrent Diverticulitis

Samuel A. Younan and Alexander T. Hawkins

Introduction

Historically, colectomy was recommended after two episodes of diverticulitis to prevent catastrophic recurrence without specific consideration of the lived experiences or preferences of patients. But recent research observes that future episodes are not more likely to be associated with perforation and emergency surgery [1–5]. Over the past decade, studies have revealed that the reduction in mortality with a prophylactic colectomy is minimal, and patients as well as professional organizations now advocate that the focus be shifted to improving quality of life [6, 7]. This requires that the values, preferences, and goals of the patient are explicitly elicited, shared between patient and clinicians, and are core to care planning for recurrent diverticulitis. As such, management guidelines now recommend an individualized approach in considering colectomy in patients with recurrent diverticulitis [8–10]. Given the significant heterogeneity in severity of disease and presentation, proper patient selection is critical for optimizing outcomes. The complexity of diverticulitis management, which includes conservative medical therapy, dietary modifications, antibiotic treatment, and surgical intervention, necessitates an approach that integrates both clinical guidelines and patient preferences. It is in this condition of heterogeneity and complexity that shared decision-making between patient and clinician is imperative.

S. A. Younan · A. T. Hawkins (✉)
Division of General Surgery, Section of Colon & Rectal Surgery, Vanderbilt University Medical Center, Nashville, TN, USA
e-mail: samuel.younan@vumc.org; alex.hawkins@vumc.org

Shared Decision-Making

Shared decision-making (SDM) in the management of diverticulitis is a patient-centered approach that fosters a collaborative partnership between clinician and patient. Unlike a traditional, paternalistic model of decision-making, where clinicians make decisions based on their expertise and present them to patients, SDM ensures that patients are central to the decision-making process. Montori and colleagues defined SDM as "a collaborative process where patients, in partnership with their clinician, are encouraged to consider the available care options and work together to choose the best course of action that aligns with their personal care goals" [11]. The SDM model involves several key components (Table 23.1) [12]. Firstly, clinicians define the problem and provide clear, evidence-based guidance on treatment options, including the benefits, risks, and potential outcomes of each choice. In parallel, patients are encouraged to express their preferences, values, and lifestyle considerations that may influence the decision. The goal is to arrive at a decision that not only

M. Boutros et al. (eds.), *Diverticulitis*, https://doi.org/10.1007/978-3-032-21720-2_23

Table 23.1 Essential elements of shared decision-making

Essential element	Notes
Define/explain problem	It is important to define the problem at hand as it lays the foundation for effective SDM and collaboration between patient and provider.
Present options	Physicians should review available options, while patients should voice the options they are aware of, as it empowers patient choice, engagement, and promotes informed decision-making.
Discuss benefits/ risks	Patient education involves discussing the pros and cons of each treatment option, promoting trust, reducing misunderstanding, and encouraging shared responsibility. This is particularly important as physicians and patients may hold different perspectives on the relative importance of benefits, risks, and costs.
Patient values/ preferences	Eliciting patient values and preferences is essential in SDM as it personalizes care and allows physicians to tailor recommendations with the patient's goals.
Physician knowledge & recommendations	Information exchange involves presenting patients with the provider's understanding of the disease and treatment recommendations in the context of patient values and preferences.
Check/clarify understanding	It is important for both parties to periodically check understanding of facts and perspectives, providing further clarification as needed.
Deliberation/ negotiation	A process of deliberation ensues that incorporates all of the above, periodically revisiting different elements as needed for further discussion or clarification
Make or explicitly defer decision	Either a final decision is made, or there is an explicit effort to defer until a later time, allowing an opportunity to discuss with family members and/or other healthcare team members.

aligns with the best available clinical evidence but also prioritizes the patient's individual needs and goals of care [13, 14].

Elwyn et al. developed a three-talk model for describing the process of shared decision-making within a patient clinical encounter [15]. The model breaks the process into three distinct phases—Team Talk, Option Talk, and Decision Talk—that are anchored on the concepts of active listening and deliberation. The initial Team Talk phase focuses on establishing a partnership between the clinician and the patient by creating a supportive environment, introducing the concept of SDM, and ensuring the patient feels empowered to participate. In the second phase, the clinician discusses potential treatment options using risk communication principles to provide evidence-based guidance to the patient. The provider should facilitate a dialog that encourages patients to ask questions, clarify any doubts, and ensure they fully understand the implications of each choice. Lastly, in Decision Talk, the patient and provider work together to decide on the most appropriate treatment, balancing evidence-based guidance with the patient's values and goals of care. Ultimately, the three-talk model simplifies the shared decision-making process by providing concrete objectives and ensuring that decisions are well-informed and patient-centered.

Why Does Recurrent Diverticulitis Require Shared Decision-Making?

SDM is crucial in recurrent diverticulitis because treatment decisions must balance medical risks, surgical complications, patient preferences, and lifestyle considerations. Within this clinical context, equipoise is present in that there is no evidence to suggest superiority between observation and surgery. Here, equipoise refers to a situation where options need to be deliberated in the setting of two or more valid treatments, and the best choice depends on how patients weigh the risks and benefits of each approach [16]. The American Society of Colon and Rectal Surgeons (ASCRS) states that "the decision to recommend elective sigmoid colectomy after recovery from uncomplicated acute diverticulitis should be individualized" [8]. In this preference-sensitive context, the ideal treatment involves trade-offs between risks, benefits, and potential outcomes that align differently with individual patient values. The need for an ostomy, infection, and mortality are among the described complications that can arise from improper patient selection for surgery [17–19]. Conversely, inappropriate observation poses risks, such as morbidity from recurrent episodes, increased likelihood of hospitalization, the possibility of emergency surgery, and a decline in overall quality of life [6, 20]. The incidence of recurrence following non-operative management of uncomplicated diverticulitis is as high as 35%, but with low rates of subsequent complicated disease or need for emergency operation [4, 8, 21–25]. Studies have demonstrated that elective colectomy does not significantly reduce the rate of emergency surgery, but may address the risk of future recurrence [4, 26–29]. One randomized trial comparing elective surgery and observation for patients with recurrent diverticulitis revealed that surgery was associated with significantly higher gastroenteric-specific quality of life (DIRECT trial) [30].

Overall, the available evidence does not definitively observe an advantage for one treatment modality over the other. One meta-analysis showed better quality of life outcomes with surgery [29]. Without clear superiority between surgery and observation for recurrent diverticulitis, the decision to pursue colectomy is highly preference-sensitive, which lends itself to the shared decision-making process and emphasizes the importance of integrating patient-focused care with clinical expertise [16]. In the case of inadequate shared decision-making, this clear equipoise can potentially lead to both high decisional conflict and regret [31].

Decisional Conflict and Decision Regret

Decisional conflict is characterized by a state of uncertainty regarding the best course of action to take. It arises in the context of complex health decisions where patients are confronted with insufficient evidence to guide treatment. They are faced with the task of weighing risks and benefits, navigating values and preferences, and evaluating goals of care without sufficient support. Decisional conflict can be quantified in the form of the decisional conflict scale (DCS), which has been tested and validated with readily available psychometric properties [32]. The scale evaluates personal perceptions of uncertainty in choosing options as well as modifiable factors contributing to uncertainty. It has been in use for over 25 years in various medical contexts and measures five dimensions of decision-making, including feeling uncertain, uninformed, unclear about values, unsupported, and ineffective decision-making [32, 33]. As patients assume greater responsibility for their health decisions, they are faced with decisional conflict, particularly when the choices involve risk, loss, regret, or challenges to personal life values. Several studies have evaluated DCS scores in colorectal disease processes such as colon and rectal cancer, but there is limited available data on recurrent uncomplicated diverticulitis [34, 35].

Reducing decisional conflict is a key goal in SDM. This can impact patient outcomes, treatment adherence, and overall satisfaction with care. There is a paucity of research on decisional conflict and its impact on the quality of life in patients with diverticulitis. This stands in contrast to the rich body of literature in surgical specialties such as otolaryngology and urology, setting a precedent for what future studies might entail [36–40]. Head and neck cancer poses a clinical dilemma similar to diverticulitis in that patients are expected to decide between treatments with equitable outcomes that vary in morbidity, all the while balancing preservation of quality of life.

High levels of decisional conflict during the decision-making process can increase the likelihood of decision regret, as uncertainty with the chosen option may lead patients to feel they made the wrong choice, particularly if outcomes are unfavorable [38]. Decision regret, as measured by the Decision Regret Scale, is defined as remorse or distress over a decision. It is often used as a tool to evaluate interventions aimed at improving the quality of preference-sensitive decisions [41]. Additionally, it is recognized as a key patient-reported outcome and a critical element of high-quality decision-making [42, 43]. A systematic review evaluating decision regret across several elective surgical disciplines found that self-reported decisional regret was present in about 1 in 7 surgical patients [44]. In diverticulitis, the prevalence of decision regret is as high as 32% and is inversely associated with value clarity, feeling informed and supported, shared decision-making, and role concordance [45]. Overall, decision regret and decisional conflict are important outcomes in assessing the quality of shared decision-making as they directly reflect the effectiveness of patient-provider communication.

Patient Perspective on Decision-Making

The decision-making process in diverticulitis can be complex and overwhelming for patients as they face uncertainty regarding the best treatment option and an unpredictable disease course with the possibility of recurrent episodes. Fear of surgery and concerns about the burden of chronic symptoms further complicate this process. A national mixed-methods study found that 17% of patients who discussed the surgical treatment of their diverticulitis with their surgeon regretted their decision to pursue colectomy or observation, which was significantly associated with bowel dysfunction [31]. Patients in this study who underwent colectomy cited disease-related factors such as a desire to live a more normal life, pain, bowel dysfunction, long-term antibiotic use, and a desire to avoid emergency surgery as major factors in the decision-making process. Psychosocial factors, such as living in a remote location, the fear and stress caused by diverticulitis, as well as the need to care for family, were also influential. Patients who elected not to proceed with colectomy cited financial or insurance concerns, fear of surgical complications, poor rapport with their surgeon, and the need to continue working as reasons not to pursue resection. Overall, the three main themes of disease-related factors, psychosocial factors, and interactions with physicians proved critical in the decision-making process regardless of treatment choice [31].

Qualitative work performed during the development and validation of the Diverticulitis Quality of Life (DV-QOL) instrument proposed several themes regarding the impact of diverticulitis on a patient's health-related quality of life [46]. These themes include intestinal and extra-intestinal physical symptoms, behavioral changes related to diverticular disease, and disease-specific cognitions and emotions. Hantouli et al. [47] classified these themes into five domains relevant to surgical decision-making, which include: physical symptoms; caretaking; restrictions to patients' ability; anxiety; and concern about permanent damage. In this study, they sought to describe how surgeons and patients in practice consider these different domains in surgical decision-making and found that physical symptoms and restrictions were most often considered important by both parties and had the highest agreement. However, caretaking, anxiety, and concern about permanent damage were domains that patients considered important but were less often considered by surgeons [47]. The findings of this study underscore key areas that surgeons should address with patients when discussing treatment options for diverticulitis.

A multi-center qualitative study evaluating the patient perspective on colectomy for recurrent diverticulitis found that patients view the decision to undergo colectomy through three major themes: their beliefs about surgery, their psychosocial context, and moderating factors that influence participant choice to undergo surgery [48]. They present a conceptual framework to summarize the patient's perspective in this decision-making process (Fig. 23.1). The two sets of contextual rings dynamically interact with each other, with the inner ring representing the participant's beliefs about surgery and the outer ring representing the patient's psychosocial context. The stacked arrows identify three moderating factors that influence a patient's choice to undergo surgery: clinical history, clinical protocols, and provider-specific factors. Eventually, patients then proceed through a stage of deliberation before finally arriving at a decision to undergo surgery. This study highlights the complexity of the decision-making process and the need for high-quality communication between patient and surgeon. Ultimately, to engage in shared decision-making, it is essential to understand the patient's perspective, colored by the diverse psychological, social, and physical symptoms they attribute to their condition.

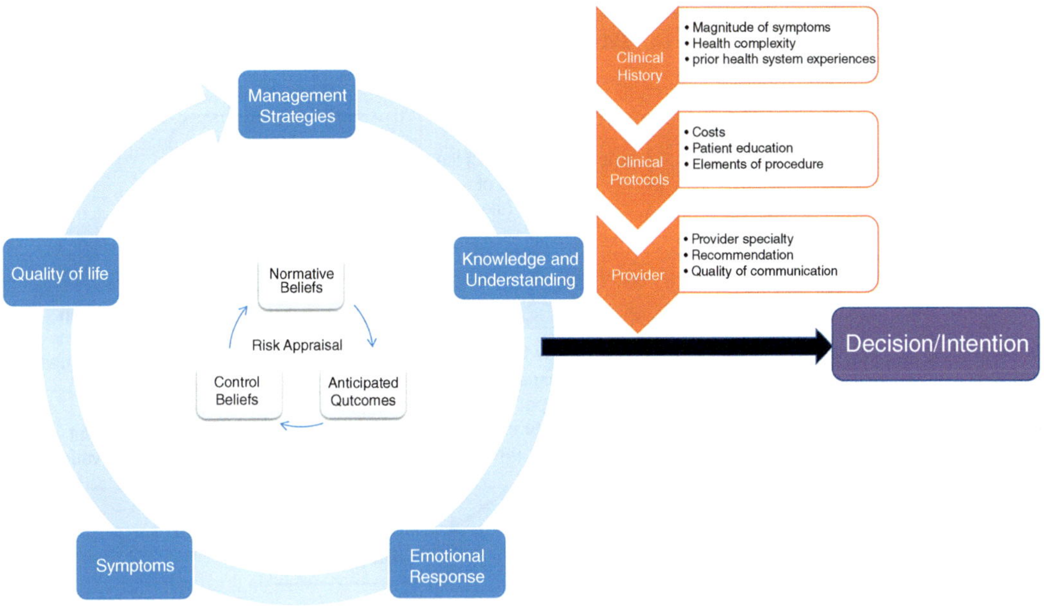

Fig. 23.1 Patient perspective on colectomy [48]. (Reused with permission © Wolters Kluwer Health, Inc.)

Surgeon Perspective on Decision-Making

Appreciating the surgeon's perspective when engaging in evaluation for colectomy is a critical step in improving the quality of the shared decision-making process. A qualitative study performed to evaluate the surgeon perspective in SDM developed a conceptual framework to summarize this thought process and included common themes that were mentioned after semi-structured interviews with a wide range of surgeons (Fig. 23.2) [49]. The results of this analysis demonstrated the complexity and heterogeneity of this process, with important common themes to include risks and benefits of both surgery and observation, patient and surgeon factors, as well as key elements in how to make a shared decision.

Risk Assessment

When considering colectomy for diverticulitis, risk assessment is one of the first steps performed by the surgeon. Findings from qualitative studies demonstrate that the risk assessment of surgery includes factors such as patient comorbidities, surgical complexity, postoperative complications, and direct cost [49]. Surgeons assess patient comorbidities and frailty in several ways. Some surgeons use formal risk calculators such as the American College of Surgeons National Surgical Quality Improvement Project (ACS-NSQIP) Risk Calculator in their preoperative assessment. Others rely on their own experience and use a Gestalt method of global assessment, evaluating a patient's perceived capacity to endure the physical demands of surgery and potential complications [49–52]. Other factors incorporated in the risk assessment are age and immunosuppression. Some surgeons feel that younger patients are more apt to benefit from elective resection with the notion that they might have a more "virulent" form of diverticulitis and have a longer life expectancy, with the potential for a cumulative improvement in their quality of life [49, 53]. This is in spite of the fact that the ASCRS guidelines recommend against including young age at diagnosis in the decision for resection [8]. Other surgeons weigh the severity of the disease and a strong family history of diverticuli-

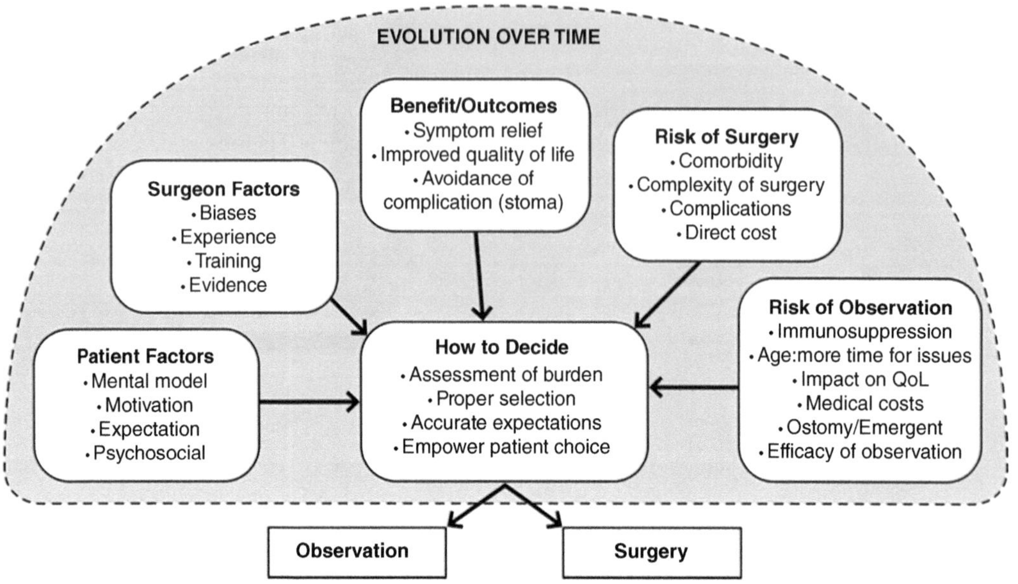

Fig. 23.2 Surgeon perspective on colectomy [49]. (Reused with permission © Wolters Kluwer Health, Inc.)

tis as important factors that may be associated with an increased risk of recurrence [49, 53].

Surgical complexity and postoperative complications are also common factors evaluated in the surgeon's risk assessment. Technical factors such as a history of extensive abdominal surgeries, obesity, and the degree of anticipated scarring are all issues that are commonly considered from the surgeon's perspective [49]. Additionally, complications such as anastomotic leak, hernia, stricture, recurrence, and mortality are all major concerns with a surgical approach and are weighed differently in the context of an emergent versus an elective operation. A systematic review and meta-analysis found that the risk of postoperative mortality following emergent surgery was 10.6% as compared to elective surgery, which was 0.5% [53]. In the same study, the total postoperative complication rate following emergent surgery was 54% vs 23% in elective resection. Additionally, they assessed the individual rates of complications such as abdominal abscess, anastomotic leak, bleeding, wound infection, pulmonary embolism, pneumonia, as well as UTI, and found that, with the exception of similar bleeding rates, all complication rates were higher for emergent procedures [54]. Finally, recurrent diverticulitis may occur in up to 15% of patients following resection, with up to 20% of postoperative patients experiencing continued chronic pain or no relief in symptoms, though this might be related to misdiagnosis [53, 55–57].

Patient and Surgeon Factors

Characterizing a patient's experience with diverticulitis and evaluating specific patient and surgeon factors is the next step after assessing fitness for surgery. The decision to pursue colectomy varies greatly depending on a patient's severity of symptoms, perception of disease, and impact on quality of life. National practice guidelines recommend that surgeons assess the frequency and severity of flares, patient preferences, and persistent symptoms when discussing treatment options [8]. Assessing the burden of disease by inquiring about the frequency of attacks, hospitalizations, complications, and lifetime episodes informs a surgeon's risk/benefit analysis of operative intervention and is a critical step in the shared decision-making process. In addition to these quantifiable aspects of disease severity, surgeons must elicit the patient's subjective experiences such as the "mental model" they use to integrate their diverticular disease into the larger sense of life [49]. For some patients, diverticulitis is just a small aspect of who they are, whereas for others, it is debilitating and greatly impacts how they live. A patient's motivation to undergo surgery, as well as their preconceived expectations for their disease course and the different treatment options, is a key part of the discussion as well. All of these elements are important to consider within the patient's large psychosocial context, which includes social networks, relationships, work, and leisure activities [49]. Several surgeon factors have been shown to influence the SDM process. The surgeon's own bias is important to consider and includes previous complications, practice environment, career experience, training background, as well as their comfort level in managing complex cases [49]. Almost all surgeons operate in a fee-for-service environment, which potentially serves as a bias toward offering surgery. Overall, the heterogeneity and number of potential factors that a surgeon must sort through with a patient in a short clinical time are the testament to the complexity of shared decision-making in diverticulitis. Educational and communication-based tools are needed to support patients and surgeons alike as they progress through this process.

Shared Decision-Making Tools

Shared decision-making tools are essential in the face of preference-sensitive decisions as they help patients and providers navigate the complexities of care options available. These tools enable patients to fully understand the risks and benefits of treatments while considering individual factors like the frequency and severity of episodes, personal preferences, and quality of life impact. One such type of intervention is patient decision aids. A Cochrane review of decision aids for people facing health treatment or screening decisions across various medical disciplines found that, compared to usual care, these aids help patients reach informed values-congruent choices [58]. They often led to increases in knowledge, accurate risk perceptions, an active role in decision-making, decreased decisional conflict related to feeling uninformed, and decreased indecision about personal values. There was no difference in the length of consultation when patient decision aids were used in preparation for the consultation, and a minimal increase in consultation length of 1.5 min was noted when decision aids were incorporated during the visit [58]. This is important to note in light of the common perception that decision aids prolong physician–patient communication and could serve as a barrier to efficient clinic workflow [59, 60]. A meta-analysis evaluating decision aids for patients facing a surgical treatment decision found similar findings. Patients in the decision aid group had greater knowledge about treatment options and experienced less decisional conflict with similar levels of anxiety and quality of life as compared to a control population receiving general patient information [61].

The literature on decision aids in diverticulitis is limited and is a field in need of dedicated research. A challenge in elective management of diverticulitis is ensuring patient understanding of the risks and benefits, which is due to preexisting patient expectations and lack of data regarding long-term treatment outcomes [52]. A national sample of colorectal surgeons notes that to combat these challenges, patient education and additional research regarding treatment outcomes are necessary in the form of diverticulitis-specific decision support tools [52]. The only such intervention for recurrent diverticulitis was recently developed as an online education decision aid to facilitate effective surgeon and patient communication about treatment options [62]. The authors used a modified design sprint methodology and engaged a multidisciplinary team to create and iteratively refine the decision aid, which has three discrete sections. The first section contains educational background information about diverticulitis and the available treatment options. The second section reviews the potential risks and benefits of each pathway (observation vs colectomy), and the third section invites patients to participate in a value clarification exercise that encourages the patient to self-reflect and come prepared to discuss personal preferences and values during their clinic appointment (Fig. 23.3) [62]. Their work highlights the development and usability phase of the decision aid, which has not yet been tested to demonstrate clinical feasibility and efficacy.

Other colorectal disease processes have also been active areas of patient decision aid development. Cohan et al. performed a qualitative study in ulcerative colitis (UC) patients who underwent surgery to understand how patients decide between end ileostomy (EI) or ileal pouch-anal anastomosis (IPAA). What they found was that

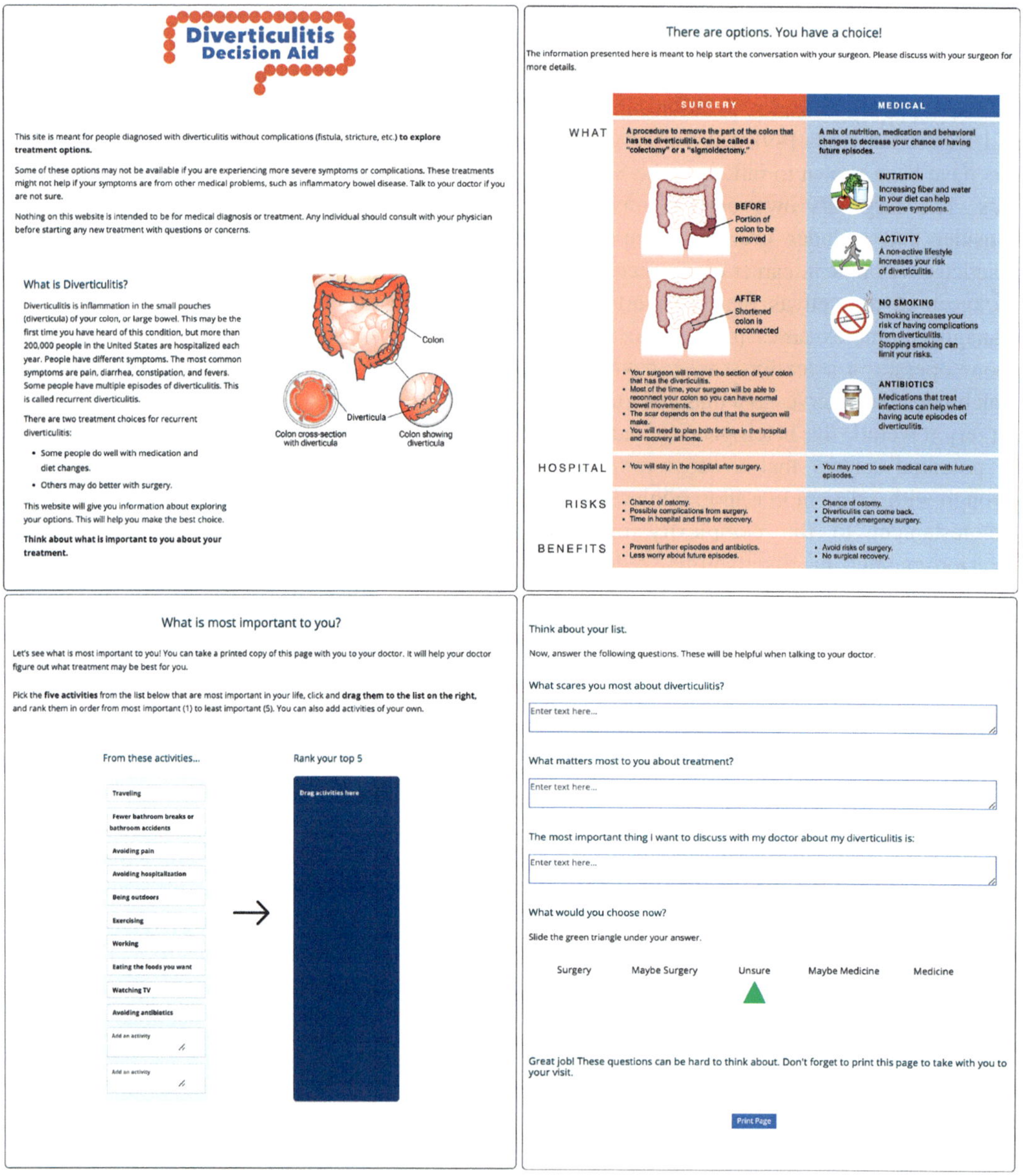

Fig. 23.3 Diverticulitis decision aid. (Copyright © 2025 by Vanderbilt University Medical Center. Used with permission. *Top left panel*: https://www.vumc.org/criss-humanfactors/node/123. *Top right panel*: https://www.vumc.org/criss-humanfactors/node/124. *Bottom left and right panels*: https://www.vumc.org/criss-humanfactors/node/125)

patients with UC struggled with inadequate educational information and social support, suggesting that they may benefit from educational materials describing surgical complications and postoperative expectations to improve decision-making [63]. The gap in shared decision-making that existed in this clinical scenario was addressed with the development of a decision aid. A pilot study was published that evaluated the efficacy of a decision aid for patients with UC who were faced with making the complex decision between EI and IPAA [64]. In this study, patients improved their knowledge scores with evidence of high patient and surgeon satisfaction with the decision aid and clinical encounter, respectively. Limitations of this study were the lack of a comparison group, indicating the importance of larger randomized trials powered to demonstrate efficacy. Similarly, in rectal cancer, a patient decision aid was developed to assist patients in picking between low anterior resection and abdominoperineal resection [34]. Results demonstrated improvement in knowledge and decreased decisional conflict, with over 96% of participants recommending the patient decision aid to others. In conclusion, patient decision aids have been studied across a variety of disease processes and demonstrate the potential for significant improvement in the shared decision-making process by empowering patients with the knowledge to make informed decisions that align with their values and preferences.

Challenges and Opportunities

Several challenges exist in the consultation and shared decision-making process for recurrent diverticulitis. Surgeons are faced with difficulty predicting outcomes of both observation and surgery, given a lack of data on long-term treatment outcomes [51, 52]. A disease-specific predictive tool that accurately measures risk and takes into consideration patient comorbidities, genetic risk, and severity of disease would be clinically valuable and offer powerful information to surgeons and patients alike. To date, there have been some advancements in this area [62, 64–66].

Bias is also a significant challenge in that patients present with preconceived notions regarding their disease due to prior experiences and desires. Moreover, surgeons rely on their clinical experience and training when treating diverticulitis and are influenced by a desire to maintain referral relationships as well as financial incentives to operate. Despite their extensive clinical training, surgeons may be less equipped to manage the psychosocial and cultural contexts of illness that are critical to understanding in the face of a preference-sensitive disease process like diverticulitis [49].

Conclusion

Coming to a thoughtful, individualized decision that is tailored to the patient's needs takes immense time, resources, support, education, and guidance. Patient decision aids have a chance at mitigating many of the challenges that are fraught in the SDM process by providing evidence-based data, considering patient values and preferences, and fostering a collaborative partnership between surgeon and patient; however, widespread use has been limited by difficulty with implementation, dissemination, and physician buy-in [58–60]. These challenges will remain until we inform existing decision aids with better longitudinal data and demonstrate their efficacy in the form of robust randomized trials.

References

1. Nguyen GC, Sam J, Anand N. Epidemiological trends and geographic variation in hospital admissions for diverticulitis in the United States. World J Gastroenterol. 2011;17(12):1600–5. https://doi.org/10.3748/wjg.v17.i12.1600.
2. Hawkins AT, Wise PE, Chan T, et al. Diverticulitis: an update from the age old paradigm. Curr Probl Surg. 2020;57(10):100862. https://doi.org/10.1016/j.cpsurg.2020.100862.
3. Chapman J, Davies M, Wolff B, et al. Complicated diverticulitis: is it time to rethink the rules? Ann Surg. 2005;242(4):576–83. https://doi.org/10.1097/01.sla.0000184843.89836.35.
4. Anaya DA. Risk of emergency colectomy and colostomy in patients with diverticular disease. Arch

Surg. 2005;140(7):681. https://doi.org/10.1001/archsurg.140.7.681.
5. Chapman JR, Dozois EJ, Wolff BG, Gullerud RE, Larson DR. Diverticulitis: a progressive disease?: do multiple recurrences predict less favorable outcomes? Ann Surg. 2006;243(6):876–83. https://doi.org/10.1097/01.sla.0000219682.98158.11.
6. Stollman N, Raskin JB. Diverticular disease of the colon. Lancet. 2004;363(9409):631–9. https://doi.org/10.1016/S0140-6736(04)15597-9.
7. Janes SE, Meagher A, Frizelle FA. Management of diverticulitis. BMJ. 2006;332(7536):271–5. https://doi.org/10.1136/bmj.332.7536.271.
8. Hall J, Hardiman K, Lee S, et al. The American Society of Colon and Rectal Surgeons clinical practice guidelines for the treatment of left-sided colonic diverticulitis. Dis Colon Rectum. 2020;63(6):728–47. https://doi.org/10.1097/DCR.0000000000001679.
9. Feingold D, Steele SR, Lee S, et al. Practice parameters for the treatment of sigmoid diverticulitis. Dis Colon Rectum. 2014;57(3):284–94. https://doi.org/10.1097/DCR.0000000000000075.
10. Stollman N, Smalley W, Hirano I, et al. American Gastroenterological Association Institute guideline on the management of acute diverticulitis. Gastroenterology. 2015;149(7):1944–9. https://doi.org/10.1053/j.gastro.2015.10.003.
11. Montori VM, Ruissen MM, Hargraves IG, Brito JP, Kunneman M. Shared decision-making as a method of care. BMJ Evid Based Med. 2023;28(4):213–7. https://doi.org/10.1136/bmjebm-2022-112068.
12. Makoul G, Clayman ML. An integrative model of shared decision making in medical encounters. Patient Educ Couns. 2006;60(3):301–12. https://doi.org/10.1016/j.pec.2005.06.010.
13. Kunneman M, Montori VM, Castaneda-Guarderas A, Hess EP. What is shared decision making? (and what it is not). Jang TB, ed. Acad Emerg Med. 2016;23(12):1320–4. https://doi.org/10.1111/acem.13065.
14. Hargraves IG, Montori VM, Brito JP, et al. Purposeful SDM: a problem-based approach to caring for patients with shared decision making. Patient Educ Couns. 2019;102(10):1786–92. https://doi.org/10.1016/j.pec.2019.07.020.
15. Elwyn G, Durand MA, Song J, et al. A three-talk model for shared decision making: multistage consultation process. BMJ. 2017;359:j4891. https://doi.org/10.1136/bmj.j4891.
16. Elwyn G, Frosch D, Rollnick S. Dual equipoise shared decision making: definitions for decision and behaviour support interventions. Implement Sci. 2009;4(1):75. https://doi.org/10.1186/1748-5908-4-75.
17. Collins D, Winter DC. Elective resection for diverticular disease: an evidence-based review. World J Surg. 2008;32(11):2429–33. https://doi.org/10.1007/s00268-008-9705-7.
18. Pessaux P, Muscari F, Ouellet JF, et al. Risk factors for mortality and morbidity after elective sigmoid resection for diverticulitis: prospective multicenter multivariate analysis of 582 patients. World J Surg. 2004;28(1):92–6. https://doi.org/10.1007/s00268-003-7146-x.
19. Simianu VV, Flum DR. Rethinking elective colectomy for diverticulitis: a strategic approach to population health. World J Gastroenterol. 2014;20(44):16609–14. https://doi.org/10.3748/wjg.v20.i44.16609.
20. Buchs NC, Konrad-Mugnier B, Jannot AS, Poletti PA, Ambrosetti P, Gervaz P. Assessment of recurrence and complications following uncomplicated diverticulitis. Br J Surg. 2013;100(7):976–9; discussion 979. https://doi.org/10.1002/bjs.9119.
21. Ambrosetti P. Value of CT for acute left-colonic diverticulitis: the surgeon's view. Dig Dis. 2012;30(1):51–5. https://doi.org/10.1159/000335717.
22. Broderick-Villa G, Burchette RJ, Collins JC, Abbas MA, Haigh PI. Hospitalization for acute diverticulitis does not mandate routine elective colectomy. Arch Surg. 2005;140(6):576–81; discussion 581–3. https://doi.org/10.1001/archsurg.140.6.576.
23. Eglinton T, Nguyen T, Raniga S, Dixon L, Dobbs B, Frizelle FA. Patterns of recurrence in patients with acute diverticulitis. Br J Surg. 2010;97(6):952–7. https://doi.org/10.1002/bjs.7035.
24. Hall JF, Roberts PL, Ricciardi R, et al. Long-term follow-up after an initial episode of diverticulitis: what are the predictors of recurrence? Dis Colon Rectum. 2011;54(3):283–8. https://doi.org/10.1007/DCR.0b013e3182028576.
25. Shaikh S, Krukowski ZH. Outcome of a conservative policy for managing acute sigmoid diverticulitis. Br J Surg. 2007;94(7):876–9. https://doi.org/10.1002/bjs.5703.
26. Simianu VV, Strate LL, Billingham RP, et al. The impact of elective colon resection on rates of emergency surgery for diverticulitis. Ann Surg. 2016;263(1):123–9. https://doi.org/10.1097/SLA.0000000000001053.
27. Morris AM, Regenbogen SE, Hardiman KM, Hendren S. Sigmoid diverticulitis: a systematic review. JAMA. 2014;311(3):287. https://doi.org/10.1001/jama.2013.282025.
28. Justin V, Uranues S, Rabl H, Fingerhut A. Quality of life in uncomplicated recurrent diverticulitis: surgical vs. conservative treatment. Sci Rep. 2020;10(1):10261. https://doi.org/10.1038/s41598-020-67094-3. PMID: 32581229; PMCID: PMC7314856.
29. Kertzman BAJ, Amelung FJ, Bolkenstein HE, Consten ECJ, Draaisma WA. Does surgery improve quality of life in patients with ongoing- or recurrent diverticulitis; a systematic review and meta-analysis. Scand J Gastroenterol. 2024;59(7):770–80. https://doi.org/10.1080/00365521.2024.2337833. Epub 2024 Apr 13. PMID: 38613245.
30. van de Wall BJM, Stam MAW, Draaisma WA, et al. Surgery versus conservative management for recurrent and ongoing left-sided diverticulitis (DIRECT trial): an open-label, multicentre, randomised controlled

trial. Lancet Gastroenterol Hepatol. 2017;2(1):13–22. https://doi.org/10.1016/S2468-1253(16)30109-1.
31. Harrison NJ, Ford MM, Wolf Horrell EM, et al. Long-term bowel dysfunction and decision regret in diverticulitis: a mixed methods study. Surgery. 2022;172(4):1194–201. https://doi.org/10.1016/j.surg.2022.04.051.
32. O'Connor AM. Validation of a decisional conflict scale. Med Decis Mak. 1995;15(1):25–30. https://doi.org/10.1177/0272989X9501500105.
33. Garvelink MM, Boland L, Klein K, et al. Decisional conflict scale use over 20 years: the anniversary review. Med Decis Mak. 2019;39(4):301–14. https://doi.org/10.1177/0272989X19851345.
34. Wu RC, Boushey RP, Scheer AS, et al. Evaluation of the rectal cancer patient decision aid: a before and after study. Dis Colon Rectum. 2016;59(3):165–72. https://doi.org/10.1097/DCR.0000000000000528.
35. Renfro LA, Zhang N, Lopatin M, Chao C, Alberts SR. Prospective evaluation of a 12-gene assay on patient treatment decisions and physician confidence in mismatch repair proficient stage IIA colon cancer. Clin Colorectal Cancer. 2017;16(1):23–30. https://doi.org/10.1016/j.clcc.2016.07.016.
36. Hoesseini A, Dorr MC, Dronkers EAC, de Jong RJB, Sewnaik A, Offerman MPJ. Decisional conflict in patients with head and neck cancer. JAMA Otolaryngol Head Neck Surg. 2023;149(2):160–7. https://doi.org/10.1001/jamaoto.2022.4269.
37. Cleveland C, Newby M, Steinman S, et al. Depression and intolerance of uncertainty: association with decisional conflict in otolaryngology patients. Ann Otol Rhinol Laryngol. 2022;131(3):252–8. https://doi.org/10.1177/00034894211018914.
38. Carr MM, Derr JB, Karikari K. Decisional conflict and regret in parents whose children undergo tonsillectomy. Otolaryngol Head Neck Surg. 2016;155(5):863–8. https://doi.org/10.1177/0194599816655996.
39. Köther AK, Alpers GW, Büdenbender B, Lenhart M, Michel MS, Kriegmair MC. Predicting decisional conflict: anxiety and depression in shared decision making. Patient Educ Couns. 2021;104(5):1229–36. https://doi.org/10.1016/j.pec.2020.10.037.
40. Heirman AN, Arends CR, De Jel DVC, et al. Decisional conflict and decision regret in head and neck oncology: a systematic review and meta-analysis. JAMA Otolaryngol Head Neck Surg. 2024;150(5):393. https://doi.org/10.1001/jamaoto.2024.0214.
41. Brehaut JC, O'Connor AM, Wood TJ, et al. Validation of a decision regret scale. Med Decis Mak. 2003;23(4):281–92. https://doi.org/10.1177/0272989X03256005.
42. Joseph-Williams N, Edwards A, Elwyn G. The importance and complexity of regret in the measurement of "good" decisions: a systematic review and a content analysis of existing assessment instruments: systematic review of regret instruments. Health Expect. 2011;14(1):59–83. https://doi.org/10.1111/j.1369-7625.2010.00621.x.
43. Oliver A, Greenberg CC. Measuring outcomes in oncology treatment: the importance of patient-centered outcomes. Surg Clin North Am. 2009;89(1):17–25. https://doi.org/10.1016/j.suc.2008.09.015.
44. Wilson A, Ronnekleiv-Kelly SM, Pawlik TM. Regret in surgical decision making: a systematic review of patient and physician perspectives. World J Surg. 2017;41(6):1454–65. https://doi.org/10.1007/s00268-017-3895-9.
45. Cohan JN, Orleans B, Brecha FS, et al. Factors associated with decision regret among patients with diverticulitis in the elective setting. J Surg Res. 2021;261:159–66. https://doi.org/10.1016/j.jss.2020.12.019.
46. Spiegel BM, Reid MW, Bolus R, et al. Development and validation of a disease-targeted quality of life instrument for chronic diverticular disease: the DV-QOL. Qual Life Res. 2015;24(1):163–79. https://doi.org/10.1007/s11136-014-0753-1.
47. Hantouli MN, Droullard DJ, Khor S, et al. Indications for surgical treatment of diverticulitis: factors that influence surgical decision-making for patients and surgeons. Br J Surg. 2022;109(12):1329–30. https://doi.org/10.1093/bjs/znac321.
48. Hawkins AT, Penson DF, Geiger TM, et al. The patient perspective on colectomy for recurrent diverticulitis: a qualitative study. Ann Surg. 2024;279:818–24. https://doi.org/10.1097/SLA.0000000000006225.
49. Hawkins AT, Rothman RL, Geiger TM, et al. Surgeons' perspective of decision making in recurrent diverticulitis: a qualitative analysis. Ann Surg Open. 2022;3(2):e157. https://doi.org/10.1097/AS9.0000000000000157.
50. Bilimoria KY, Liu Y, Paruch JL, et al. Development and evaluation of the universal ACS NSQIP surgical risk calculator: a decision aid and informed consent tool for patients and surgeons. J Am Coll Surg. 2013;217(5):833–842.e3. https://doi.org/10.1016/j.jamcollsurg.2013.07.385.
51. De Roo AC, Vitous CA, Rivard SJ, et al. High-risk surgery among older adults: not-quite shared decision-making. Surgery. 2021;170(3):756–63. https://doi.org/10.1016/j.surg.2021.02.005.
52. Williamson AJH, Cain BT, Hoggan TJ, et al. Challenges and opportunities in the elective management of diverticulitis: perspectives from a national sample of colorectal surgeons. Dis Colon Rectum. 2024;67(2):264–72. https://doi.org/10.1097/DCR.0000000000002941.
53. Regenbogen SE, Hardiman KM, Hendren S, Morris AM. Surgery for diverticulitis in the 21st century: a systematic review. JAMA Surg. 2014;149(3):292. https://doi.org/10.1001/jamasurg.2013.5477.
54. Haas JM, Singh M, Vakil N. Mortality and complications following surgery for diverticulitis: systematic review and meta-analysis. United Eur Gastroenterol J. 2016;4(5):706–13. https://doi.org/10.1177/2050640615617357.
55. Strate LL, Morris AM. Epidemiology, pathophysiology, and treatment of diverticulitis. Gastroenterology.

2019;156(5):1282–1298.e1. https://doi.org/10.1053/j.gastro.2018.12.033.
56. Bolkenstein HE, Consten ECJ, Van Der Palen J, et al. Long-term outcome of surgery versus conservative management for recurrent and ongoing complaints after an episode of diverticulitis: 5-year follow-up results of a multicenter randomized controlled trial (DIRECT-trial). Ann Surg. 2019;269(4):612–20. https://doi.org/10.1097/SLA.0000000000003033.
57. Santos A, Mentula P, Pinta T, et al. Quality-of-life and recurrence outcomes following laparoscopic elective sigmoid resection vs conservative treatment following diverticulitis: prespecified 2-year analysis of the LASER randomized clinical trial. JAMA Surg. 2023;158(6):593. https://doi.org/10.1001/jamasurg.2023.0466.
58. Stacey D, Lewis KB, Smith M, et al. Decision aids for people facing health treatment or screening decisions. Cochrane Database Syst Rev. 2024;1(1):CD001431. https://doi.org/10.1002/14651858.CD001431.pub6.
59. Légaré F, Ratté S, Gravel K, Graham ID. Barriers and facilitators to implementing shared decision-making in clinical practice: update of a systematic review of health professionals' perceptions. Patient Educ Couns. 2008;73(3):526–35. https://doi.org/10.1016/j.pec.2008.07.018.
60. Graham ID, Logan J, Bennett CL, et al. Physicians' intentions and use of three patient decision aids. BMC Med Inform Decis Mak. 2007;7(1):20. https://doi.org/10.1186/1472-6947-7-20.
61. Knops AM, Legemate DA, Goossens A, Bossuyt PM, Ubbink DT. Decision aids for patients facing a surgical treatment decision: a systematic review and meta-analysis. Ann Surg. 2013;257(5):860–6. https://doi.org/10.1097/SLA.0b013e3182864fd6.
62. Hawkins AT, Fa A, Younan SA, et al. Decision aid for colectomy in recurrent diverticulitis: development and usability study. JMIR Form Res. 2024;8:e59952. https://doi.org/10.2196/59952.
63. Cohan JN, Ozanne EM, Hofer RK, et al. Ileostomy or ileal pouch-anal anastomosis for ulcerative colitis: patient participation and decisional needs. BMC Gastroenterol. 2021;21(1):347. https://doi.org/10.1186/s12876-021-01916-0.
64. Cohan JN, Ozanne EM, Sewell JL, et al. A novel decision aid for surgical patients with ulcerative colitis: results of a pilot study. Dis Colon Rectum. 2016;59(6):520–8. https://doi.org/10.1097/DCR.0000000000000572.
65. Covino M, Papa V, Tursi A, Simeoni B, Lopetuso LR, Vetrone LM, Franceschi F, Rapaccini G, Gasbarrini A, Papa A. Development and validation of predictive assessment of complicated diverticulitis score. J Pers Med. 2021;11(2):80. https://doi.org/10.3390/jpm11020080. PMID: 33572940; PMCID: PMC7911244.
66. De Roo AC, Chen Y, Du X, et al. Polygenic risk prediction in diverticulitis. Ann Surg. 2023;277(6):e1262–8. https://doi.org/10.1097/SLA.0000000000005623.

Correction to: Symptoms and Diagnosis

Andrea Petrucci and Sebastien Lachance

Correction to:
Chapter 3 in: M. Boutros et al. (eds.), *Diverticulitis*,
https://doi.org/10.1007/978-3-032-21720-2_3

The original version of Chapter 3 was inadvertently published with the omission of the co-author, Sebastien Lachance, which has now been corrected.

The updated version of this chapter can be found at
https://doi.org/10.1007/978-3-032-21720-2_3

M. Boutros et al. (eds.), *Diverticulitis*, https://doi.org/10.1007/978-3-032-21720-2_24

Index

M. Boutros et al. (eds.), *Diverticulitis*, https://doi.org/10.1007/978-3-032-21720-2

GPSR Compliance

The European Union's (EU) General Product Safety Regulation (GPSR) is a set of rules that requires consumer products to be safe and our obligations to ensure this.

If you have any concerns about our products, you can contact us on ProductSafety@springernature.com

In case Publisher is established outside the EU, the EU authorized representative is:

Springer Nature Customer Service Center GmbH
Europaplatz 3
69115 Heidelberg, Germany

Batch number: 10731395

Printed by Printforce, the Netherlands